BE WISE! BE HEALTHY!

BE WISE! BE HEALTHY!
Morality and Citizenship in Canadian Public Health Campaigns

Catherine Carstairs
Bethany Philpott
Sara Wilmshurst

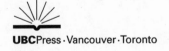
UBCPress · Vancouver · Toronto

27 26 25 24 23 22 21 20 19 18   5 4 3 2 1

Printed in Canada on FSC-certified ancient-forest-free paper (100% post-consumer recycled) that is processed chlorine- and acid-free.

Library and Archives Canada Cataloguing in Publication

Carstairs, Catherine, author
Be wise! Be healthy! : morality and citizenship in Canadian public health campaigns / Catherine Carstairs, Bethany Philpott, Sara Wilmshurst.

Includes bibliographical references and index.
Issued in print and electronic formats.
ISBN 978-0-7748-3718-7 (hardcover). – ISBN 978-0-7748-3720-0 (PDF). – ISBN 978-0-7748-3721-7 (EPUB). – ISBN 978-0-7748-3722-4 (Kindle)

1. Health promotion—Canada—History—20th century. 2. Public health—Canada—Marketing—History—20th century. 3. Public health—Moral and ethical aspects—Canada—History— 20th century. 4. Public health—Canada—History—20th century. 5. Canada—Moral conditions—History—20th century. I. Philpott, Bethany, author II. Wilmshurst, Sara, author III. Title.

RA427.8.C37 2018   613.097109′04   C2018-900318-9
                                                        C2018-900319-7

Canadä

UBC Press gratefully acknowledges the financial support for our publishing program of the Government of Canada (through the Canada Book Fund), the Canada Council for the Arts, and the British Columbia Arts Council.

This book has been published with the help of a grant from the Canadian Federation for the Humanities and Social Sciences, through the Awards to Scholarly Publications Program, using funds provided by the Social Sciences and Humanities Research Council of Canada.

UBC Press
The University of British Columbia
2029 West Mall
Vancouver, BC V6T 1Z2
www.ubcpress.ca

Contents

Illustrations

Figures

Table

Acknowledgments

Catherine Carstairs

This project has been a joy to complete: historical work is usually a solo endeavour, but it has been so much more fun to do it alongside the brilliant, thoughtful, and hardworking Bethany Philpott and Sara Wilmshurst. I greatly enjoyed our many trips to Ottawa, gossiping about the Health League along the way. And I am grateful to both of them for their ongoing passion for the project, even while they both moved on to other, highly worthy activities. I also want to make special mention of Shawn Goodman and Caitlin Fendley, whose work was vital to Chapters 1 and 2, respectively.

My own history with the Health League is a long one. As a graduate student, I came across *Health* magazine in the gorgeous stacks of Gerstein Library. Sitting on the translucent floor and shifting through the magazine's later issues, I was shocked and amused by its pervasive moral tone. Later, when I turned my attention to the history of water fluoridation, I became aware of the important role that the Health League had played in that campaign. Curious, I spent a few Saturdays in Gerstein going through issues of the magazine from the 1950s and became convinced that the Health League was a worthy story in and of itself.

Soon afterwards, I was teaching a class on the history of disability, which attracted a number of extremely bright, engaged students. When the class ended, Shawn Goodman asked to do a senior thesis with me. I suggested that he might be interested in the Health League. I approached some of the other high-performing students in the class to see if they also wanted to work on the Health League. In this way, Bethany Philpott and Sara Wilmshurst joined the project. Little did they know what a commitment it would be! Bethany and Sara would stick around for their MA degrees and would ultimately produce two outstanding masters theses. These theses became the backbone of this book. Sara would also publish an article on the Health League, "Tobacco Truths: *Health* Magazine, Clinical Epidemiology and the Cigarette Connection" in the *Canadian Bulletin of Medical History*. Both Sara and Bethany would continue to work on the project as research assistants after they completed their theses. Shawn's work on the Health League's venereal disease campaigns would provide the underpinnings for the first chapter of this book.

Bethany, Sara, and I (and occasionally Shawn) would make many trips to Library and Archives Canada over the next few years to collect material. We put all of the photos we'd taken in the Cloud, allowing us to share research resources. A few other students became involved as well. Nicki Darbyson took photos of *Health* and created a database for the magazine. Kelly Wiley assisted with photos, while Sheilagh Quaile helped to complete the database and did some additional research on milk pasteurization. Alexandria Marriot wrote a senior thesis on the Health League's approach to pollution. Caitlin Fendley wrote a senior thesis on the campaign of the Canadian Social Hygiene Council/Health League against diphtheria, which provided the basis for the corresponding section of Chapter 2. Melissa Micu, my undergraduate research assistant in the summer of 2015, did additional research on industrial health and provided a careful edit of the manuscript. Paige Schell's work on milk pasteurization, done for a senior thesis long before this project was conceived, helped me write the section on pasteurization in Chapter 2. Jeremy Istead's work on sexually transmitted diseases between 1960 and 1980, funded by a Hannah summer studentship, provided valuable background for Chapter 8. Linda Mahood provided valuable comments on a draft. Our copy editor, Barbara Tessman, did a fantastic job of cleaning up the manuscript. I am very grateful for all this support, and I take full responsibility for any remaining errors.

We are very grateful to the president of the Health League of Canada, Ray Gibson, who allowed us to reproduce the archival images found in this book. Pippa Wysong, Gordon Bates' granddaughter and a science writer and public health activist herself, graciously invited us to her home to share her memories of Bates, regularly provided us with updates and photos, and got Sara and I involved in her quarantine tent project. Gordon Bates' son, John Bates, and his family – including his wife, Connie, and daughter Susan

Conlin – also invited us to their home, where they regaled us with family stories and history. Another granddaughter, Wendy Schrama, shared her memories of Bates in an interview at the University of Guelph.

We are also very grateful to the Social Sciences and Humanities Research Council of Canada and to the University of Guelph for providing us with the funding necessary to complete this work.

I owe a huge debt to my parents, Sharon and John Carstairs, who not only provide me with a place to stay when I'm at Library and Archives Canada, but also cook my meals and ply me with wine. They are always interested in what I found at the archives that day. They also hosted Shawn, Bethany, Sara, and Melissa for dinner on various occasions, and were delighted to get to know the students that I'm so proud of. It has been a gift to have spent so much time with them.

Tim Neeb will probably never read this book, but he has filled my life with joy and laughter, and has put up with my many absences in Ottawa.

Bethany Philpott

First and foremost, my thanks to Catherine Carstairs and Sara Wilmshurst. Without them, this book would never have come into existence, let alone have been the enjoyable educational experience that it was. Catherine's knowledge, guidance, and dedication carried this project to completion while allowing me to pursue other education. I so appreciate her support and kindness over the years. Sara set the standard for what an exceptional learner looked like, inspiring me to achieve and providing me with tea, trivia, and friendship along the way.

I am thankful for all the wonderful teachers and mentors I found at the University of Guelph and through the Tri-University History Program. In particular, I thank my MA committee, Heather MacDougall, Tarah Brookfield, and Alan Gordon. Their questions and wisdom pushed me and no doubt enhanced my work.

The Social Sciences and Humanities Research Council generously supported my MA with their CGS Master's Scholarship. I am thankful to SSHRC for allowing me to focus my time on the Health League and for bolstering my confidence as a fledgling learner.

Between them, my parents studied both history and medicine. They have inspired and influenced me more than they know, both personally and professionally. The love and encouragement of my family has allowed me to dream and to succeed, through this project and in all the time before and since. Alex Wideman has been steadfast in his support for all my undertakings. I cannot thank him enough for sharing in the struggles and the joys and keeping me smiling through it all.

Sara Wilmshurst

I must start by thanking Catherine Carstairs and Bethany Philpott. I learned so much and benefited from their support and advice at every turn. It was a privilege and a pleasure to work with them, and I will use this project as a model of collaboration for the rest of my career.

I would also like to thank Alan Gordon and Cynthia Comacchio, who sat on my M.A. committee and provided guidance and refinement to my ideas. I am grateful to the University of Guelph's excellent educators, who equipped me to contribute to this project. I am particularly thankful to Catharine Wilson, Ian Mosby, Matthew Hayday, and Kevin James.

I would like to thank the Social Sciences and Humanities Research Council. Parts of this book draw from my MA thesis, which the council supported with a CGS Master's Scholarship.

This project would not have been possible without the expert staff at Library and Archives Canada and the City of Toronto Archives.

On a personal level, I am grateful to my parents, to my sister, and to the Telfords for their unending kindness and support. Thanks also to my friends for forming a valuable network of support, especially Renée Worringer, Stephen Rowell, and their four-footed colleagues Sulu, Arrow, Gem, and Khan.

Finally, thanks and love to Fraser Telford. I feel like I can figure anything out as long as I have Fraser to brainstorm with. Thanks for keeping me going with encouragement and perfectly timed cups of tea.

BE WISE! BE HEALTHY!

Introduction
Creating Healthy Citizens

Over the past decade, Canadians have seen an explosion of public health messages telling us to lose weight and to exercise more. Parents are urged to follow the full vaccination schedule and put aside their concerns about the (discredited) link between vaccines and autism. And, of course, public health officials continue to warn us about the risks of smoking. Such messages are part of a long tradition. For well over a century, governments and voluntary groups have run educational campaigns to encourage Canadians to adopt health habits that promise to prolong our lives, increase our quality of life, cost the state less money, and make us more efficient workers. Mostly, these messages are helpful. As a result of public health education, fewer people die of infectious disease, fewer children are maimed in accidents, and fewer people die prematurely because of smoking. But public health is not without its costs. Smoking and drinking, for all the harm they can cause, are also pleasurable. High-fat foods taste good (and may not be as harmful as nutrition professionals once believed). Riding a bike without a helmet is a lot more fun. Excessive concerns about health can lead to anxiety, eating disorders, and feelings of worthlessness.[1] Public health campaigns often further stigmatize marginalized populations, implying that they take inadequate care of their own health, even though poorer health outcomes of marginalized groups have clearly been linked to the experience of poverty and trauma.[2] Some public health interventions, such as vaccinations, are not without risk, even if that risk is very small. And while not all public health interventions involve compulsion, some do, and this raises complex issues about people's rights over their own bodies versus the rights of others to be safe from harm. Partly as a result of such issues, public health has always been controversial.

This book will explore the history of public health in Canada from the 1920s to the 1970s, a period that saw a massive expansion of public health education programs, through the lens of the Health League of Canada, one of Canada's leading organizations promoting public health. During these decades, the Health League of Canada and its precursors urged Canadians to protect their health by drinking pasteurized milk, immunizing their children, guarding themselves against winter colds and sore feet, avoiding extramarital sex, improving their nutrition, embracing the fluoridation of the water supply, and educating themselves about chronic diseases. The league instructed Canadians that it was their responsibility as citizens to keep themselves safe from disease, and it encouraged them to look to doctors and dentists as the experts who would guide them along the path of health. The Health League was a pioneer in what many have described as the "new public health," which shifted the focus away from the environmental causes of disease (polluted water, poor housing conditions, inadequate sanitation) towards the individual, encouraging citizens to change their health habits and behaviours to help prevent disease.[3]

The Health League was not Canada's largest public health organization – indeed, it was dwarfed by federal and provincial departments of health, as well as numerous other voluntary groups, but it was the only voluntary group dedicated to pushing a broad public health agenda, as other groups pursued particular diseases or causes. It is of interest to historians because its many campaigns provide us with a window into the broader world of public health education in the middle decades of the twentieth century. The Health League was involved in all of the leading public health issues of the day, ranging from immunization and water fluoridation to nutrition education, venereal disease prevention, and industrial health. It was well connected with federal and provincial public health bodies, and most Canadians would have encountered its publicity at one point or another, whether through National Health Week, National Immunization Week, or educational campaigns about milk pasteurization or the dangers of sexually transmitted infections. The Health League also provides an interesting case study of the role of voluntary organizations in Canadian society. Groups such as the Red Cross, St. John's Ambulance, Big Sisters/Big Brothers, and many others have played a vital role in civil society, but, in general, these groups have not been as well studied as governmental organizations.[4]

The Health League began life in 1919 as Canadian National Council for Combatting Venereal Disease (CNCCVD), led by a young Toronto physician, Dr. Gordon Bates. In 1922, it changed its name to the Canadian Social Hygiene Council (CSHC), a title it thought would be more acceptable to potential supporters and one that reflected the fact that Bates and his organization wanted to be involved in a broader program of health prevention.[5] The term "social hygiene" can encompass many different things: neither contemporaries nor historians of the movement have agreed on a definition. In the United States, contemporaries and historians generally use the term to describe the crusade launched by the American Social Hygiene Association (ASHA) to fight against venereal disease and prostitution.[6] The ASHA was an alliance of female moral reformers and physicians. One historian has described its work as a "quintessentially Progressive blend of moral zeal and technical expertise."[7] In Britain, the term has been used more expansively. David Evans describes social hygiene as combining social purity, feminism, and public health to condemn the "racial poisons" of venereal disease, alcoholism, and feeble mindedness.[8] British historian Greta Jones goes even further. She only peripherally includes venereal disease and sex education in her discussion of social hygiene. She argues that the movement aimed to regulate the working classes through a wide range of projects including "scientific eating," the compulsory detainment of the so-called mentally deficient, and maternal education. She contends that it provided an alternative to the welfare state by suggesting that biology, rather than poverty, was at the root of most health and social problems.[9] Despite differences in definitions, the social hygiene movement in both the United States and Britain was strongly linked to venereal disease prevention and was highly influenced by the eugenics movement that was sweeping the Western world at the time. Part of what distinguished social hygiene from previous reform efforts was its emphasis on biology and its faith in medical expertise. At the same time, social hygiene advocates believed that citizens' voluntary action had the power to improve the nation's health and well-being.

The Canadian Social Hygiene Council started as an anti–venereal disease group that, like its American namesake, combined medicine and morality. But, reflecting the British definition of "social hygiene," the CSHC quickly moved into a broader program of health education. Bates believed that social hygiene involved not just physical health, but also moral, mental, and social health.[10] Nonetheless, by 1935, feeling that "social hygiene" had become too closely associated with venereal disease and sex education, the CSHC decided to adopt a name that would better reflect the scope of its ambitions, and it became the Health League of Canada.[11] Despite the broader mandate implied by the name change, this book will argue that the social hygiene roots of the organization would persist throughout the history of the league. Over the course of its existence, it would aim to prevent disease by trying to change individuals' behaviour. It would build alliances between doctors and voluntary organizations, believing that health should be the concern of all citizens. While the explicitly racialized language of eugenics faded away, the organization's emphasis on health as a duty of citizenship reflected the ongoing influence of "positive eugenics," which had long drawn connections between proper living and population health. While historians usually see positive eugenics as being about promoting the reproduction of the "fit," it also promoted health among children and families, by publicizing the importance of improved eating habits, sanitary homes, and particular health and moral behaviours.[12] As Frank Dikötter has noted, the historiography on eugenics has long focused on the more "extreme expressions of race improvement." He makes the point, however, that "eugenics belonged to the political vocabulary of virtually every significant modernizing force between the two world wars" and has a legacy that extends well beyond the Second World War.[13] The *Oxford Handbook of the History of Eugenics* also stresses the degree to which the eugenics movement in many countries strove to "bring about fitter life" through environmental reforms, public health, and education about the training and rearing of children.[14] We argue in this volume that there are important continuities between the social hygiene movement of the early decades of the twentieth century and the "health promotion" movement of the 1970s.

In their influential book, *The New Public Health: Health and Self in the Age of Risk*, Australian scholars Alan Peterson and Deborah Lupton argue that the new public health that emerged in the 1970s drew on the concept of the "entrepreneurial self" – the individual who is expected to be self-monitoring and to take account of risks and adjust behaviour accordingly.[15] Peterson and Lupton take the view that the rise of the entrepreneurial self has to do with the retreat of welfare state liberalism. Our work on the Health League suggests that models for the entrepreneurial self predate the retreat of welfare state liberalism, at least in the Canadian context. From its inception, the league counselled Canadians to avoid health risks and urged individuals to take responsibility for their choices – an indication that this model of public health could exist alongside expanding welfare state provisions. Indeed, as

James Colgrove argues in *State of Immunity*, Progressive Era health reformers in the United States differentiated themselves from their counterparts in earlier eras of public health reform by locating health risks in individual behaviour and urging people to take individual responsibility for their well-being, again suggesting that the entrepreneurial self has deep roots in the field of public health.[16] At the same time, the Health League of Canada encouraged Canadians to defer to doctors and dentists in all matters of health, helping to consolidate the prestige of medicine in this period.[17] Our book shows the considerable power of medical expertise in the middle decades of the twentieth century, as Canadians learned to adopt new health behaviours and were urged to think of health as a duty to themselves, their families, and their nation.

The ideology of social hygiene fed the CSHC's expansion into other health education work, including on the pasteurization of milk and diphtheria immunization, by the second half of the 1920s. The organization began presenting lectures and producing radio broadcasts on subjects ranging from child health to smallpox. In 1933, the council launched a magazine, *Health*, which covered a diverse array of health topics. Despite its innovations in the late 1920s and early 1930s, the organization barely survived the difficult years of the Great Depression, but an infusion of funds during the Second World War allowed it to launch new ventures. It started an Industrial Health Division to educate workers on how to improve their health and avoid absenteeism, renewed its anti–venereal disease program, significantly expanded its immunization activities, and partook in the campaign to educate Canadians about new developments in the field of nutrition. In 1944, the league launched National Health Week, a yearly crusade that drew Canadians' attention to preventive health through an exhaustive array of public talks, advertisements, radio broadcasts, and posters. Reflecting the fact that rates of death from infectious disease were declining, the organization began to put more effort into educating the country about the perils of chronic diseases like heart disease and cancer and encouraged Canadians to eat properly, avoid stress, exercise regularly, avoid excessive use of alcohol and other drugs, and pay attention to their mental health. In the 1950s, the league also became a major force in the campaign for water fluoridation.

Although most Health League activities were geared towards changing behaviour, a few of its initiatives, most notably its advocacy of milk pasteurization and water fluoridation, aimed to achieve legislative reform. But these initiatives, at least in Bates' view, were also about modifying behaviour. Bates wanted to convince people of the merits of these measures, and he hoped that, once people understood their benefits, they would demand that the law be changed. Such advocacy was part of the active democratic citizenship required in a society that put health first. Bates believed that health and the duties of citizenship were intimately connected.

The Health League focused its efforts on public education: it distributed pamphlets, developed radio programming, showed films, mounted exhibits, created posters, and issued a constant stream of press releases. Gordon Bates, who was director during most of the years of the active operation of the league, was a vigorous (some might say obstreperous) leader with a talent for generating media coverage. As a result, the league's influence stretched beyond its small size. The Health League provides us with a window on how public health messages were constructed, the controversy that these messages sometimes generated, and how Canadians learned

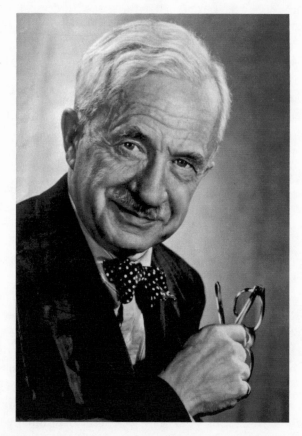

Figure 1 Gordon Bates. | LAC, MG28, I332, vol. 202.

to regulate their bodies and behaviours in new ways as they adopted the health habits advocated by the league, governments, and other organizations. Moreover, because it left extensive records – more than 250 boxes at Library and Archives Canada contain newspaper clippings, publicity materials, meeting minutes, and correspondence – the league constitutes a valuable case study. These records give a clear idea of the league's reach: clipping files, for example, show the significant publicity that its campaigns and educational programs generated across Canada.

During the years the Health League and its predecessors operated, enormous strides were made in the fight against disease. There is a fierce historical debate as to whether rising incomes (with concurrent improvements in living conditions and nutrition), public health interventions, or medical treatments made the biggest contribution to reducing mortality. Regardless of the weight assigned each factor, as living conditions improved and new vaccines and treatments were developed, deaths from infectious disease plummeted.[18] For parents, the tragedy of having a child die became an increasingly rare event. New treatments such as insulin for diabetes, sulpha drugs and antibiotics for infections, and surgical improvements, as well as important public health interventions such as better sanitation and the pasteurization of milk, also enhanced child and adult health. In the fifty years between the early 1920s and early 1970s, life expectancy increased by ten years for men and fifteen years for women.[19] While their cities became more sanitary and their food safer, Canadians gained better access to medical advice and care (or, depending on one's perspective, were more likely to be exposed to the medical "gaze"). Beginning in the late nineteenth century, the number of hospitals began to increase rapidly, and, by the 1920s, Canadians of all social classes sought hospital care for a wide range of procedures, including delivering babies.[20] As incomes rose, and access to private insurance increased after the Second World War, Canadians became more likely to see a physician if they became ill.[21] By 1961, all Canadians were entitled to free hospital care; by 1972, all Canadians had access to free primary physician care. Throughout these decades, Canadians also became better informed about health through pamphlets, exhibits, advice manuals, and the media.

The Health League and other non-governmental organizations as well as the government urged Canadians to consciously take care of their bodies (and, increasingly, their minds) for the good of themselves, their children, and their nation. British historian Dorothy Porter has used the term "health citizens" to describe the responsibilities of citizens to be healthy in, and for, the modern state.[22] Canadians increasingly think of citizenship in terms of rights and entitlements, but, in the middle decades of the twentieth century, there was a much greater focus on the responsibilities of citizenship.[23] Bates was very much of this school: for him, being a good Canadian meant listening to health authorities, adjusting one's behaviour accordingly, and saving the state money that it would otherwise have to spend on treatment for preventable conditions. Citizenship also meant being involved: he consistently urged Canadians to join committees promoting health in their communities. Throughout his career, Bates would be a "joiner" – his affiliation to the Rotary Club would be dear to his heart, and he was also an active member of the Alliance Française. Bates was what Robert Putnam would describe in his groundbreaking book about community and social capital, *Bowling Alone*, as a "macher" – an individual who makes things happen in a community.[24]

As numerous historians have noted, Canadians intensively debated the duties and meanings of citizenship in the middle decades of the twentieth century, as Canada participated in and then recovered from two world wars, gradually drew away from Britain, and slowly and incompletely moved towards adopting bilingualism, multiculturalism, and tolerance as important components of Canadian identity.[25] The Health League participated in this conversation. It argued that taking measures to protect one's own health and the health of one's children was an essential component of Canadian citizenship. Editorials in *Health* badgered Canadians about the importance of health in a democratic society. In 1941, for example, Bates quoted Benjamin Disraeli, the nineteenth-century British prime minister, as saying that the "first duty" of the statesman was "the care of public health."[26] Bates insisted that health was a matter of national interest, not just a personal or local matter. In 1952, he called on all citizens to partake in Health Week because health was not just the concern of the individual. Individual health behaviours could affect the whole community, and he urged Canadians to talk about health in their churches, service clubs, and schools.[27] Bates believed strongly in the importance of voluntary groups in democracy and, under Bates, the league continually reached out to women's organizations and service clubs such as the Rotary, Kiwanis, and Lions Clubs. In short, for Bates, health was the bedrock of democracy and the way forward to a stronger nation. And yet, as the discussion on Bates and medicare in Chapter 8 will reveal, he came to believe that health should be maintained not by the state through the provision of medical care, but by the individual actions of all citizens, who would keep themselves healthy by adopting the rules of health. He felt considerable unease about the increasing involvement of government in public health infrastructure, believing that public health work could best be done through voluntary organizations.[28] Of course, this perspective was self-interested: he believed that the Health League should receive more funding, and that, if it had adequate resources, it would be better able than government agencies to provide health education.

During these decades, Canadians came to have much higher expectations for their own health and that of their children, but they also learned to examine and control their bodies in new ways and to engage in what for many were new duties, such as visiting their doctors and dentists for regular check-ups, getting their children vaccinated, and monitoring their diets. As Alison Bashford has described for Australia, "hygiene was a responsibility, a duty."[29] It was far easier for middle- or upper-class and urban Canadians to meet these responsibilities. Poorer Canadians and those living in remote regions had a much harder time fulfilling the duties of health citizenship. Not only did they have limited access to physicians, but the medical profession treated them with much greater condescension, often assuming ignorance and apathy on the part of the poor, especially poor women.

The Health League did nothing to address these inequalities, declining to address the greater difficulties faced by certain Canadians in pursuing health citizenship and failing to represent them in their profiles of the ideal health citizen. The league did attempt to reach out to working-class Canadians through its workplace programs, but these were often condescending and assumed that employers had their employees' best interest at heart. For the most part, the league represented Canadians as white and middle class. While a large literature has drawn attention to the racialized nature of many public health campaigns, the Health League is particularly striking for its unthinking whiteness. Except in its early years, when it was focused on venereal disease, the organization rarely addressed immigrants or people of colour. This is surprising, given that these population groups were often regarded in public health circles as sources of contagion.[30] Bates did express fears that recent Italian immigrants might defeat fluoridation in Toronto (see Chapter 7), but that itself is an indication that immigrants would have to work hard to fit into his model of the idealized health citizen. Mostly the league ignored racialized "others," including Indigenous people and the large number of "New Canadians" who were transforming Canadian life in the period after the Second World War, preferring instead to focus on its idealized (white) health citizen. This meant that racialized citizens and new immigrants were denied the oftentimes-valuable education that the league gave to other Canadians on how to improve their health.

While most Canadians believed that science and medicine had done much to improve health and prolong life, and many willingly adopted the practices promoted by the league, there were always pockets of resistance. Not everyone agreed that vaccination was worth the risks to themselves and their children. Some believed that raw milk had benefits over pasteurized milk, and others felt that health agencies and governments had no business interfering in their health and with their bodies – arguments very similar to those used in present-day debates over vaccination, pasteurization, and other issues.

The Strengths and Weaknesses of the League

Bates and his allies liked to define the Health League as a national organization, but it is more accurate to call it a local agency with national aspirations and some national programs. Its headquarters were in Toronto, and, in spite of efforts to create branches in other regions and to appoint board and committee members from across Canada, Torontonians played a dominant role in daily operations, often to the dismay of people from outside the city.[31] There was an active Health League organization in Vancouver, but, much to Bates' frustration, it functioned fairly separately from the main league (and will, consequently, not be examined in any detail in this book).[32] The league also had a Quebec branch, which cooperated more closely with the "national" organization, although over the years it had some significant organizational challenges.[33] The closer relationship with the Quebec branch undoubtedly was due partly to geography (it was much easier for Bates and other league employees to travel to Montreal than to Vancouver), but it also related to Bates' vision of Canada. Bates was a francophile and, beginning in his late sixties, he regularly travelled to Paris to take courses at the Sorbonne.[34] *Health* often ran editorials on the benefits of bilingualism and, from 1958 onwards, included a regular feature entitled "Learning French." This column was a somewhat odd addition to a magazine purportedly about health, but it does illustrate the league's broad vision for health citizenship. Bates also hoped that the league would be able to raise funds in Quebec at a time when many of Canada's leading corporations were headquartered in Montreal. However, these fundraising campaigns met with little success, and one of the main roles of the Quebec branch appeared to have been translating the material that emerged from the Toronto office.

The league wanted to represent and to speak to the nation, but branch offices outside Quebec and Vancouver were haphazard and short lived. People from other parts of Canada had few opportunities to shape the message, and the Health League often remained ignorant about the challenges and opportunities that existed outside Toronto. As the director of health education in Saskatchewan and a former league employee, Christian Smith, put it in 1945:

> the League is far from reaching its potentialities in Canada. The liaison with national organizations, the distinguished names on its literature and the press service do not make it a national association. It will be truly national when it involves the common people across the country, not just as paid members or readers of the magazine, but as active participants in activities.[35]

The league often put forward strategies for organizing in other parts of the country, but it fully expected that what worked in Toronto would work elsewhere and then could not grasp why local communities failed to respond enthusiastically.[36] As a result, branch organizing was rarely successful. Instead, the league developed publicity materials in Toronto and circulated them to the rest of the country. Sometimes provincial health units embraced and used these materials; sometimes they did not. Many newspapers ran articles provided by the league, but others chose not to. Reflecting the league's reach and influence, this book has a strong focus on Toronto and Ontario, although as much as possible we have tried to outline the extent of league activities elsewhere in the country. The Health League, of course, is far from being the only central Canadian organization with illusions of representing the country as a whole. Indeed, the history of the league arguably parallels that of Canadian nationalist ambitions more broadly, from the Group of Seven to the Committee for an Independent Canada.[37] Yet, while the Health League failed to integrate the concerns and perspectives of different regions of the country, many of its campaigns had a remarkably broad reach.

The Health League was not a grassroots organization. As we will show in subsequent chapters, it was never particularly successful at recruiting members. It occasionally mobilized a network of female volunteers, most obviously in the social hygiene work of the CSHC in the 1920s and in the league's nutrition work during the Second World War.[38] There were also female staffers, although usually not in the most prominent roles. For the most part, the league was dominated by male voices. It was organized into divisions, which supported particular activities, such as milk pasteurization, water fluoridation, and food handling. Each division had a voluntary committee associated with its work. These committees were nearly always chaired by male volunteers, and most committee members were male. This skewing reflected Bates' preference for drawing supporters from the medical and dental communities and from among business leaders and politicians, all fields dominated by men. For similar reasons, the national executive and the Honorary Advisory Board were also male dominated.[39] While the league did attempt to include representatives from other parts of the country on its committees and boards, meetings were held in Toronto, which limited the input of people from outside Toronto and Quebec.

Bates' strong personality and his control over the board ensured that the Health League operated according to his command, which had both positive and negative consequences for the organization. Bates had a talent for generating publicity. Always confident of the righteousness of his causes, he wooed doctors and politicians to pursue his agenda. Opinionated and headstrong, he often made enemies as well as allies. Throughout his long career, he did not shrink from insulting or defying those who stood in the way of his vision. As journalist Sidney Katz put it in a profile of Bates for *Maclean's* in 1955, his "formula for getting results was to frighten, shock, anger and educate."[40] Bates had less talent for organizational work. Over the years, the league was criticized for starting too many projects without finishing them and for failing to test new ideas before implementing them.

Even so, the league and its predecessor organizations can be credited with several significant achievements. In the 1920s, the CSHC played a key role in educating Canadians about venereal disease and encouraging them to seek treatment. Over the course of the decade, the number of people infected with venereal disease in Canada fell substantially. The council encouraged parents to talk to their children about sex, although, like other organizations involved in sex education at the time, it significantly downplayed the pleasurable aspects of sexuality to focus on the role of sex in reproduction and the dangers of premarital sex.[41] Another success was the league's magazine, *Health,* which published continuously from 1933 to 1980, with only a brief pause from 1969 to 1972. While the magazine never enjoyed a large subscription base, it was widely available in medical and dental waiting rooms, and the league also used its articles as press releases. The magazine helped encourage a national conversation about public health. The Health League also had a voice in Ottawa. In the mid-1920s, in an effort to stave off an attempt to cut a government grant for venereal disease education and treatment, the Canadian Social Hygiene Council created the Voluntary Committee on Health of the Senate and House of Commons, which organized regular luncheon talks on health issues. This committee lasted until the 1970s.[42] All members of Parliament who were doctors, dentists, pharmacists, as well as female members of Parliament, were invited to join; Bates served as the secretary of the committee, giving him a powerful audience.[43]

The league also mounted large-scale education campaigns, such as Toxoid Week, National Immunization Week, and National Health Week. Starting in 1931, the CSHC helped conduct the Toronto Department of Health's Toxoid Week to promote diphtheria prevention. In 1943, the league independently established National Immunization Week, an annual campaign to promote vaccination against numerous preventable diseases. A year later, the league began to organize National Health Week, establishing and consolidating collaborative relationships with schools, churches, voluntary groups, and service clubs around Canada to execute this yearly publicity blitz. The league played an important role in lobbying for milk pasteurization and water fluoridation, and, along with other organizations, it encouraged Canadians to learn more about the role of nutrition in health. It played an important supportive role in educating Canadians about child and maternal health and about the growing threat of chronic diseases. In 1953, the league received a kind of international recognition when it was chosen by the World Health Organization (WHO) as the Canadian Citizens' Committee of the WHO.[44]

Given all of these accomplishments, why did the Health League not survive? Even while the league expanded its activities, there were signs that it was being overtaken by other organizations. During its years of operation, the federal and provincial governments significantly expanded their public health activities. By 1962, Ottawa employed more than 5,000 people in the field of public health, producing pamphlets, films, radio programs, and exhibits on a variety of health topics.[45] At the same time, the health-related activities of the government of Ontario cost over $136 million per year and employed over 11,000 people. The provincial government had a large publicity branch, which addressed topics such as nutrition, dental hygiene, child health, and industrial hygiene.[46] The league's work increasingly overlapped with services provided by provincial governments, and, over time, these governments came to the conclusion that they could do this work better themselves. Also, in the years after the Second World War, several voluntary organizations, often focused on a single disease or disability, either sprang up or expanded their operations. These organizations, which could tug at the heartstrings of people who had had friends or family members affected by the disease or disability, were far more successful at raising funds and at organizing local and provincial branches than was the Health League, which always took a preventive and general approach to health. Organizations like the Canadian National Institute for the Blind (founded in 1918), the Canadian Tuberculosis Association (1900), the Canadian Cancer Society (1938), and the Canadian Diabetic Association (1953), outpaced the Health League in size and budget. Even smaller organizations like the Canadian Paraplegic Association, the Muscular Dystrophy Association, and the Ontario Heart Foundation had larger annual budgets than the Health League, much to Bates' despair.[47]

Crucially, Bates also failed to adapt to changing times. He had started his career as a progressive voice. Along with feminists and like-minded medical men, he was eager to open up the discussion about venereal disease and to educate people about sex. Drawing from the message of first-wave feminists, he criticized the sexual double standard and upheld the importance of confining sex to marriage. As the years passed, his views changed very little – indeed, perhaps they became more conservative. By the 1960s, when Canadians were debating the merits of legalizing birth control and the possibility of decriminalizing homosexuality, and young people were asserting that there was nothing wrong with having sex before marriage, his views seemed increasingly outdated.[48] At the same time, many decades of working in public health had increased his frustration with Canadians who refused to adopt the health measures that he saw as being in their best interests, and his tone became increasingly shrill, especially when it came to water fluoridation. Moreover, after initially being sympathetic to publicly funded physician care, Bates eventually became an opponent of the measure, even as it quickly gained strong support from Canadians. In short, by the 1960s, Bates was increasingly out of touch with a Canada that was adopting new ideas about morality, citizenship, and the role of the state.

The Health League was also losing strength with respect to its collaborators and networks. It had successfully worked with many of the leading medical figures of the first half of the twentieth century, including Alan Brown, the autocratic physician-in-chief at Toronto's Hospital for Sick Children; J.J. Heagerty, who had a long and illustrious career in the federal Department of Health and played a crucial role in some of the early studies that led to medicare in Canada; J.W.S. McCullough, Ontario's first chief provincial health officer; and Charles Hastings, Toronto's activist medical officer of health. The Supreme Court judge and prominent author William Renwick Riddell served as the president of the Canadian Social Hygiene Council and, later, the Health League until he passed away in 1945. Bates was less successful at building connections with the physicians and other leading citizens who obtained prominence after the Second World War. Moreover, he failed to build positive links with rapidly expanding government health services at both the provincial and federal level in the postwar period. His connections with the business community also faltered.[49] Although he was able to renew the National Board of Directors and the Honorary Advisory Board in the 1950s, when the first wave of long-term allies of the league began to retire or pass away, he was not able to replace this new generation when they began to disappear in the 1960s and 1970s. This failure contributed to the gradual decline in the league's influence.

The Health League's demise can be attributed to a number of factors. Its financial security was seriously compromised when it lost United Community Fund support in the mid-1960s. Furthermore, despite Bates' protestations to the contrary, much of the organization's initial work was complete by then. Routine vaccination had become a norm, rates of child and maternal mortality had declined, and pasteurization was widespread. By the 1950s, the Health League was often fighting battles that had largely been won.[50] In addition, the general preventive approach to wellness and public health supported by the league seemed outdated. Moreover, with the passing of the Hospital Insurance and Diagnostic Services Act in 1957 and the Medical Care Act in 1966, governments had taken over much of the responsibility for their citizens' health and sickness.[51] Also, by the 1970s, the type of civic engagement encouraged by Bates was already in decline: people were attending church less regularly, were voting less often, and were drifting away from service clubs.[52] Crucially, the league was really the creation of a single individual. When Gordon Bates passed away in November 1975, the league had no succession plan, and the organization gradually withered away, although efforts are currently underway to revive the organization to focus on the dangers of spreading communicable diseases through international air travel.[53]

The League, Morality, and Public Health

Our history of the Health League emphasizes that public health campaigns in this period encouraged Canadians to adopt an entrepreneurial view of themselves and their bodies, to become aware of health risks, and to take appropriate measures to avoid these risks. Advocates presented this as a moral project and depicted Canadians who did not undertake these measures as failing in their responsibilities of citizenship. Despite the intransigence of its views, we acknowledge the real improvements that resulted from the work of the Health League and other organizations: widespread vaccination greatly reduced childhood mortality, improved sanitation practices led to fewer cases of food- and water-borne illness, and the introduction of fluorides greatly reduced tooth decay.

Yet, public health reformers, including Bates, often passed judgment on other people's health-related behaviours, leading to stigmatization and creating new forms of regulation. Thus, such reformers depicted parents who refused to vaccinate their children as lazy, uncaring, or negligent. They viewed people who opposed water fluoridation as ignorant and anti-scientific. Public health advocates demonstrated little understanding of why people might choose not to follow the recommendations of "experts" and showed little tolerance for other points of view. Such reformers gave little consideration to the fact that people living in poverty might not be able to follow the nutritional guidelines promoted by organizations such as the Health League or that working people might not have the time or financial resources to take annual holidays and exercise regularly. As American historian Allan Brandt has argued, the language of "risk" not only makes individuals responsible for their own health, it also erases the social factors that we know have a critical impact on health outcomes, such as race and class.[54] The Health League's outlook and approach was shaped by a capitalist society that concentrated power in the hands of the wealthy and well educated. In this environment, it was easy to assume that the poor needed to be pulled out of ignorance for their own good and for the good of the nation, that women needed to be counselled on how to feed and care for their families, and that workers needed to be advised on how to avoid spreading colds throughout the factory.

While the Health League was a small organization, its history parallels the history of public health in Canada and has much to teach us about the history of health education and, in particular, the connections that were made between health and citizenship in the middle decades of the twentieth century. To date, the history of public health in English Canada is not extensive. There is a much stronger tradition of public health history in Quebec.[55] Broad overviews in English include Christopher Rutty and Sue C. Sullivan's *This Is Public Health*, a celebratory book produced for the hundredth anniversary of the Canadian Public Health Association.[56] Heather MacDougall's *Activists and Advocates* examines Toronto's Health Department between 1883 and 1983. She shows how the bacteriological revolution and increasing interest in health education transformed public health in the twentieth century, and illustrates the diversity of public health endeavours in Toronto, including those related to sanitation, housing, food safety, disease prevention and treatment, and water and air quality.[57] Canadian scholars have contributed to an excellent literature on the history of child and maternal health in the first half of the twentieth century, including Cynthia Comacchio's *Nations Are Built of Babies*, Katherine Arnup's *Education for Motherhood*, Denyse Baillargeon's *Babies for the Nation*, and most recently Mona Gleason's *Small Matters*, which examines health history from the perspective of sick children.[58] There is also a significant literature on the history of venereal disease control, although much of it is very dated. Jay Cassel's book *The Secret Plague* examines the history of venereal disease control in Canada, while several articles examine the gender and class biases of the anti-VD campaigns before and during the Second World War.[59] Recently, the history of the Spanish flu epidemic has attracted significant attention from historians, while two outstanding works on the history of nutrition education have been published.[60] The campaign for milk pasteurization has generated a small literature.[61] With the exception of the broad overviews by Rutty and Sullivan and by MacDougall, little attention has been paid to public health in the years after the Second World War, which were arguably the years of the Health League's greatest successes. Nor has the history (with the exception of the remarkably good work on infant and maternal health and some of the recent work on nutrition) focused on how public health campaigns sought to shape people's health habits, their sense of self, and their feelings of responsibility towards their country.

This book provides a new perspective on the history of immunization, pasteurization, water fluoridation, anti-VD work, and nutrition education. It describes some of the health work that was done in factories and other workplaces, and it outlines the educational efforts that were made to combat chronic disease in the years after the Second World War. At the same time, the history of the Health League has much to teach us about the changing landscape facing voluntary organizations in a period when the role of the state was expanding rapidly. Several books have examined the history of voluntary fundraising and the growth of the United Community Funds across the country, but they have generally examined these subjects from the perspective of the funders and not the organizations being funded.[62] Although the Health League was supported by Toronto's United Community Fund and its earlier incarnations, Gordon Bates carried out a long campaign against the federated fundraising movement, which helps cast light on the tensions involved in such fundraising. As noted above, Bates also became an opponent of medicare, believing that it would transfer responsibility for health from the individual to the state. Our discussion of the Health League and medicare helps elucidate the role of voluntary organizations in this important transition in the provision of health care in Canada.

Finally, this study of the Health League helps us understand how health, morality, and citizenship were constructed in the middle decades of the twentieth century. For public health advocates, being a good citizen involved adopting a wide range of health behaviours, from vaccinating one's children and eating nutritiously to wearing proper footwear. Bates' view that Canadians who fell ill were failing in their duty to themselves, their families, and their country was an extreme perspective, but it continues to echo today in the debates over smoking and obesity. While there is much to celebrate in the history of public health, there is also much to criticize. Public health organizations like the Health League frequently targeted women and the working classes and accused them of being ignorant and apathetic about their health. They created a culture of judgment that encouraged Canadians to look disparagingly on fellow citizens who refused or failed to fulfil the multitudinous duties of health citizenship. Ultimately, the league and other health bodies did not address many of the underlying causes of poor health, including poverty, social marginalization, and mental distress. Instead, their rhetoric blamed individuals for their own health problems, failing to recognize that, while much disease is preventable, sickness is also inevitable and cannot be avoided simply by following the rules of health citizenship.

"Tell Your Children the Truth"
The Canadian Social Hygiene Council and Venereal Disease Education

In the early 1920s, half a million Canadians flocked to see *The End of the Road* (1919), a silent film about syphilis, sponsored by the Canadian National Council for Combatting Venereal Disease (CNCCVD). *The End of the Road* featured Mary, whose mother educates her about sex through a careful introduction to the birds and bees, and Vera, whose mother tells her that good girls do not ask questions about such matters.[1] Her mother's evasion leads Vera to seek information from neighbourhood children. When the girls reach adulthood, Mary becomes a nurse, a profession that exposes her to the tragedies caused by sexually transmitted infections and premarital intercourse. When her long-term boyfriend asks her to have sex with him before he enlists, she refuses. By contrast, Vera's mother encourages her to go to the city to seek out a wealthy spouse. She finds a job in a department store (a place notorious for the mingling of the sexes).[2] She becomes the mistress of a wealthy man and contracts syphilis. Panicked, she contacts Mary, who introduces her to her employer, Dr. Bell. After the physician educates Vera about the consequences of syphilis by showing her a range of patients suffering severe symptoms, she agrees to undergo treatment. In the end, Mary and Dr. Bell marry, while Vera turns over a new leaf and devotes her energies to the war effort.[3] While Vera is portrayed as exhibiting serious lapses in judgment, the truly guilty parties in the film are her mother, for failing to provide her with a moral upbringing and honest instruction, and the cad who infects and leaves her. The film also shows that a woman such as Mary can be exposed to social problems like premarital pregnancy and venereal disease without jeopardizing her own virtue, thereby emphasizing the importance and rectitude of bringing these issues into the open. Indeed, Dr. Bell likes Mary that much more for her willingness to provide succour to the fallen.

In the first two decades of the twentieth century, rapid changes in the diagnosis and treatment of venereal disease, along with shocking revelations about the high rates of VD among the troops during the First World War, made Canadians far more aware of sexually transmitted infections. The CNCCVD, which was formed in 1919, became the leading organization urging Canadians, especially Canadian men, to adopt higher moral standards to combat the venereal disease menace. The organization, which would soon change its name to the Canadian Social Hygiene Council (CSHC), urged those infected with venereal disease to seek treatment at the free clinics that were being established throughout Canada as part of a cost-sharing agreement between the newly established federal Department of Health and the provincial governments. In its publications, exhibits, and many public lectures, the CSHC instructed men and women to marry young and to refrain from sex before marriage. It told men that no harm could come to them from abstinence, and it warned that strong drink could diminish inhibitions and lead men to do things they might regret. The CSHC encouraged parents to have open discussions with their children about sexuality, to ensure that curious children would learn about sex in the home instead of the streets, and it urged that wholesome entertainment be provided to young people.

The organization attempted to reduce the stigma associated with venereal disease as part of its efforts to convince people to seek treatment. Yet, the organization's efforts to lessen stigma were undermined by its insistence that the failure to live up to proper moral standards was behind the venereal disease problem. Even so, considering the degree to which any discussion of sexuality was morally fraught in the early decades of the twentieth century – and in comparison with later Health League campaigns, which blamed parents for childhood diseases and condemned people for failing to listen to the doctors – the CSHC's venereal disease campaign took a somewhat less judgmental tone.

The CSHC, like the Social Hygiene Councils in Britain and the United States, with which it was well connected, was strongly influenced by the eugenics movement.[4] The recent literature on eugenics has stressed the diversity of that movement: while some eugenicists supported immigration restriction and the sterilization of the "unfit," others emphasized "positive eugenics" and believed that improving the environment (often through changing individuals' health behaviour) would produce stronger, healthier babies and citizens.[5] The motto of the CSHC's journal *Social Health,* "The Race Is to the Strong," demonstrates the clear influence of social Darwinism, but, on the whole, the CSHC was more concerned with environment than heredity.

Venereal Disease in Early Twentieth-Century Canada

The most comprehensive examination of the history of venereal disease treatment and activism in Canada remains Jay Cassel's *The Secret Plague* (1987).[6] In addition, a significant literature has rightly tied the interest in venereal disease in the early decades of the twentieth century to a broader project of moral regulation. This project, as Tina Loo, Carolyn Strange, Mariana Valverde, Joan Sangster, and others have pointed out, disproportionately targeted the working classes, whose morals were regarded as in need of improvement.[7] Influenced by the nineteenth-century social purity movement, these moral reformers assumed that the majority of women desired sex only for the purposes of reproduction. For them, the villains of the venereal disease epidemic were men who infected their wives, although they also blamed, to a lesser degree, prostitutes and "feeble-minded girls." Many anti–venereal disease campaigners believed that prostitutes had been forced into the work through "white slavery" or low wages and tragic family circumstances. Even so, they believed that such women were in need of rehabilitation and moral guidance. The true victim of venereal disease was the innocent woman, infected as a result of her husband's premarital or extramarital affairs, and the young child born with congenital syphilis or blindness caused by gonorrhea. Doctors drew attention to the degree to which venereal disease caused sterility, preventing women from fulfilling their maternal destiny. While venereal disease often did result in infertility and frequently led to long-term health problems, couching the problem in this way also emphasized that all women were expected to want to be mothers, and that a failure to fulfil this maternal destiny was catastrophic for women.

These moralizing and frequently maudlin eugenic discourses deserve criticism, but it is important to recognize that venereal disease was a very real problem in Canada. Shortly before the outbreak of the First World War, researchers estimated that somewhere between 5 and 15 percent of Canadians were infected with syphilis and that an even greater number had contracted gonorrhea at some point in their lifetime.[8] Today, these diseases are usually easily treated, but at the turn of the century syphilis could be a death sentence. The complications of tertiary syphilis included insanity, difficulty in controlling movement, and heart disease. Gonorrhea could lead to pelvic inflammatory disease, which could lead to infertility and a form of arthritis. Doctors such as Gordon Bates observed the complications of these diseases first hand: they saw patients who had difficulty walking as a result of syphilis and they encountered women who required hysterectomies or the removal of their fallopian tubes due to pelvic inflammatory disease. Doctors also saw how the disability or death of a breadwinner could leave a family in poverty.[9] Bates himself completed a study of fifty women who attended his venereal disease clinic at Toronto General Hospital. Collectively, the women had 192 pregnancies: 53 ended in miscarriage and 24 in stillbirths, 36 infants were born with congenital syphilis, and 42 of the babies died in early infancy. Only 37 babies were born healthy. Bates declared that this was an example of "mass murder."[10] Indeed, it takes little imagination to understand the pain and suffering involved for the women who miscarried, gave birth to stillborn children, or had a child born with congenital syphilis.

A number of groups spoke out about venereal disease in Canada prior to the First World War, but the widespread testing and treatment of soldiers made it clear how common such disease was and how much manpower was being lost as a result.[11] By 1915, testing revealed that 28.7 percent of the men in the Canadian Expeditionary Force were infected with venereal disease, the highest rate among troops in the Western theatre.[12] In the early stages of the war, nearly half of the men hospitalized were there because they had been infected with VD.[13] At the same time, rapid changes were taking place in the world of venereal disease treatment. In 1905, German researchers identified the spirochete that caused syphilis.[14] The first serological test for the disease (the Wassermann test) emerged a year later, although it did not come into widespread usage in Canada until the war. The first effective treatment for syphilis appeared in 1909, when Paul Ehrlich and his team discovered the antimicrobial drug arsphenamine, which was patented under the name Salvarsan.[15] Salvarsan treatment was an ordeal: repeated injections were necessary, and the drug caused nausea and vomiting, as well as liver disease and changes to the blood, but it could cure syphilis. The patient was usually given injections every three to five days for two months; then potassium iodide was given to keep the disease in check while the patient recovered. More rounds of Salvarsan would follow until repeated Wassermann

tests showed that the patient was completely free of the disease. Not surprisingly, patients often failed to complete the full course of treatment. Neo-
salvarsan, introduced in 1912, reduced the side effects, but it was somewhat
less effective, and arsphenamine seems to have been more commonly used
in Canada, at least in the 1920s.[16] David Evans argues that the introduction
of Salvarsan increased medical interest in venereal disease in Britain and led
doctors to demand action.[17] This seems to have been true in Canada as well.

The war drew attention to the seriousness of the venereal disease problem, but it also made it more difficult to simply blame philandering men.
Young men were being sent overseas to serve their country, and many contemporaries believed that they were being placed in the way of temptation
as a result.[18] Lucy Bland has argued that, in Britain, the fiery prewar feminist critique of male sexuality was displaced by the idea that men's sexual
needs should be met as safely as possible.[19] The critique of male sexuality
remained in Canada (as it did in Britain), but it softened. Politicians, jour-
nalists, and public health officials were aware that prostitution, venereal
disease, and war had long gone hand in hand. At the same time, they were
concerned that infected soldiers would spread the disease to their wives,
or future wives, back home.[20] The initial response was to give lectures to
the troops, with illustrated slides outlining the dire consequences of venereal disease infection, and to urge them to be sexually continent. But such
advice was difficult to follow when sex was readily available: according to
Cassel, women offered sex in canteens and railway stations, and sometimes even in soldiers' tents. Reportedly, women were especially interested
in Dominion troops, as they had more money to spend.[21] Eventually, the
army started organizing more wholesome entertainments to keep the men
occupied. A few units undertook to distribute prophylactic kits, but army
medical officers were not convinced that prophylaxis was effective.[22] Eventually, they came to recognize its merits, and, by 1916, the army had made
arrangements with the City of London National Guard Volunteer Corps
to establish prophylactic centres in London for men on leave. Later, the
army began offering prophylactic washes at brigade hospitals and in medical officers' huts. By December 1916, the army started distributing "preventive kits" with ointment in them, which medical personnel considered
to be more effective than condoms in combatting venereal disease. They
army does not appear to have distributed condoms. According to Cassel, giving out condoms, which could also prevent pregnancy, would have
made it seem as if the army were condoning promiscuous sex. Also, as
Andrea Tone makes clear in Devices and Desires, the quality of condoms

left something to be desired.[23] At the end of 1917, military authorities in Canada attempted to trace the contacts of infected men, but with limited success.[24] In 1918, the Canadian government passed an addition to the Defence of Canada Order, stating that it was an offence for a woman suffering from venereal disease to invite any member of the armed forces to have sex with her. Interestingly, in light of a long history of feminist action against the sexual double standard in Britain, Canadian feminists did not oppose the new legislation, probably reflecting the more conservative nature of the feminist movement here.[25] Cassel explains that Canadian feminists probably believed that these new regulations would help protect their own health, while British feminists saw them as a sign of blatant discrimination against all women.[26]

During the war, Gordon Bates was the VD Officer for Military District no. 2 (Toronto). Bates had been born in 1885 into a medical family. His father, Frank Dewitt Bates, was an eye, ear, and nose specialist.[27] His was not a happy family: his parents split up when he was young, and his strong-willed mother raised him on her own. This family history may have spurred Bates' interest in feminism and family life education.[28] His younger brother, Kendal, would also become a doctor, while his sister, Mona, would become a renowned pianist, who sometimes put on fundraising shows for the league. Gordon Bates entered medical school at the University of Toronto in 1903.[29] His grades were unremarkable, but, in the last two years of his degree, he became the medical representative on the newly formed Students' Parliament. According to the student yearbook, *Torontonensis*, he distinguished himself as a "a politician of no small fame."[30] Within a few years of graduation, he was serving as an instructor in medicine at the University of Toronto. He was also active in social causes, and, in 1912, he became secretary of the Provincial Association for the Care of the Feeble-Minded, an organization that included several people who would become prominent in the CNCCVD and the CSHC. That organization was undoubtedly important in informing Bates' views about the role that the "feeble minded" played in spreading venereal disease.[31] Later, he became a member of the Canadian National Committee on Mental Hygiene, a group formed from the ashes of the dissolution of the Provincial Association for the Care of the Feeble-Minded.[32] He also chaired the State Medicine section of the Toronto Academy of Medicine in the 1910s.[33] In short, in a brief period of time, he became an active member of the Toronto medical scene, building his networks and contacts with physicians and social reformers, including many people with eugenic inclinations.

Bates was also becoming well known as an expert in the diagnosis and treatment of venereal disease. He was doing research involving the Wassermann reaction as far back as 1912.[34] In 1914–16, he was an assistant pathologist at the Toronto Hospital for the Insane, and, in this role, he published at least one article on the use of Salvarsan treatment for general paresis.[35] Bates continued to run a venereal disease clinic after the formation of the CSHC. His close professional involvement with the disease may help to account for the fact that he does not appear to have been a supporter of negative eugenics: he was well aware that venereal disease affected both the rich and the poor and those of both high and low status.

In his military role, Bates took an activist approach to venereal disease: he created a committee of more than one hundred volunteers, including doctors, lawyers, newspaper editors, judges, the heads of women's organizations, and clergy. This committee organized VD education in churches and schools, created women's patrols to police the streets of the city, established a Recreation Committee for Soldiers to keep them out of trouble, and put out press releases drawing attention to the issue.[36] As the war came to a close, Bates launched a campaign to continue his venereal disease work, stressing that VD was not just a military problem and that moral conditions in Canada were far from ideal. He noted that, when the army decided to give all members of a draftee regiment a Wassermann test, it found that 5.7 percent of the men had syphilis. Since the majority of the men had been in the army for just one week, it was clear that they had acquired the infection prior to enlistment. Likewise, in the Toronto General Hospital, 12 percent of all ward patients had syphilis, and most of them were unaware that they were infected.[37] Bates was further inspired by a trip to the United States, which allowed him to observe the US Army's extensive anti-VD program.[38] Back in Canada, he urged government authorities to look to what he had accomplished in Military District no. 2 as a starting point and recommended that a national committee for combatting venereal disease be formed and receive government endorsement.[39]

The federal Ministry of Health was created in 1919 and included a Venereal Disease Division headed by J.J. Heagerty. The division's main objective was to provide matching funds to provinces that agreed to establish free VD clinics.[40] This was one of the first examples of a federal-provincial cost-sharing program, an initiative that would arguably help lead to far more extensive publicly funded health care in Canada in future decades.[41] In the interim, Bates had created the CNCCVD, and the division hoped that the CNCCVD would do most of what was required in terms of education activities. To that end, it provided the organization with a yearly grant that started at $5,000 but increased over time to $20,000.[42] This reliance on non-governmental groups was not an unusual strategy, as the newly created Department of Health was small. It did develop an extensive library of educational material in child and maternal health under the leadership of Helen MacMurchy, but it was inclined to turn to voluntary groups to work on more sensitive topics. The department also gave funds to the Canadian National Committee on Mental Hygiene to help it conduct its work.[43] The provinces took action against venereal disease as well. In 1918, an order-in-council mandating the reporting of venereal disease passed in Saskatchewan. The Ontario government followed suit. Eventually, similar legislation passed in every province in Canada, except Quebec, which did not require compulsory notification.[44] The legislation could be draconian. In Ontario, for example, if the medical officer of health in a community suspected someone of being infected with venereal disease, that person could be ordered to undergo an examination and, if infected, could be served with a form requiring him or her to seek medical treatment and report monthly to the medical officer. While under treatment, the person was to avoid sexual intercourse, marriage, or any other conduct likely to infect another person. Abandoning treatment could result in a fine of $25–$100 or three months' imprisonment, while infecting someone else could result in a fine of $500 or twelve months' imprisonment.[45] That said, in most provinces, compulsory treatment was not generally enforced for most of the population.[46] It was different for prisoners. Because all residents of provincial prisons were tested, many underwent compulsory treatment while incarcerated, and some were detained beyond the period of their sentence to ensure that they were free of disease upon release. In her memoir, *Incorrigible*, Velma Demerson describes undergoing painful treatments for sexually transmitted infections while in the Mercer Reformatory in Toronto – treatments that were likely mandated under Ontario's Venereal Disease Control Act.[47] In her study of the Mercer, Carolyn Strange discovered that the physician at the reformatory, Edna Guest (who also served as a speaker for the Canadian Social Hygiene Council and was on the national executive of the Health League of Canada for many years), gave women treatments far in excess of what was required to render them non-infectious and detained infected women for longer than their original sentence. She regarded her patients as "filthy."[48]

Establishing the CNCCVD/CSHC

Bates successfully recruited a wide range of individuals to participate in the CNCCVD/CSHC. These included Florence Huestis, already well known for her public health work with the Toronto Local Council of Women; Barnett Brickner, a progressive young rabbi who sat on the Toronto Committee of the CSHC; and Andrew S. Grant, a Presbyterian minister involved in moral and social reform, especially temperance.[49] Many prominent doctors served on the Executive Committee of the CNCCVD/CSHC, including J.G. Fitzgerald, the founder of the influential Connaught Laboratories;[50] J.W.S. McCullough, Ontario's chief medical officer; C.K. Clarke, a well-known psychiatrist and dean of the Faculty of Medicine at the University of Toronto; and Antoine-Hector Desloges, general medical superintendent for the insane asylums of the province of Quebec, who also led that province's anti–venereal disease campaigns.[51] Dr. William F. Roberts, Canada's first provincial minister of health (for the province of New Brunswick) was also involved with the council.[52] Bates also enlisted businessmen, such as J.J. Gibbons, a pioneering advertising executive, and the financier Lewis Wood – the latter was also a key player in the formation of the Canadian National Institute for the Blind.[53] The wide diversity of people involved in the organization is a testament to Bates' networking skills, and may have kept the CNCCVD/CSHC fairly moderate in its orientation, since Bates needed to appeal to a broad constituency even within his own organization.

One of the first organized activities of the CNCCVD was working with a commercial firm to show *The End of the Road,* the movie described at the beginning of the chapter. By the early 1920s, Canadians were flocking to movie theatres to see Hollywood features, but they also saw educational films, especially if they had to do with sex. Martin Pernick has shown that, before the end of the silent era in 1927, more than 1,300 health-related films had been produced in the United States.[54] The CNCCVD believed that the showing of *The End of the Road* increased attendance at venereal disease clinics; it also provided the council with opportunities to distribute educational pamphlets to audience members.[55] The council may have been right: a study of the effectiveness of First World War VD films in the United States concluded that, although they had little impact on behaviour, audience members retained the information, had more faith in medical science, and went to the doctor more frequently.[56] A few years earlier, a much-cited study revealed that most young men learned about sex from older peers, not parents. Social hygienists feared that such information was "unwholesome," and they supported the film's message about the benefits of parents speaking to their children about sex.[57] Throughout his career, Bates regarded *The End of the Road* as the best anti-VD film ever made, even better than *Damaged Lives* (1933), which he helped to create.[58]

In the early 1920s, the CNCCVD arranged for the British suffrage leader Emmeline Pankhurst to give lectures across Canada. Pankhurst, well known to Canadians who had followed the protests and hunger strikes of the British campaign for suffrage, was short of funds and was thinking of moving to Canada. Feminists in the United Kingdom, including Pankhurst's daughter and political ally Christabel Pankhurst, had long been interested in venereal disease. In 1913, Christabel had published *The Great Scourge*, a tract that blamed venereal disease on prostitution. Her cure was reflected in the slogan "Votes for Women and Chastity for Men."[59] Bates recruited Emmeline to become the vice-president of the CNCCVD, and she agreed to a long series of speaking engagements.[60] In her first six weeks in Toronto, Pankhurst spoke to church groups, the Imperial Order Daughters of the Empire (IODE), the Canadian Manufacturers' Association, and private gatherings.[61] The speeches stressed the dangers of venereal disease for women and for "the race." In a 1921 speech to a large audience in Massey Hall, Pankhurst stressed, "It is the right of every child to be born healthy, of healthy and intelligent parents." She warned that venereal diseases threatened to destroy the human race, and that to conquer them it was necessary to inculcate "high ideals of marriage and life."[62] She was not unique in these views: many British feminists drew links between venereal disease and the decline of the race.[63] Pankhurst recommended that everyone have a certificate of health before marriage. She announced that she had moved to Canada with the goal of making the country an example to the rest of the world, by making "its people pure."[64]

In 1923, Bates and Pankhurst conducted a national speaking tour across Canada. Over 60,000 people attended the lectures.[65] In January, they made a two-week trip across New Brunswick, addressing audiences in twelve cities. At the final meeting, at the Imperial Theatre in Saint John, the lieutenant governor, William Pugsley, claimed that he had never addressed a larger crowd in the province.[66] Between May and August, Bates, Pankhurst, and J.J. Heagerty, the director of the Venereal Disease Division of the federal Department of Health, made sixty-three speeches in Manitoba, Saskatchewan, and Alberta.[67] These lectures typically began with a screening of *The End of the Road* and concluded with Bates and Pankhurst discussing the medical and social implications of VD. Pankhurst stressed the "need for a higher moral standard, improved home conditions, leisure time, and an end to white slavery.["68] She blamed the sexual double standard for the sex trade and told tragic stories of innocent women and children who had been infected with VD by family members. Pankhurst also embarked on an automobile tour of thirty-six towns and cities in Ontario, chauffeured by the secretary of the Ontario branch of the CSHC, Estelle Hewson. In an age when car travel was still an adventure, they drove as far as Sault Ste. Marie and Manitoulin Island, suffering numerous blown tires and one near miss by a train along their way.[69]

By 1924, Pankhurst had grown tired of the long hours lecturing and travelling across the country and she resigned from the CSHC. In a farewell letter, she wrote that Bates' "enthusiasm and unselfish devotion" had been a "constant inspiration."[70] Certainly, the experience of lecturing with Pankhurst left a deep impression on Bates. In later speeches and articles, he would reminisce about their tours together, claiming she was "a great and sincere woman" whose work with the CSHC had "made a wonderful contribution to the cause."[71] He would continue to cite her as an inspiration for years to come, especially when he argued in favour of women taking a greater role in political and community life.[72] Indeed, Bates professed feminist principles throughout his life, even while his organization assumed that women's primarily responsibilities would be in the home.

By 1921, the CNCCVD had organized committees in every province, with the exception of Prince Edward Island. In general, the CNCCVD/CSHC found it very challenging to organize branches in the Maritime provinces. In the rest of Canada, many cities had CSHC branches, including Montreal, Ottawa, Kingston, Hamilton, Brantford, London, Windsor, Winnipeg, Edmonton, and Vancouver. These branches ran more or less independently from the main Toronto office, although their activities were very similar, with a few regional differences. The Winnipeg branch (which called itself a Health League, rather than a Social Hygiene Council) distributed literature to adolescents and their parents on venereal disease and hosted a venereal disease exhibit, including wax models that showed the ravages of syphilis, but it also hosted radio talks on an array of health topics.[73] More unusually, it also delivered lectures in Yiddish, Polish, and Ruthenian and launched an investigation into unsanitary mattresses and upholstery.[74] In Montreal, the Social Hygiene Committee was created as part of the Montreal Tuberculosis and General Health League.[75] In northern Alberta, the Social Hygiene Council distributed literature, argued for the teaching of social hygiene in Alberta normal schools (schools to train teachers), and, in a departure from regular CSHC activities, lobbied for the compulsory testing of restaurant workers

for VD.[76] This branch also fought for special classes for "mentally defective" children.[77] In 1923–24, the Ontario secretary reported that there were
twenty-one different branches of the CSHC in the province, fourteen of
which were active. In the middle of the 1920s, the CSHC added two doctors to do organization work in both the eastern and western provinces and
hired C.P. Fenwick to work in the Toronto council and to serve as Bates'
assistant.[78] In 1924, the CSHC began publishing a magazine, *Social Health*,
which bore the motto "To Advocate the Knowledge and Practice of Social
Hygiene as the One Way to Racial Improvement." *Social Health* provided
educational articles along with an overview of CSHC activities. In 1925, the
CSHC moved offices to Elm Street in downtown Toronto and took over
a neighbouring church, which gave the organization an auditorium that
seated 1,650 people. The council called its new headquarters Hygeia House,
evoking the classical goddess of health and hygiene.[79] Members initially
voiced some unease about that name, which some said reminded them of
underwear and hydrotherapy, but it eventually won out over less evocative
names such as Elm Street Hall, highlighting the organization's attachment
to the principles and ideology of social hygiene. In 1925, the CSHC received
a $15,000 grant from the Metropolitan Life Insurance Company, adding to
the significant sums that it received from the Venereal Disease Division of
the federal Department of Health and from the Ontario government.[80] Metropolitan Life had an extremely active health education program, making
them an obvious contributor to the CSHC.[81]

The Toronto Social Hygiene Council was particularly active; indeed, it
shared and helped fund the CSHC's offices at Hygeia House.[82] The Education Committee of the Toronto council gave frequent talks to parent groups
about sex hygiene. Speakers included the top names in social welfare and
sex education in Ontario, including Dr. Margaret Patterson, a judge on the
Women's Court; Dr. Edna Guest; Peter Sandiford, a professor at the Ontario
Institute for Studies in Education and a well-known proponent of intelligence testing (which he believed revealed important racial differences); and
J.J. Heagerty.[83] In 1924, a social hygiene exhibit (including wax models) was
shown for six consecutive weeks in Toronto, with two to three showings
each day at the St. Charles Hotel. Over 17,000 people attended the exhibit,
and over 100,000 pamphlets were distributed.[84] Other CSHC branches had
short bursts of activity. The Welland committee hosted Social Hygiene
Week in January 1924. As part of that event, *The Gift of Life* (a beautifully
animated film about reproduction in plants and animals) was shown to the
local Women's Institute, the Catholic Women's League, girls and boys in

the high school (in separate showings), the IODE, the Navy League, and the Girls' Auxiliary to the Navy League. In Fort William, Ontario, nearly 5,000 people attended a social hygiene exhibit, an impressive number in a city with a population of just over 35,000 people. The exhibit was shown separately to men and women, and when it opened to women, police had to be called in to manage the crowds. The CSHC then moved the exhibit to Wayside House, a settlement house, where they proudly reported "42 nationalities are being Canadianized" (that is, being taught English, civics, history, and so-called Canadian ways).[85] Another thousand people attended. In Peterborough, the social hygiene exhibit attracted 4,711 visitors – almost a quarter of the city's total population. The CSHC hosted additional exhibits at the Kiwanis Fair and the Peterborough Exhibition. While local Social Hygiene Councils initially had success with speakers and exhibits, enthusiasm often petered out, and few of the councils in smaller cities and towns existed for more than a few years. By the end of the decade, all of the branches in Ontario except those in Toronto and Ottawa had folded.[86] Keeping local branches active would prove to be a perennial problem for the CSHC and the Health League in the decades to come.

Eugenics, Morality, and the CSHC

Feminist historians have drawn attention to the degree to which the social hygiene movement was responsible for the sexual policing of women. As Kristin Luker puts it, female moral reformers involved in the social hygiene movement wanted to end the sexual double standard, but, in doing so, they created a world in which female sexual behaviour was more regulated than ever before.[87] As several historians have shown in the Canadian context, women were often institutionalized for sexual offences.[88] Moreover, the venereal disease acts that passed around the country in the aftermath of the First World War forced people, including many women, to undergo treatment against their will. While the CSHC did not spend much time lobbying for legislation to control venereal disease or prostitution, probably because it believed that the current legislative framework was sufficient, its education efforts certainly supported repressive existing legislation.

As previously mentioned, the Canadian Social Hygiene Council was highly influenced by the eugenic movement, although it tended to embrace "positive eugenics." American historian David Pivar notes that, although the American Social Hygiene Association was influenced by eugenic ideas, it represented a mix of views: a number of organizers were strict hereditarians and supported sterilization, while others opposed it.[89] The Canadian Social

Hygiene Council had a similar mix. Some people involved in the organization were supporters of negative eugenics. C.K. Clarke, who served on the
Executive Committee, was Canada's leading psychiatrist and a well-known
proponent of immigration restriction.[90] Emily Murphy, who had supported
the passage of the Sexual Sterilization Act in Alberta, served as one of the
many vice-presidents of the CSHC, although she did not take a particularly
active role in the organization.[91] Charles Hastings, an enthusiastic member
of the CSHC and of the Eugenics Society, lobbied the federal government
to restrict immigration.[92] Although many people involved in the CSHC also
belonged to the Eugenics Society of Canada, there is no evidence that Bates
was a member.[93]

The CSHC occasionally published items in *Social Health* that were out-
right racist. One issue featured an image captioned "The Fit and the Unfit
to Carry on the Race." It foregrounded a healthy young white couple cra-
dling a baby, while, in the distance, a darker, presumably African Canadian,
man sat in a chair holding a cane, while his white wife or nurse held an
infant. The white couple looked lovingly into the infant's eyes, while the
other woman looked up, seemingly in despair (see Figure 2).[94] The journal also expressed support for immigration restriction: in 1924, an article
complained about the quality of British children being sent to Canada on
subsidized schemes; C.K. Clarke had long been concerned about what he
saw as the "poor quality" of the Home Children.[95] A 1925 article, written by
Clarence Hincks of the Canadian National Committee on Mental Health,
warned that "we cannot be too careful in connection with the prudent
selection of our immigrants."[96] In 1928, the CSHC passed a resolution at its
annual meeting supporting the dominion government in its effort to expand
the medical inspection of immigrants.[97] But, for the most part, the organization focused its efforts on sexual education and venereal disease exhibits.

The council's educational program for women focused on ensuring wom-
en's health for the sake of future generations. Its pamphlet (originally produced by the ASHA) *Healthy Happy Womanhood* urged women to walk,
swim, and skate, to get plenty of fresh air and sleep, to eat well, and to stand
up straight. It warned that "the future of the race depends on the children"
and told women that, by keeping themselves healthy and by choosing a
physically fit spouse, they could give their children "a clean bill of health."[98]
In such ways, the council promoted the values of positive eugenics, stressing the role that environment could play in producing strong and healthy
children.[99] By the end of the 1920s, the concern with parental health led the
organization to support the idea of compulsory premarital medical exams,

SOCIAL HEALTH

To Advocate the Knowledge and Practice of Social Hygiene as the One Way to Racial Improvement

ORGAN OF THE CANADIAN SOCIAL HYGIENE COUNCIL

HON. MR. JUSTICE RIDDELL, *President*   DR. GORDON BATES, *Gen.-Secretary*

"The Race is to the Strong"

VOL. 1 No. 2   TORONTO, MARCH, 1924   507 YORK BLDG., 146 KING ST. W.

Re-making Men's Lives

Those who saw the Exhibit of soldiers' work at the Canadian National Exhibition last year must have been amazed at not only its variety and excellence but at the background of governmental care of the lives of our returned men which it implied.

Toys, pottery, wood carving, modelling, weaving, basketry, embroidery, leather work, furniture, painting, brooms were only some of the things shown. These were the work, in innumerable cases of convalescent or partially disabled men, who had been helped to self expression and some measure of self support through vocational training provided by a government which "cares." Thousands of men who, in less enlightened times, and under a less generous government, might have been just so much human driftwood have been turned into useful craftsmen. Lives have been re-made. Many totally blind men, unable to pursue former vocations have been trained into expert masseurs, piano tuners, or other wage producing professions and trades. Even hospital cases have been provided with useful crafts. Unhappy invalids have been enabled to reach comparative contentment through productive occupations. Effort, imagination, money, have all been expended on our returned men to rehabilitate them comfortably in civil life. Our Canadian Government has not left its broken soldiers to shift for themselves. Pensions used to be the limit of help afforded national "heroes" by after-war governments. Nowadays this is seen to be only the first of our responsibilities. Soldiers' lives when not lost or broken are often driven from old moorings by war. Life may remain, but what of training uncompleted in trade or profession, placing gone, or aptitude changed? Our Canadian Governments have tried hard to answer these questions in terms of an actual re-making of men's lives.

The Fit and the Unfit to Carry on the Race

Pick up last year's Blue Book from the Department of Soldier's Civil Re-Establishment and note not only the large sums spent for hospitals, medical, dental, orthopaedic or ophthalmic care, but for soldiers' comforts, farm and garden expenses, vocational instruction, allowances to the sub normal, training pay and allowances or unemployment relief. Through a system of inspired doles, numbers of men, you will find, have been set up in business, and have with few exceptions, succeeded. Out of 203 totally or partially blinded soldiers 171 have been given full training at productive work. So successful have been the rehabilitation measures taken for blinded soldiers that there has resulted a noticeable improvement in the possibilities for all blinded people, so that civilian as well as soldier, blind are now being assisted to become self supporting.

All this is known to be constructive work of a high order. It has its counterpart among the civil population in our public health work. For if wounds cripple the soldier, disease cripples the civilian and lessens enormously his productive value in the community.

Recently Dr. Vincent, President of the Rockefeller Foundation congratulated Canada on being in the very forefront of public health work in the after-war world. An enviable reputation to enjoy among our neighbors.

Yet there are now rumors that as our national expenditures must be reduced, both in rehabilitation and public health, estimates may be seriously curtailed. We have faith, however, that these are only rumors, and that the Federal Government which has already shown so fine a vision regarding the welfare of its people, both soldier and civilian, will find ways and means to continue grants which cannot be regarded as liabilities but as assets.

At present among other grants the Dominion Government gives to the provinces a sum of $200,000

Figure 2   The images on this CSHC newsletter provide a clear example of the racism espoused by the league. | *Social Health*, March 1924, LAC, MG28, I332, vol. 124, file 6.

although it did not lobby for them, believing that an extensive educational campaign was required to enhance support for such tests.[100] Premarital medical exams were first required in some American states in the early years of the twentieth century, although at that time they were required only for grooms, as it was believed that it would be too humiliating for a woman to undergo such an examination.[101]

In all of its activities, the CSHC stressed the importance of proper housing and healthful recreation. The organization believed that there were clear links between overcrowded housing conditions and sexual immorality, and it argued that the state should license boarding houses to prevent them from being used as houses of assignation.[102] The CSHC thought that boarding houses should have to provide drawing rooms where boarders could receive guests instead of having to take them to their rooms. At the same time, drawing on a long tradition of recreation reform, the CSHC urged social workers to provide wholesome entertainment activities such as folk dancing, debates, and plays. The council wanted young people to spend leisure time outdoors and hoped that organized sports activities would combat immorality and promote health, not just for young people, but also for future generations. To this end, the Toronto Social Hygiene Council put on regular dances and hosted bridge nights at Hygiea House.[103]

Although the CSHC was morally opposed to prostitution, it was not involved in any campaigns to close down brothels or rid the streets of prostitutes: instead, it focused its attention on preventing casual sex through education and improving housing and recreational activities. This approach likely reflected the council's belief that there was relatively little organized prostitution in Toronto at this time. It believed that most venereal disease was spread through casual contacts or "occasional prostitution." The group acknowledged that organized prostitution was more widespread in Montreal and some Western cities.[104] Certainly Montreal contributors to *Social Health* were far more adamant about the need to eradicate red-light districts.[105]

In its work around VD, the CSHC also emphasized the importance of treatment. It urged venereal disease clinics to create social case sheets that would allow doctors and social workers to trace the source of the infection. Such a practice would bring more people into treatment and allow authorities to better understand the factors behind the spread of the disease, although it also represented a serious infringement of people's privacy. The organization also emphasized the economic and social costs of failing to treat venereal diseases. The organization stressed that venereal disease reduced the birth rate by causing sterility. It cut short the lifespan, ensuring that many productive work years were lost, leaving the state to care for the dependants of the deceased.[106] One of the cases Bates cited almost incessantly was that of a man in Brantford, Ontario, who had applied for relief. The immediate cause was rheumatism, but a blood test found that he had syphilis. He had seven children: all were infected. The first child was deaf and visually impaired, the second child was reportedly "dumb," the third had a bone infection caused by syphilis, the fourth was "mentally backward," and yet another was "an idiot."[107] The case illustrated the eugenic implications of venereal disease but also underlined the extent to which illness created poverty, which would become one of the Health League's major themes. It also echoed the family histories favoured by eugenicists, like those of the Jukes and the Kallikak families, which were supposed to illustrate how poverty, crime, and feeble-mindedness ran in families.[108]

Above all, Bates believed lack of education was to blame for sex work and venereal disease. More than once he cited the case of a young prostitute who told him that she would never have entered the sex trade if her mother had told her anything about men or about venereal disease.[109] In a lecture to the Theosophical Society of Toronto in 1919, he claimed that "10,000 immoral women in Montreal ... had fallen from virtue because they had not been taught sex hygiene at school."[110] One of the pamphlets circulated by the Social Hygiene Council was Edith Hooker's *The Scapegoat*. It told the tragic tale of a farm worker who discovered that his five-day-old son was blind as a result of a gonorrheal infection that he believed was long gone. Hooker blamed not the man who had acquired the infection but the doctor who had not told him that he was contagious.[111] The pamphlet stressed the importance of educating people about venereal disease. Throughout its VD work, the CSHC believed that people needed to be educated about their bodies, and they needed to understand how venereal disease was spread. In its films and lectures for both adolescent and adult audiences, the CSHC taught people about the reproductive system, using scientific language and terms. Two of the films it used, *How Life Begins* (1916) and *The Gift of Life* (1920), featured detailed discussions of reproduction in plants and animals.[112] The organization encouraged parents to speak openly and accurately about sex to their children, although it felt that these discussions should be subordinated to broader conversations about morality, relationships, and health habits. The CSHC's pamphlet on sex education, *Tell Your Children the Truth*, urged parents to abandon "foolish lies" about the cabbage patch and the doctor's black bag but also encouraged them to put sex education second to the "training of character, the development of fondness for good literature, the creation of frank, friendly companionships between parents and children" and the "formation of definite health habits" such as personal cleanliness, wearing loose hygienic clothing, exercising regularly, eating wholesome food, and avoiding constipation.[113] The Social Hygiene Council circulated stories that featured factual, age-appropriate information about where babies came from, such as Edith Howes' "The Cradle Ship" (a fairy tale for children aged seven to ten), and D.B. and E.B. Armstrong's "Sex in Life" (for children entering puberty).[114]

The council also carried out an extensive campaign against the sexual double standard. Its oft-printed pamphlet *An Open Letter to Young Men* (initially published by the British Social Hygiene Council) urged men to practise self-restraint, characterizing it as the "basis of law and order," "a necessity in the service of god," and a "keynote of civilization." *An Open Letter* told men that premarital or extramarital sex degraded them, as well as women, and it advised men to marry young to avoid temptation. The pamphlet observed that intercourse was not necessary for health. The author, Douglas White, argued that regulated prostitution did nothing to diminish venereal disease and that the only solution was to abolish the sex trade entirely. He urged men to avoid alcohol in their quest for self-control and continence, arguing that "disease and alcohol go largely hand in hand," and he advocated that dirty books and pictures be off-limits.[115] Like most of the council's educational material, *An Open Letter to Young Men* assumed that men were to blame for the spread of venereal disease. But, on occasion, the CSHC could also blame women. In its early years, the council sometimes showed the First World War film *Fit to Fight.*[116] The lead character, Billy Hale, a brave, outstanding soldier, refuses to have anything to do with drink or with prostitutes. A boxer, Kid McCarthy, realizes the evil of his ways thanks to Hale's influence and decides to abstain from alcohol and illicit sex for the remainder of the war. The other three men featured in the film are all infected with venereal disease – the innocent country boy becomes infected through just one kiss "with an immoral woman." In contrast to the *End of the Road*, which regarded women as the innocent victims of venereal disease, *Fit to Fight* treats women as temptresses whom good soldiers need to stay away from. It is in keeping with the CSHC's feminist principles that it emphasized *The End of the Road* rather than *Fit to Fight*, although it may also have based this decision on the fact that *The End of the Road* is a more entertaining and less didactic movie.[117]

Venereal Disease Campaigns of the 1930s

By the early 1930s, the sense of crisis around venereal disease had diminished. It was clear that syphilis was being caught and treated much earlier, leading to fewer cases of tertiary syphilis. Across the country, 102 clinics had been established to treat venereal disease, and more than 350,000 people had been treated.[118] In 1929, the Toronto Social Hygiene Council and the Toronto Academy of Medicine undertook a survey of venereal disease in Toronto.[119] All of the city's venereal disease clinics, and 98 percent of its physicians, responded to the questionnaire. These respondents were treating nearly three thousand cases of syphilis and over two thousand cases of gonorrhea. Although the numbers were alarming, the rates of VD in Toronto appeared to be significantly lower than in most US cities – in Toronto, there were 8.44 cases per 1,000 population, compared to 11.67 cases per 1,000 in a group of fourteen US cities.[120] Another survey, carried out by the Health League of Winnipeg, suggested that prevalence rates in Winnipeg were considerably lower than in Toronto – approximately 6.45 per 1,000, although the league felt that the low rate reflected inadequate diagnosis.[121]

By 1937, when the Health League of Canada carried out another survey in Toronto, venereal disease rates appeared to be stable, and had dropped considerably since the war. The rate of infection of both syphilis and gonorrhea in Toronto was 9.59 per 1,000.[122] In Ottawa, another survey showed an infection rate of 9.95.[123] More significantly, routine Wassermann tests at the Toronto General Hospital showed that positive tests for syphilis had declined from 10.4 percent in 1916 to 1.7 percent in 1936. Other hospitals in Ontario were also showing low rates of disease: between 1932 and 1937, at Kingston General Hospital, only 1.3 percent of patients had tested positive; and in Hamilton, between 1927 and 1937, the positive test rate was 3.4 percent.[124] There was also a significant reduction in the number of people suffering from general paralysis of the insane (a complication of syphilis) in asylums. In Ontario, it had decreased from 1.5 percent in 1920 to 0.71 percent in 1928. In Saskatchewan, the rate had fallen from 2.7 percent in 1920 to 1.8 percent in 1928.[125] Because venereal disease clinics continued to see large numbers of patients, the decrease in positive routine Wassermann tests suggests that people were being diagnosed and getting treated earlier than they had before.

In 1931, the CSHC received the devastating news that the federal government was cancelling its venereal disease grant, which had sustained the organization since its beginnings in 1919. (The federal grant also included money to the provinces to fund treatment clinics.)[126] The cancellation of the grant marked the end of a long battle. In 1924, when the Liberal government had threatened to cut it, Bates had launched a major offensive, putting on a display on Parliament Hill (including the wax models illustrating the effects of VD), sending packages to every member of Parliament on the problem of venereal disease, and urging health officers across the country to write their parliamentary representatives in support of the continuation of the grant. Progressive and Labour MPs supported Bates, and the grant was continued, although it was significantly reduced. In 1925, when the grant was once again in jeopardy, Bates organized an all-party committee to urge for its continuation – the Voluntary Committee on Health of the House of Commons and the Senate. Bates served as secretary to this committee for several decades, and it provided an effective mechanism for the CSHC, and later the Health League of Canada, to inform parliamentarians of its views. Despite the influence of the committee, in 1925, the VD grant was cut, but by less than had previously been anticipated, before being eliminated entirely in 1931.[127] The Division of Venereal Disease of the federal Department of Health was disbanded in 1932.[128]

By this time, the Canadian Social Hygiene Council had branched into other activities, as we will discuss in Chapter 2, and it received other grants, most notably from the government of Ontario, the city of Toronto, and the Metropolitan Life Insurance Company. Even so, its revenues dropped precipitously in the early 1930s. The number of staff fell from fourteen to three, and it had to move out of Hygeia House.[129] Fortunately, a new opportunity arose. In 1933, Bates was asked to be a consulting physician on the production of a venereal disease film called *Damaged Lives* (an obvious play on Brieux's famous 1911 play on the subject, *Damaged Goods*).[130] Bates and his long-time secretary, Mabel Ferris, drove down to Hollywood for the production of the film.[131] The movie featured Donald Bradley Jr., the young heir of a shipping company, and his long-term girlfriend, Joan. They plan to marry, but Joan wants to wait until Donald is more settled. To advance his career, Don cancels a date with Joan to go out with a business associate. To Don's frustration, the event is a party, not a business dinner. The business associate brings along his long-term mistress, Elise Cooper, an attractive blonde, but he gets drunk, ignores Elise, and flirts with another woman. Brought together by the boorish behaviour of the business associate, Donald and Elise visit a speakeasy. Thoroughly drunk, they return to Elise's apartment, where they have sex. Donald confesses this transgression to Joan, and she realizes that she has been wrong to delay the marriage. They wed that night. Several months later, Elise calls and frantically demands that Don come to her apartment. When he arrives, she tries to explain that she has syphilis and that he might be infected as well. As he exits the apartment, the hysterical Elise shoots herself. Don visits a doctor to see if he was infected, but the doctor turns out to be a quack.[132]

The Bradleys' closest friends are a physician and his wife. One day, his doctor friend comes by Don's office and demands that he come with him right away, telling him that Joan is pregnant and needs to be treated for VD. His physician friend brings Don to a specialist so that he can observe the destructive impact of the disease if left untreated. (This scene parallels that in *The End of the Road* when Vera seeks treatment from Dr. Bell.) The specialist takes Don through a series of rooms containing patients with different symptoms of VD. The doctor is sympathetic towards some of these patients, such as a woman who was unknowingly infected by her husband and has passed the disease on to her children. Other individuals, such as a man who contracted VD after having sex with a prostitute, are judged as "not so innocent." After observing the patients, Don is reunited with Joan, who collapses after learning the news of her infection. The specialist explains that they were fortunate the condition was discovered early and assures them they can expect to be cured within two years if they follow the treatment. After the couple leaves the office, the physician expresses concern for Don and the fear that the discovery of his condition, along with having to deal with a "hysterical wife," could be mentally stressful. (This sympathy for men who had strayed only once appears in other CSHC material as well. Overall, the movie suggests that it would be best if the shame associated with venereal disease were diminished, while at the same time it reinforced the stigma of the disease by underlining that there were both innocent and guilty victims of VD.) Joan later becomes so distraught that she attempts to kill herself and Don by filling their apartment with gas from the oven. Don intervenes in time, and the couple is saved from Elise's fate. As they console each other, Joan receives a phone call from a friend who is distraught because she is pregnant and has just eaten a pickle and is worried about the impact that this might have on her baby. Don and Joan laugh together, showing that in the end they are a "modern" couple who believe in the power of science. It becomes clear that they will follow the necessary course of treatment and survive as a couple. Christabelle Sethna has argued that *Damaged Lives* portrays both Joan and Elise as threatening "new women" who emasculate Donald and are therefore responsible for the couple's fate. We disagree. Elise is a "good-time girl" but she is also a victim, infected by the cad who took her as his mistress. Joan is the good girl next door – she has no career and dreams only of motherhood. Although she errs in delaying the marriage (the CSHC consistently promoted early marriage as a venereal disease preventive), she realizes her mistake as soon as Donald strays. In many ways, Elise and Joan are very similar to Vera and Mary from *The End of the Road*, with the exception that, unlike Mary, who became a nurse, Joan does not work.[133]

Screenings of social hygiene films like *Damaged Lives* or the *End of the Road* were often followed by lectures. *Damaged Lives* broke new ground by including a filmed lecture by Bates at the end of the feature. Although the footage itself has been lost, the scripts remain in the archives. Bates' lectures (one for men and one for women) were long, scientifically complex, and dull.[134] At their conclusion, he emphasized the importance of early marriage to avoid the temptation of premarital sex and imparted a eugenic message. He proclaimed that "to conserve the family is to conserve the race" and argued that each generation should be better morally, mentally, and physically than the generation preceding it.[135] To Bates' chagrin, the American version of the film did not feature his lecture; instead, there was a new lecture by Murray Kinnell, the actor who played the doctor in the movie.[136]

Bates wrote to health officers and theatre owners all over Ontario in the hopes of convincing them to show *Damaged Lives*. The associate director of the Canadian Medical Association, the national commissioner of the Canadian Red Cross, members of the IODE and the Toronto Council of Women, and numerous clergymen in Toronto endorsed the film.[137] The picture attracted large audiences in towns and cities across Canada, with showings usually segregated by gender.[138] The *Charlottetown Guardian* reported that *Damaged Lives* "is probably the finest picture of its type ever produced. The photography is first-class, the acting is excellent, and the sets all that could be desired."[139] The *Toronto Star* declared that it was a "very gripping drama" and added that it was "splendidly acted and produced." The *Saskatoon Star-Phoenix* urged parents to take their adolescents to see the film, saying that "it accomplishes more in two hours than any number of well-meant parental talks."[140] In some cities, the film had quite a dramatic effect: one correspondent from Vancouver revealed that during the showings about fifty people fainted – twenty-nine men and seventeen women.[141] By 1935, *Damaged Lives* had been shown to nearly a million people in Canada.

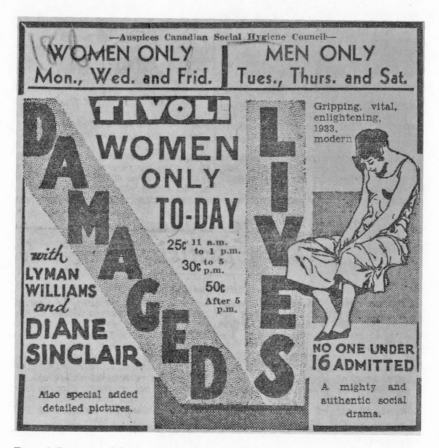

Figure 3 Promotion for *Damaged Lives* advertised showings segregated by gender. | *Toronto Globe*, 24 May 1933, 151.

The film was a significant success outside Canada as well. It received widespread publicity in Australia, where the showings included Bates' lecture. Approximately 5 million people saw it in Britain. The film was mentioned by name during a debate in the House of Lords about the need for medical examinations before marriage.[142] The British Social Hygiene Council reported that the film also prompted increased attendance at treatment clinics wherever it was shown. Spanish and French versions of the film were made and shown in South America, Mexico, and a number of European countries.[143] The film encountered greater difficulties in the United States. In 1933, the American Social Hygiene Association endorsed the film.[144] But, the following year, it removed its name as a sponsor, reporting that the producer, Weldon Picture Corporation, had been unable to control the "unauthorized activities" of distributors who were emphasizing the salacious features of the film."[145] This tendency to publicize the prurient had been a growing problem with sex hygiene films in the United States.[146]

The income generated by *Damaged Lives* helped the CSHC survive the bleak years of the early 1930s. In 1935, the Health League (as the CSHC had by then become) once again began receiving $5,000 per year from the federal government for venereal disease education.[147] In 1938, the league lobbied heavily for the renewal of the grant to the provinces and succeeded in persuading Ottawa to give $50,000 to the provinces for the purchase of arsenical drugs for the treatment of VD.[148] The following year, the league persuaded Ottawa to increase its grant to $10,000.[149] Bates' powerful supporters, including physician Alan Brown, Mrs. Edgar Hardy (the corresponding secretary of the National Council of Women), and R.Y. Eaton (the head of Eaton's department store), wrote letters to the minister of pensions and welfare, Chubby Power, asking for an increase in the grant.[150] The Voluntary Committee on Health of the Senate and House of Commons also lobbied in favour of the grant. Bates was putting twenty years of experience to good effect: while interest in venereal disease education had waxed and waned, he had built up a highly successful network of contacts, honed his lobbying skills, and ushered the organization through some difficult times. Significantly, he had also taken the CSHC well beyond the issue of venereal disease. By the 1930s, the council was also involved in campaigns for immunization and the pasteurization of milk.

***

The anti–venereal disease work of the Canadian Social Hygiene Council focused on education and advocacy: the organization urged Canadians to get tested and treated for venereal disease, it stressed the importance of parents educating their children about sex, it promoted early marriage, it condemned the sexual double standard, and it emphasized the importance of staying continent before marriage for the good of the race. In its support for positive eugenics, its belief in the value of compulsory treatment, its concern about the danger posed by the feeble minded, its opposition to sex before marriage, and its stress on the importance of healthy recreation for young people, the organization was in step with many other social reformers of the era. As a result, it was able to build strong relationships with other organizations, including women's groups, and social reform leaders across Canada. Such relationships contributed to the success of the CSHC. Because it was interested in reaching as broad an audience as possible, the council veered away from what might have been the more controversial aspects of the movement: it took no stance, for example, on the compulsory sterilization of the "unfit," it only rarely addressed the question of immigration restriction, and it did not fight for compulsory medical examinations before marriage.[151] But as time went on, as subsequent chapters will show, the organization would become less flexible, more dogmatic, and more judgmental, with respect to venereal disease as well as other issues.

2

Expanding the Mission
Publicizing Public Health

Tuning into their radios in the 1930s, many Canadians would have heard the first radio drama sponsored by the Health League of Canada. It featured a farm couple who disagreed on the merits of pasteurized milk – the father argued that farmers have been "healthy and happy" for years without pasteurizing their milk, a process that took "the goodness out of it and kills the nice flavor." His wife thought that all the doctors couldn't be wrong and that cities wouldn't be pasteurizing their milk if there were not some advantages to it. A few months later, the father anxiously called a doctor about his young daughter, who had fallen going up the stairs. For a month, her leg had been sore and she had been limping. Liniment and rest had not helped. When the doctor arrived, he determined that the child was suffering from bovine tuberculosis and he warned that she could die. He scolded the farmer: "It could have been prevented if you'd only had some sense in that thick skull of yours." The drama urged listeners to follow the advice of doctors and medical science and warned of dire consequences if the rules of healthy citizenship were not followed.[1]

By the late 1920s, interest in venereal disease as a pressing social problem was declining. Public health authorities tended to focus their energies on infant and child health. At the same time, they were increasingly acknowledging that infectious disease was declining as a cause of death and that chronic diseases like heart disease and cancer were having a bigger impact on overall mortality. At the helm of the Canadian Social Hygiene Council

(CSHC), Bates was worried about declining interest in venereal disease, and he was keen to expand the work of the council into other areas of disease prevention.[2] The fact that the CSHC saw its venereal disease work as part of a larger social hygiene project to "improve the race" also made it easy for it to justify taking on other health topics. During the late 1920s and through the 1930s, the council (which would become the Health League of Canada in 1935) repositioned itself as a general-interest preventive health organization. It used its media savvy to get involved in the early years of radio, delivering talks on a wide range of topics. It launched a consumer magazine, *Health,* which aimed to educate Canadians about how to remain healthy over the life course. And it participated in two of the leading health crusades of the era – immunizing children against diphtheria and the pasteurization of milk.

The council involved itself in these campaigns despite its increasingly dire financial situation. As discussed in the preceding chapter, the federal government had discontinued the CSHC's financial grant in 1931 and, while the council made some money from movie receipts, such income did not make up for the loss of the grant. The council had to negotiate a substantial decrease in its rent for Hygiea House and eventually was forced out of its lavish headquarters and into a more modest office on Bond Street in Toronto.[3] Bates and his loyal secretary, Mabel Ferris, both took salary cuts.[4] Even in these reduced circumstances, the CCSHC/Health League would play an important role in several important victories: by the end of the 1930s, childhood diphtheria was no longer a significant threat in the city of Toronto, and the province of Ontario had passed legislation mandating the pasteurization of milk. The league had built important alliances with major figures in public health in the city and the province: the organization could easily gain an audience with leading provincial politicians, and it was recognized as one of the leading voluntary groups in the city. Bates himself had a high profile – as the *Globe* put it, he was one of "Toronto's personalities" – and the work of the Voluntary Committee on Health of the Senate and House of Commons meant that he was well known in Ottawa as well.[5] In addition, the league's radio programs and news releases raised the profile of the organization across the country. When the Depression ended with the beginning of the Second World War, the league was quickly able to take advantage of new funding opportunities to pursue its public health agenda.

In its new work, the organization applied the same passion and sense of moral righteousness that it had used in its anti–venereal disease campaign.

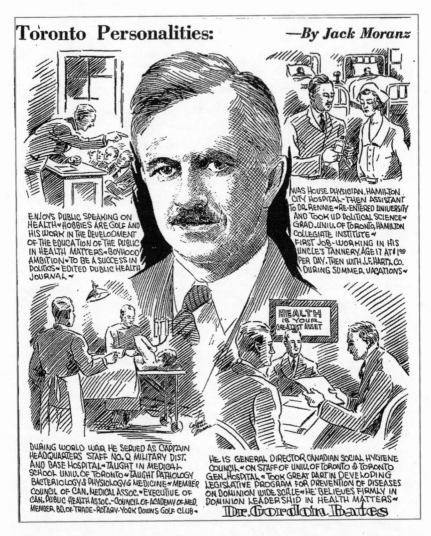

Figure 4 Gordon Bates as a "Toronto personality," reflecting his status in the city. | Jack Moranz, "Toronto Personalities," *Globe and Mail*, 5 December 1932, 9.

The CSHC told parents who failed to immunize their children that they were ignorant and irresponsible, and that they were putting the lives of their children and other people's children at risk. It dismissed people who opposed milk pasteurization as ill informed and often accused them of putting their financial interests ahead of their concern for the health of children. When it came to chronic diseases like heart disease, arthritis, or cancer, where there was more uncertainty about what people could do to prevent illness, the organization was far less dogmatic. For the most part, however, the CSHC/Health League hectored Canadians to take responsibility for their own health and for the health of their children. Although the Great Depression was having a dire impact on many Canadian families, the CSHC/Health League paid no attention to hunger and poverty as causes of disease, nor did it appear to make any special effort to address the needs of poorer or immigrant Canadians. This approach differs significantly from that in the United Kingdom, where Dorothy Porter argues that emphasis on individual behaviour emerged only in the 1950s: in the 1930s, people trained in public health/social medicine were more concerned about the impact of class status on health.[6] The difference is likely due to the origins of the Health League in venereal disease eradication, which meant that it was always concerned with individual behaviour, and the fact that class-based politics have never been as dominant in Canada as they were in the United Kingdom.

Educating Canadians: Media Campaigns

The Canadian Social Hygiene Council had long been adept at getting its message out. Lectures, social hygiene exhibits, and movie showings all received extensive press coverage. In 1927, the council started a news service, issuing regular articles to more than nine hundred newspapers and magazines across the country in both French and English.[7] From the beginning, the news service covered a broad range of health topics, including smallpox and typhoid, in addition to information about sex hygiene. At the time, the council reasoned that addressing an expanded range of topics would overcome the opposition of editors who were uncomfortable running articles about social hygiene, but this approach was also in keeping with the organization's broadening mandate.[8] The news service, sometimes titled "The Health League of Canada Presents Topics of Vital Interest," would remain a vital aspect of the league's program for the next forty years, and would ensure that the league received regular publicity in newspapers, both small and large, over most of its existence.[9]

The CSHC also made excellent use of the new medium of radio. Commercial radio got its start in Canada in the early 1920s. Initially, it served the few radio buffs who were willing to construct their own sets, but, by the late 1920s, nearly half a million Canadians had a receiving licence and the number of stations was growing. The CSHC released its first radio talks in 1927. The council estimated that some 43,000 people heard the talks in Toronto, which were also delivered on radio stations in Winnipeg, Vancouver, and Halifax, and in the province of Alberta.[10] The talks, which were less than fifteen minutes long, concluded by encouraging listeners to order additional educational materials. Judging by subsequent appeals for literature, the most popular topics were infant care and information on specific diseases such as smallpox and diphtheria.[11] In 1928, the council produced a thirty-program series on social hygiene, with the last six lectures focusing on parent education. The council reported that eleven radio stations aired these talks.[12]

In 1929–30, the CSHC hosted weekly talks on CKCL (the Dominion Battery station, one of just a handful of radio stations in Toronto at the time), many given by extremely high-profile speakers, including J.H. King, the federal minister of pensions and national health, and Franklin Roosevelt, then governor of the New York and a polio survivor and activist. As well, a variety of prominent doctors spoke on topics including bacteria, X-rays, sunlight and health, and tuberculosis.[13] By 1931, the council reported that eleven stations across the country were airing the radio talks.[14] After they aired, the talks were circulated to the press.[15] They were also translated into French and broadcast on CKAC, a station owned by *La Presse*, a Montreal newspaper.[16] In 1937, the Health League provided thirty radio addresses that aired on twenty-nine stations.[17] In the mid-1930s, the league added radio dramas to the straightforward lectures it had been producing. Popular topics included diphtheria, nutrition, tuberculosis, infant feeding and care, and mental hygiene. By the late 1930s, talks focused on chronic disease, including regular lectures on arthritis, heart health, and cancer. In the early 1940s, the league completed another set of radio dramas, authored by Rai Purdy, who had been the head of drama at the Toronto radio station CFRB and who would go on to a successful broadcasting career in Canada, the United States, and Scotland. These plays focused on the heroes of medicine, including Louis Pasteur, Edward Jenner, Lord Lister, Paul Erlich, and Frederick Banting.[18] By 1945, these talks were being aired on more than three dozen radio stations from Kelowna to Charlottetown.[19]

In typical Health League fashion, the radio dramas emphasized the importance of recognizing the expertise and heroism of doctors and the value of health. The one on polio opened with a brilliant young surgeon completing a difficult operation. When his older mentor praises his skill, he complains that it would be better to prevent infantile paralysis than to ameliorate the resulting disabilities. The young surgeon persuades his mentor,

Dr. Powell, to begin research on a preventive measure, but Dr. Powell soon finds himself in trouble with his wife, who resents the time that the research is taking away from their social life. She is also angry that the research is detracting from his successful surgical practice and is making the family poorer in the process. Ultimately, their own son comes down with polio, and Dr. Powell is able to save him with the serum he has been developing. His wife realizes her mistake and apologizes.[20] Another play, whose goal was to warn listeners about the dangers of spreading germs, focused on a busy female doctor who has been neglecting her husband and child. As a result, her husband is having an affair. The mistress inadvertently gives the daughter a septic sore throat by kissing her on the lips. The daughter recovers and the husband realizes the errors of his way.[21] (Interestingly, given that there was considerable unease about working women in the 1930s when this play was broadcast, it was the father and not the working mother who needed to be reformed. This likely reflects the glory that the Health League attached to doctors, Bates' admiration for accomplished women, and his critique of the sexual double standard.)[22] A third on goiter (an enlargement of the thyroid gland, usually caused by lack of iodine in the diet) revealed that rates were highest among the "foreign population." It told the story of a Ukrainian widow who learns that her son is suffering from goiter. Her husband has just passed away in a threshing accident and she is reluctant to send the boy away for treatment. Eventually, the doctor persuades her that her son will regain his love of the land only if he goes away for treatment. He is returned back to her energetic and bright.[23] Here immigrants are represented as hard working but ignorant of modern medical progress and as more prone to disease than Anglo-Saxon Canadians. Such a perspective, of course, reflects a long tradition of seeing immigrants as a public health threat.[24]

These dramas encouraged the public to respect doctors' knowledge and wisdom, and to have sympathy for their busy lives. At the same time, they urged listeners to recognize that health was more important than money or time. Occasionally, the dramas and lectures took a scolding tone. The lecture on typhoid declared that, "when a case of typhoid occurs someone should be hanged." It blamed the spread of typhoid on inadequate sanitation and careless food handlers, and it warned summer visitors or travellers to faraway lands to be careful of food and drink that might have become contaminated.[25] The talk on diphtheria stressed the need for parental responsibility, saying, "the only things which still makes diphtheria possible is the apathy, indifference or negligence of parents."[26] A play about tonsils focused on a family who delayed having their son's tonsils out because they feared the expense. As a consequence of the delay, he came down with a mastoid that seriously endangered his health.[27]

Other talks, especially on chronic disease and childcare, were more informative. A radio talk on teeth, for example, provided a detailed description of how teeth developed and when a parent could expect various teeth to erupt. It urged parents to take their children to the dentist before they reached the age of two and instructed parents that children should brush their teeth three times a day, using three different toothbrushes to allow the brushes to dry between cleanings.[28] A talk on arthritis clearly delineated between rheumatoid arthritis and osteoarthritis, emphasizing that rheumatoid arthritis in particular could produce "an appalling toll of disability and suffering." It suggested that many cases of arthritis started with a devitalized tooth, or an infected tonsil, and recommended that people with infected teeth or tonsils have them removed. (This talk reflected the theory of focal infection, which was popular in the interwar years. It fell out of fashion in the 1940s, but Bates continued to be a life-long believer, as we will discuss in Chapter 7.)[29] The talk urged sufferers to eat a diet rich in green vegetables, cod liver oil, wheat germ or baker's yeast, and fruit juices, to get lots of rest, and to avoid emotional strain. It pointed out that a change of climate might be helpful.[30] A lecture on mental hygiene declared that mental disabilities had been neglected for too long because of fear and prejudice. It emphasized that mental disorders were far more widespread than most Canadians realized, and that they lowered "personal and national efficiency" and contributed to "dependency, delinquency and other forms of social failure." It argued that more research was necessary and that promising new treatments were in the process of being developed.[31] Here again, we see the CSHC's emphasis on improving the quality of the Canadian race.

Radio broadcasts and press releases were not the organization's only tools for getting its message out. In 1933, the council began publishing *Health*, a health magazine for a general audience, modelled on the American Medical Association's "family health magazine," *Hygiea*.[32] The idea for *Health* may also have been inspired by the nationalist campaign in support of Canadian magazines in the 1920s.[33] *Health* advertised its existence through the Women's Institutes of Ontario, encouraging group subscriptions.[34] It initially published sporadically, but by 1935 it was producing four issues each year.

When establishing the magazine, Bates enlisted several influential allies, demonstrating the extent of his networks. *Health*'s board of management included Bates as well Alan Brown, the physician-in-chief at the Toronto

Hospital for Sick Children; C.O. Knowles, the managing editor of the *Toronto Evening Telegraph;* and B.K. Sandwell, the editor of *Saturday Night,* which was then one of Canada's most respected magazines.[35] All of the members of the board of management were based in Toronto, as was half of its editorial board. By 1935, *Health* had a circulation of 10,000 and was generating substantial revenue from advertising and subscriptions, although not enough to cover costs.[36] The magazine was reformatted in 1941 with the goal of increasing its popular appeal. Advertising revenue and subscriptions temporarily increased, although subscriptions fell to 5,000 by 1946, when the magazine was forced to reduce publication due to paper shortages caused by the war.[37] In 1947, *Health* relaunched with a new format and began publishing six times per year instead of quarterly. Although circulation increased to 12,500, the magazine cost the league almost three times as much as it made back in advertising and subscriptions.[38] By 1950, circulation had increased to 25,000. While respectable, this paled in comparison with Canada's leading magazines, *Maclean's* (404,000) and *Chatelaine* (374,000). By 1956–57, *Health's* circulation was 30,000, and by the early 1960s it was up to 35,000.[39] Readers were overwhelmingly located in Ontario.[40] As a result of the organization's financial decline that began in the mid-1960s, the league started cutting back on the number of issues produced each year, and in the early 1970s publication was suspended altogether. It attempted to bring the magazine back in 1972, but was able to publish only sporadically for the rest of the decade. The final issue was released in 1981.

From the very beginning, *Health* attempted to make money through advertising, but this was never a notable success. Frequent advertisers included insurance companies, banks, and railways as well as a range of health food companies. One of the most frequent advertisers was the Rosell Bacteriological Institute, which sold yoghurt and kefir. Advertisements often appeared for Squibb cod liver oil, Vi-Tone (a vitamin supplement), Hovis bread, and Roman Meal. More mainstream food products such as Heinz baby foods, Ritz crackers, Ovaltine, and Shredded Wheat were also advertised. The other major category of advertisements were for drugs and health aids, such as aspirin and cold medicines, support shoes, and hearing aids. The advertisers suggest a readership composed largely of women responsible for the health and feeding of their families. Pepsi and Coke both advertised in the magazine from the 1940s onwards, which occasionally provoked angry letters from readers who did not regard these as healthy beverages.[41] Interestingly, in the 1950s, the magazine accepted advertisements from numerous cigarette companies. These ads raised the ire of some readers and were eventually discontinued as the evidence of the link between smoking and lung cancer mounted.[42]

Even though *Health* continuously lost money, it was a valuable mouthpiece. The Health League distributed it to every member of Parliament, helping to keep the league in the minds of parliamentarians. In the 1960s, it was distributed to every physician in Canada free of charge. As a result, many non-subscribers saw the magazine while they were waiting to see their doctor.[43] In 1960, doctors reported that between two and fifty patients read it every week.[44] Articles initially published in *Health* were often used in other Health League activities – condensed versions were sent out by the news service, and some were reworked into pamphlets.

Many of the articles in *Health* were written by staff contributors, such as Gordon Bates, Mabel Ferris, Margaret Smith (of the league's Nutrition Division), and Christian Smith (of the Venereal Disease Division). But Bates was also able to recruit leading figures in Canadian medicine and politics to write. Toronto's Hospital for Sick Children was prominently represented. The nutrition expert and co-inventor of Pablum, Frederick Tisdall, was a frequent contributor in the late 1930s.[45] Elizabeth Chant Robertson, another nutrition researcher at the Hospital for Sick Children, who wrote a column for *Chatelaine* as well as several books on childcare and nutrition for a general audience, wrote numerous articles in the 1950s and 1960s.[46] Another regular contributor, Gordon Bell, was Canada's leading expert on alcoholism.[47] J.D.M. Griffin, one of Canada's leading mental health experts and the director of the Canadian Mental Health Association (1950–71), served as the magazine's consulting editor for mental health and wrote many articles for the magazine on health worries, psychiatry, and the importance for children of love and affection.[48] Political leaders contributed as well. The minister of national health and welfare, Brooke Claxton, published an article in 1945, while Paul Martin, Sr. (who succeeded Claxton as head of the ministry in 1946) contributed an article in 1947 on possible changes to Canada's health services.[49]

Bates occasionally drew on international experts as well. Thomas Parran, the surgeon general of the United States, contributed two articles – one on the eradication of syphilis and another on food issues during the Second World War.[50] The internationally recognized family life expert and well-known eugenicist Paul Popenoe contributed an article entitled "First Aid for Unhappy Marriages" in 1946.[51] Henry Sigerist, a medical historian who played a vital role in the campaign for national health insurance in the United States and who chaired a health commission in Saskatchewan in

1944 that was crucial to the creation of that province's hospital insurance program, also wrote an article for *Health*.[52] Louis Dublin of the Metropolitan Life Insurance Company, who was famed for his groundbreaking studies on mortality, contributed several articles.[53] So, while *Health* never had a particularly large circulation, it had influential authors and readers and was frequently cited or reprinted in other Canadian publications, ensuring that its importance extended beyond mere circulation figures.

Over the years, the Canadian Social Hygiene Council/Health League's media program was crucial in educating Canadians about the care of infants and children, infectious and chronic disease, nutrition, and other health issues. The message focused on duty and responsibility and often threatened Canadians with dire consequences if they failed to behave as responsible health citizens. It is possible that a more positive message might have resonated more strongly, but, in any case, Canadians do seem to have listened to the Health League and other public health bodies, as increasingly large numbers arranged to have their children immunized, purchased pasteurized milk, and called a doctor when they felt ill.

"Someone Should Be Held Responsible": Diphtheria and Toxoid Week

One of the most important activities of the Canadian Social Hygiene Council/Health League in this period was Toxoid Week. Diphtheria has been all but forgotten today, but at the turn of the twentieth century it was a leading cause of infant death and an important factor in the high infant mortality rates.[54] Until 1930, one in every seven or eight children in Canada got diphtheria, and more children aged two to fourteen died from diphtheria than any other disease.[55] Diphtheria acts quickly: children who fall ill can die within a week. Symptoms start with a mild fever and sore throat, but, eventually, a "diphtheric" membrane forms in the throat (*diphtheric* being the Greek word for leather), which can lead to suffocation and death. The disease also releases a toxin that sometimes harms other organs in the body, especially the heart.[56] The first effective intervention against diphtheria was an antitoxin that was first introduced in 1895.[57] By 1916, the antitoxin was available to any health department or physician in Ontario who requested it. The province of Saskatchewan provided the antitoxin free of charge, as did two municipalities in Quebec.[58] But even with the antitoxin, death rates were high, because the initial symptoms were often dismissed as a simple sore throat, and by the time the membrane developed, it was too late.[59] In 1925, Gaston Ramon of the Pasteur Institute developed an effective vaccine (toxoid) against diphtheria, which became available for use in Toronto at the end of 1926.[60] Toronto's Health Department began using the toxoid soon thereafter.[61] Injections received from the Health Department were free of charge. After a brief interruption in Toronto's toxoid program in 1929, the number of cases of diphtheria almost doubled (from 593 in 1928 to 1,022 in 1929), and the number of deaths increased from forty-eight to eighty. The Toronto Academy of Medicine and the Toronto Social Hygiene Council urged the medical officer of health, Dr. Gordon Jackson, to renew the toxoid program.[62] As a result of the increased mortality, the Toronto Diphtheria Committee was established in 1931 under the leadership of John Patterson. Patterson, an advertising executive and prominent member of the Rotary Club, chaired the committee until his death in 1944.[63] Other members included Bates, Jackson, Dr. L.A. Pequegnat (Jackson's deputy), C.P. Fenwick (the associate director of the Canadian Social Hygiene Council), a representative of the Toronto Board of Education, as well as number of people from the media.[64] Together, this group launched a concerted crusade, using billboards, radio, church pulpits, and schoolrooms to convince parents to have their children toxoided against diphtheria.

For the next twenty-two years, Torontonians would be cajoled, guilted, and scolded into having their children toxoided. The results of the campaign were remarkable: the death rate in Toronto from diphtheria would fall from a few dozen children a year in the early 1930s to none. The success of the campaign, as Jane Lewis details in her article comparing diphtheria immunization in Ontario to that in Britain, had much to do with the ready supply of vaccine in Ontario, the important role played by the Ontario Board of Health, and the positive attitude of Canadian physicians towards vaccination.[65] It likely also had to do with the extensive campaign that was put in place to encourage parents to immunize their children. It was a remarkable accomplishment that would earn Toronto international renown for its public health work.

One part of the anti-diphtheria campaign was Toxoid Week; it was a major affair, and most Torontonians must have been aware of its existence. During the week, City Hall was adorned with an anti-diphtheria banner.[66] The Toronto Diphtheria Committee arranged for Toronto streetcars to display advertising cards promoting toxoid.[67] The E.L. Ruddy Company donated substantial billboard space, which featured posters of happy babies with slogans like "Parents ... TOXOID prevents DIPHTHERIA."[68] The Diphtheria Committee also used a variety of posters, initially purchasing them from the United States.[69] The three leading newspapers in Toronto usually published editorials in favour of having

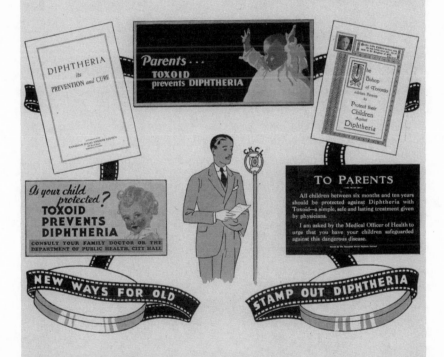

Ammunition For The War Upon Diphtheria

The educational material illustrated below has been used by The Health League of Canada.

Upper left, an educational pamphlet, written in popular style, for general distribution. **Top centre,** a 24-sheet billboard poster. **Top right,** a leaflet containing a special message to church members. These messages are issued by individual denominations to their members. **Lower left,** a street car card. **Lower right,** a notice to be posted up in physicians' offices. The figure in **lower centre** indicates prepared radio addresses. The Health League of Canada is willing to supply all material of this type in any part of Canada at actual cost.

Figure 5 The Health League of Canada promoted the use of a variety of educational materials, which it called "ammunition for the war upon diphtheria," c. 1935–36. | LAC, MG28, I332, vol. 89, file 12.

children toxoided.[70] They also featured daily tallies of the number of
children innoculated in the city. In the 1930s, the Diphtheria Committee put together a short movie featuring Jackson and Patterson as well
as the mayor of Toronto, Bill Stewart, and Dr. J.M. Robb, the minister
of health for Ontario. In 1933–34, it ran in sixteen theatres in Toronto
during Toxoid Week.[71] Members of the Diphtheria Committee organized
lectures delivered to a variety of groups in Toronto.[72] The committee
also authored and circulated a detailed pamphlet on diphtheria with the
tagline "Someone must be held accountable for every death from diphtheria." In a long list of questions and answers, the pamphlet explained
that, even with toxoid, not every child would be protected, as the vaccine was effective only 90 percent of the time. It elaborated on what else
could be done to protect children who had been stricken with the disease, and it explained the process by which one could determine whether
or not someone had acquired immunity to diphtheria (the Shick test).[73]
The pamphlet addressed what was then the most prominent reason for
opposing the toxoid, the mistaken belief that it was derived from animal products and was therefore unethical.[74] The pamphlet explained that
the toxoid was not a serum (meaning that it was not made using animal blood) but that it was produced from de-activated germs that were
cultivated in the laboratory.[75] While the language was clear and easy to
understand, the information was much more extensive than what would
be provided in many of the league's later pamphlets. This level of detail
may have been provided because the CSHC had more faith in the public's ability to comprehend the information than the Health League would
have later. Additionally, it might reflect the general tendency over the
period of the Health League's existence towards shorter and less detailed
public health information in the hopes of more clearly getting the message across.

The Toronto Diphtheria Committee made extensive use of radio,
including short announcements and longer lectures. Every year, prestigious
people involved in Toxoid Week, including Jackson, Fenwick, and Bates,
gave daily radio talks. The mayor often spoke, as did various city council-
lors.[76] Bates sent out letters to each radio station in Ontario, asking them
to make brief statements about diphtheria immunization and providing
them with a list of messages.[77] The announcements told parents how they
could get their children immunized and reinforced the urgency of doing
so. Longer radio programs often warned parents that people who did not
appear to be sick could endanger the health of their children. One radio

program listed possible threats: "the seat mate, in school, in Sunday school, at the children's party; perhaps the older brother or sister, or aunt or uncle or grandparent may bring the bug into your family circles."[78] The message of responsibility was strongly enforced: "No one who cares for children, for their health and happiness – even for their lives – can be disinterested in or can disregard toxoid."[79]

The Diphtheria Committee worked in close collaboration with churches in Toronto. The Catholic archbishop produced a letter endorsing toxoiding for distribution in Catholic churches.[80] The moderator of the United Church, Albert Moore, gave permission to the Canadian Social Hygiene Council to publish a leaflet that included a letter from him endorsing toxoid.[81] Many churches in Toronto included announcements about Toxoid Week and diphtheria immunization in their printed bulletins, and many clergymen drew attention to Toxoid Week during church service.[82] Moreover, a number of the toxoid clinics were set up in places of worship.[83] This partnership marked the beginning of the Health League's long cooperation with churches, which would continue with National Immunization Week and National Health Week.

The schools were probably the most important site for Toxoid Week advertising and propaganda. The Toronto Diphtheria Committee was part of a much larger effort in the early decades of the twentieth century to improve the health of children. Public health and educational reformers sought to educate children on health issues and how to prevent sickness, in the hope that they would bring these messages home to their parents and that eventually they could pass these lessons on to their own children.[84] In Toronto, health education was reinforced by an extensive program of medical inspections in schools. One of the first activities of the Toronto Diphtheria Committee was to produce scribblers for school use that had messages on the importance of toxoiding against diphtheria. In the 1930s the message read, "The Only sure way to protect against diphtheria is the Toxoid Road ... A Good Rule – Toxoid for all ... A message for parents: Make no exceptions and have no regrets."[85] Every year, the Diphtheria Committee encouraged teachers to provide daily lessons on diphtheria during Toxoid Week and provided them with a folder of material that included a letter expressing the importance of toxoid and the promotion of Toxoid Week, a chart showing the prevalence of diphtheria in Toronto, and cards (and later bookmarks) listing the immunization centres and radio programs to be scheduled that week (these were to be sent home with the children). In addition, the school materials included suggestions for messages that teachers could write on classroom black-boards.[86] These messages were explicit:

> Everyone going to school should be protected against diphtheria. Last year there were 20 cases of diphtheria in Toronto and two children died. This year 5 children have already died from this disease. Your parents can protect your life by taking you to your doctor or to one of the Clinics to be toxoided. Tell them what has happened to the other children who have not been protected. TOXOID PREVENTS DIPHTHERIA.[87]

The Diphtheria Committee hoped that frightened children would convince their parents to have them toxoided.

It is clear that the Diphtheria Committee used guilt and hyperbole to get its message across. This approach was similar to the strategies used by anti-diphtheria campaigns in the United States.[88] In this vein, Dr. Charles Hastings, Toronto's medical officer of health and a long-time collabora-tor with the Canadian Social Hygiene Council, declared in 1928 that there should be a coroner's inquest for every childhood death from diphtheria in Toronto, implying that any such death was preventable, even negligent.[89] The Toronto Diphtheria Committee approvingly quoted Hastings in its radio talks and press releases.[90] In 1932, a radio talk for Toxoid Week blared: "If your children die of diphtheria, it is your fault because you prefer not to take the trouble to protect against it."[91] Other talks emphasized the suffering of children with diphtheria: "One can imagine no more heart rending sight than this of a child struggling, fighting for breath, his little face gradually becoming darker as his blood is affected by the process, with death ever and ever nearer." Such messages implied that any parent who would let a child suffer like this by failing to toxoid him or her was cruel.[92] One of the oft-reported stories of the campaign was that of a happy family who had a successful farm in an isolated district. The children were all healthy and enjoyed the rural life – swimming and fishing in the summer, skating and sleighing in the winter. But one day two of the children fell ill. The mother, thinking it was an ordinary sore throat, kept them warm and comfortable and hoped that it would pass. But they grew worse and the other children came down with the same illness. Eventually, a doctor was called, but it was too late. Within the week, all five children had died.[93] The story underlined the suffering that diphtheria could cause and the urgency of ensuring that one's children were toxoided. Other approaches stressed the danger that untoxoided children poised to others. One radio program asked, "Is your child toxoided? If not," it scolded, "he is a definite menace to himself" and to other children. The talk compared the untoxoided child to the spark that starts a raging forest fire.[94]

During the Second World War, officials expressed fear that diphtheria and other diseases would spread as a result of the increased movement of troops and people, coupled with interrupted public health programming. This was a legitimate concern: wars frequently lead to epidemics. For example, the Nazi invasion of Norway in 1940 led to a significant increase in diphtheria in that country.[95] Moreover, during wartime, home, family, and children are often held up as the reason for the fighting and sacrifice.[96] The Health League was quick to use patriotic sentiment to its advantage. A poster promoting Toxoid Week in 1940 counselled, "The health of a nation at peace is of paramount importance, but the health of a nation at war is even more vital. Every unnecessary loss of life in Canada during wartime means a slackening of Canada's war effort. Make sure your own pupils are protected."[97] In fact, Toronto did see a resurgence of diphtheria during the war. In 1939, there were only seven cases and one death from diphtheria. In 1940, there were no cases and no deaths – the first time that a city of Toronto's size had gone a year without a death from diphtheria (although Toronto's proud recitation of its success garnered a few snide comments from smaller centres in Ontario, such as Hamilton and Brantford, that had wiped out diphtheria much earlier).[98] The news of Toronto's success reached as far as Britain, where posters circulated with the slogan "Toronto Canada Stamped out Diphtheria, If They Can Do It, We Can Do the Same."[99] But then, in 1941, Toronto had twenty cases and two deaths. Some speculated that the disease may have come from soldiers visiting Toronto or from recently arrived war workers and their families.[100] In 1942, the numbers looked even worse, with fourteen cases in January alone. The epidemic was centred in the industrial district of Moss Park, leading city officials to mount extra clinics in that neighbourhood.[101] That same year, the local Board of Health and Ontario's deputy health minister expressed concern that Toxoid Week was no longer having an impact on the public and that "a more dynamic approach" was needed. Gordon Jackson pointed out that approximately 60 percent of the Toronto population had been immunized, suggesting that Toxoid Week was, in fact, a success.[102] While Jackson and the Health League hoped that the majority of children would be vaccinated, they were likely aware that "herd immunity" could protect the population as a whole, even if not everyone was vaccinated.[103] Even so, the wartime campaigns warned against the dangers of complacency, arguing that, even if children seemed healthy, they could quickly be struck down by diphtheria. Using a military metaphor, Bates pleaded that failing to use toxoid was like "throwing away a rifle when confronted by a savage foe."[104] While the direct patriotic appeal lessened once the war was over, Toxoid Week continued to instruct Torontonians that they needed to remain on guard against diphtheria.

Soon after the war began, Toxoid Week was expanded to include all of Ontario, and there were attempts to reach out to the rest of the country as well.[105] Beginning in 1941, Montreal hosted a Toxoid Week, with the full support of the Montreal Department of Health. In 1942, Quebec City, Halifax, and many other communities also participated. The governor general of Canada, the Earl of Athlone, gave a national radio address on CBC inaugurating Toxoid Week across the nation. In 1943, Montreal and Quebec City again hosted Toxoid Week, this time joined by Sherbrooke.[106] The Health League put together a Toxoid Week manual that described the activities that had been undertaken in Toronto, in the hopes of replicating them elsewhere in the country.[107] Not all provinces were enthusiastic about a national campaign, feeling that their own strategies were effective enough, and that the week chosen (in April) was not particularly appropriate, as the roads in some provinces were still too rough for travel.[108] For the time being, Toronto's Toxoid Week continued as usual, with promotion in schools and on radio programs. At the end of the war, the Toronto Department of Public Health estimated that 25,000 children in Toronto still needed to be protected against diphtheria and stressed that those aged six months to six years old were still especially vulnerable.[109] A new pamphlet proclaimed "25,000 Toronto Children to Be Toxoided" and urged parents to vaccinate their children before they went to school.[110] In 1951, more than 90,000 bookmarks promoting vaccination were distributed to schools along with additional "blackboard messages" for teachers. Churches continued to be encouraged to make announcements.[111] Despite the continuation of such activity, it was clear that, by the late 1940s, diphtheria was not the threat it once was. By April 1949, Toronto had not had a single case of diphtheria for eighteen months.[112] In 1953, Toxoid Week was folded into National Immunization Week, which will be discussed in Chapter 6.[113]

In many respects, Toxoid Week was a remarkable success. By the early 1930s, the incidence of diphtheria had plummeted, and while the disease was not completely eradicated, it became increasingly rare for a Toronto child to die of diphtheria (Figure 6). That city's success was not reflected in the rest of the country. In 1948, when Toronto had no cases of diphtheria, there were still nine hundred cases nationwide.[114] In 1939, the *Canadian*

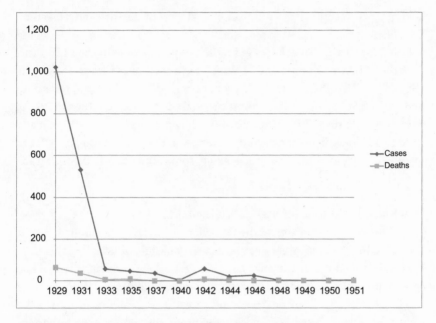

Figure 6 Diphtheria cases and deaths in Toronto, 1929–50
Source: "Facts about Toronto's 22nd Annual Toxoid Week," Library and Archives Canada, MG28,
I332, vol. 92, file 16.

Public Health Journal complained that, in many places, immunization was
carried out "spasmodically"; in some communities only schoolchildren were
vaccinated, while other places had no immunization program at all.[115] Rates
of diphtheria in Canada fell substantially in the late 1920s and early 1930s
after the initial introduction of the vaccine and then underwent another
dramatic drop in the late 1940s.[116] The success of Toronto compared to
other Canadian locales might be due to the city's relatively extensive public
health infrastructure. It is possible that diphtheria would have declined in
Toronto even without Toxoid Week. But there are some signs that that event
did make a difference. The number of immunizations skyrocketed after Toxoid Week began in 1931. In 1930, 5,385 immunizations were given. In 1931,
this jumped to 21,089, and in 1932 it increased to 27,456. The rate fell substantially in 1933, but this may reflect that fact that fewer children needed
to be immunized.[117]

Toxoid figures from the 1930s and early 1940s suggest that children
were significantly more likely to be toxoided in April, May, and June than
in the other months of the year, suggesting that Toxoid Week (which was

held in April) was having an impact.[118] A survey of doctors undertaken by the Health League in 1947 indicated that more than half of respondents believed that Toxoid Week had led more people to come to their offices to have their children immunized.[119] While it is impossible to know for sure, it seems likely that the yearly publicity blitz helped to remind parents of the importance of having their children vaccinated. At the same time, it seems worth asking if the tactics of shame and guilt were successful. Could equally good results have been achieved by a campaign that stressed the benefits of toxoid and assumed that parents would automatically do what was best for their children?

"Raw Milk Is Poison": The Campaign for Pasteurization

The second major campaign of the Canadian Social Hygiene Council/Health League in this period was for compulsory milk pasteurization. By the turn of the century, it was clear that many diseases, especially tuberculosis, could be spread through milk, and that pasteurizing milk could destroy the organisms that caused disease. But not everyone agreed that pasteurization was the right approach. In the early decades of the twentieth century, even some doctors and sanitary inspectors believed that pasteurization allowed dairies to take sanitation shortcuts, they worried that pasteurization was not always carried out correctly, and they expressed concern that pasteurized milk was less digestible for babies.[120] By the 1920s, the vast majority of doctors and inspectors had come to support pasteurization, but it still encountered widespread opposition from small producers and dairies that could not afford pasteurization equipment and from people who felt that keeping cows and barns clean, and culling tubercular cows, was a better way of preventing disease. Many people continued to believe that raw milk was a nutritionally superior product, despite research showing that pasteurization had a minimal effect on the nutritional value of milk.[121] As a result of such resistance, legislation mandating pasteurization was slow to pass. In 1914, Toronto and Saskatoon became the first cities in Canada to mandate pasteurization. Other cities in Ontario adopted mandatory pasteurization in the 1920s and 1930s, as did a handful of cities in Quebec.[122] Ontario implemented compulsory pasteurization in 1938, although, even then, there were exemptions for outlying regions that lacked pasteurization facilities. The only other province to mandate pasteurization, Saskatchewan, did so in 1949, although the measure was limited to towns with over one thousand people.

Economics rather than the law drove many dairies to begin pasteurizing their milk. Rates of pasteurization were particularly high in urban areas, where long transit times allowed the bacteria in milk to multiply, making it far more dangerous to consume raw milk. Pasteurization made the milk last longer, which was advantageous for both producers and consumers. By the early 1930s, 72.4 percent of the milk sold in Canada's twenty-four largest cities was pasteurized.[123] A study in the *Canadian Public Health Journal* in the late 1930s indicated that in Montreal 95 percent of all milk was pasteurized, while in Winnipeg, Edmonton, and Vancouver more than three-quarters of all milk sold was pasteurized.[124] None of these cities had compulsory pasteurization laws. The spread of pasteurization went hand in hand with consolidation in the dairy industry – as fluid milk plants grew in size, there were fewer of them, and they were more likely to pasteurize.[125]

Pasteurization debates have to be understood in the context of the importance of milk to the North American diet in the first half of the twentieth century. As many scholars have pointed out, doctors and nutritionists promoted milk as a vital food, especially for children. This was a fairly new development. Historically, even societies that consumed a lot of dairy products tended to use fermented milk products, such as yogurt, which lasted longer and contained less lactose. But beginning in the mid-nineteenth century, fresh milk began to assume an important place in the North American diet.[126] Cow's milk had long been regarded as a substitute for mother's milk, and as wet-nursing declined (due in part to concerns about venereal disease) and more working-class women began working outside the home, the sale of fluid milk grew.[127] At the same time, temperance supporters were encouraging the consumption of non-alcoholic beverages, including milk.

By the interwar years, Canadian doctors and nutritionists were recommending that Canadians, and especially children, drink enormous quantities of the white beverage. In a 1921 pamphlet entitled *Canadians Need Milk*, Helen MacMurchy, the well-known author of the Canadian government's "blue books" on childcare, told parents that children needed at least a quart of milk a day and that "more children are delicate and sickly from the want of milk than from any other cause." She claimed that parents who were not giving their children enough milk were "wronging their children and depriving them of their indispensable food."[128] She strongly asserted that all milk should be pasteurized. E.W. McHenry, one of Canada's best-known nutritionists, declared that pasteurized milk was the most valuable "protective food." He explained that nutritional surveys showed that the most common dietary defects were a lack of protein and calcium and suboptimal supplies of vitamins. Foods that made up these deficits were called "protective" foods. Milk, which is high in protein and calcium and is easily digested (or so he thought), was the best food for combatting the most common nutritional deficiencies. He pronounced that "every scientific expert in nutrition would agree that a liberal use of milk improves health, provided the milk is safe and does not spread infectious disease."[129] A widely circulated 1930s nutritional pamphlet, *What to Eat to Be Healthy*, had a prominent place for pasteurized milk on its cover and recommended that children drink one and a half pints of milk every day and that adults consume at least half a pint.[130] While milk consumption never rose to recommended levels, there was a steady increase in the consumption of fluid milk, from 320 pounds per person per annum in 1880 to 360 in 1900 and 370 in 1920.[131] It gradually rose to a high of 460 pounds per person at the end of the Second World War but fell to just under 400 pounds per person (approximately four-fifths of a pint per person per day) in the early 1950s.[132]

Yet, the experts acknowledged that milk could be a dangerous food. Bovine tuberculosis was a real risk, especially to children: in the 1920s, medical authorities believed that at least 10 percent of extra-pulmonary tuberculosis in Canada in children under fourteen years of age was of the bovine variety. Research done in England and Germany suggested that somewhere between 6 and 10 percent of the deaths from tuberculosis in children under the age of five were likely due to bovine tuberculosis.[133] When it attacked the bones, bovine tuberculosis could lead to significant disability, including deformations of the spine. But thanks to the culling of tubercular cattle and the increased incidence of pasteurization, bovine tuberculosis was rare in Canada by the end of the 1930s.[134]

A survey of milk-borne disease across Canada stretching from 1912 to 1937 determined that there had been almost 9,000 cases of illness and 703 deaths, although it is worth pointing out that more than two-thirds of the deaths could be traced to a typhoid epidemic in Montreal in 1927, which actually originated in a dairy that sold pasteurized milk: much of the milk had mistakenly passed through the plant without being pasteurized.[135] Another, likely underreported, problem was undulant fever, which caused very high fevers, headaches, and weakness for several months. The number of deaths caused by undulant fever was low, but the consequences for the adults who contracted it could be severe, especially in terms of work time lost to illness.[136] In 1938, the federal Department of Agriculture estimated that approximately 2 percent of all cattle under supervision were positive for *Brucella abortus*, the organism that caused undulant fever.[137]

In the 1930s, when there was still strong evidence of significant illness being caused by unpasteurized milk, the Canadian Social Hygiene Council adopted pasteurization as one of its key issues. As was typical of the CSHC/

Health League, it modified its rhetoric little over the next two decades, even as rates of pasteurization increased and evidence of milk-borne illness declined. While the major campaigns in favour of pasteurization took place in the 1930s and 1940s, *Health* continued to publish warnings on the dangers of unpasteurized milk well into the late 1950s, when most of the milk drunk in Canada was already pasteurized. Indeed, the league continued to tout the importance of mandatory pasteurization throughout its existence. Moreover, the Health League continued its campaign even when local officials warned that promoting pasteurization might do more harm than good. In Nova Scotia, for example, the deputy minister of health, P.S. Campbell, suggested in 1946 that pasteurization was progressing well in the absence of agitation and that "stirring up interest" might have the opposite effect from what was intended, by provoking the opponents of pasteurization.[138]

The CSHC's work on pasteurization built on what it had done in the field of venereal disease. In the early 1930s, the council developed an exhibit entitled "The Value of Pasteurization," which travelled to health exhibits and fairs. (As discussed in Chapter 1, the council had success with a similar social hygiene exhibit in the 1920s.) At a typical event, children were shown health films, toured exhibits, and were given a glass of (pasteurized) milk.[139] The council also circulated articles touting the value of pasteurization to weekly newspapers across the country.[140] In the mid-1930s, as the Social Hygiene Council became the Health League of Canada, the organization took over the pasteurization campaign from the Ontario Committee for Safe Milk. That committee had been a broad organization that encompassed public health workers, social service organizations, insurance companies, milk producers, milk distributors, women's organizations, and the Canadian Public Health Association. It distributed more than 100,000 pamphlets promoting pasteurization, paid for primarily by the Metropolitan Life Insurance Company of Canada and the Ontario Milk and Cream Distributors Association.[141] The Safe Milk Committee of the Health League included representatives from the dairies, Metropolitan Life, and the Ontario and Toronto Departments of Health. This work on the pasteurization campaign showed, once again, that both government public health workers and business leaders alike regarded the Health League as a valuable ally.[142] As in his other areas of interest, Bates had several influential allies in the pasteurization campaign. A key player was J.W.S. McCullough, who had been the chief public health officer in Ontario from 1910 to 1935. Under McCullough, the distribution of diphtheria anti-toxin and the establishment of provincial laboratories and travelling VD clinics reduced infant mortality and increased life expectancy in the province. McCullough had been involved with the CSHC since its earliest days, and he became a vice-president of the CSHC and the Health League. Among other tasks, he headed the league's Cancer Committee, which was eventually taken over by the Canadian Medical Association. In retirement, he wrote articles and radio programs for the Health League, including many on pasteurization, until he passed away in 1941.[143] The head of the Pasteurization Committee for many years was Dr. Alan Brown, the influential physician-in-chief at the Hospital for Sick Children who turned the hospital into a research powerhouse.[144]

As shown in Chapter 1, the Health League strongly believed in promoting health messages through new media. In 1936, it received permission from Famous Players to distribute pamphlets on the need for the pasteurization of milk at the showings of the Hollywood blockbuster and Academy Award–winning film *The Story of Louis Pasteur*.[145] As Susan Lederer and John Parascandola argue, the popularity of this film is indicative of the strong public interest in films about doctors and medicine at this time.[146] The film portrayed Pasteur as a heroic man of science who saved the world from anthrax and rabies, while carrying out a principled fight against the doctors of France who refused to accept that microorganisms caused disease. The league pamphlet reprinted Pasteur's final speech from the film, taken from a talk at the Academy of Medicine in Paris, in which he urged young doctors and scientists to work for the welfare and progress of humankind. On the back page, the pamphlet noted that compulsory pasteurization had eliminated bovine tuberculosis in Toronto, "yet a great percentage of towns and cities in the Dominion fail to safeguard public health and still expose children and adults to the dangers of raw milk."[147] It was typical of the league's Toronto-centrism that it would promote that city's achievements in public health without much understanding of how boosterism was perceived in the rest of the country. It was also typical that at least some of these pamphlets may have been distributed only in Toronto, a place where mandatory pasteurization had already been achieved: the Health League believed in reinforcing victory.

The league also delivered radio addresses on the value of pasteurized milk and mounted large exhibits at the Canadian National Exhibition in 1938 and 1939 and at the Royal Winter Fair in 1938. The league encouraged teachers to order educational materials such as food charts, colouring activities, and booklets that emphasized the importance of consuming pasteurized milk.[148] It carried out an annual campaign on the dangers of drinking unpasteurized milk while on summer holiday (see Figure 7).[149]

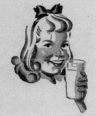

Vous partez en

VILLÉGIATURE??

Faites que vos vacances soient saines, en vous
rendant à des endroits où vous pourrez
vous procurer du

LAIT PASTEURISÉ

Ne courez aucun risque!

**Protégez vos enfants
et vous-même**

LE LAIT EST LE PLUS NUTRITIF
DE TOUS LES ALIMENTS

mais à l'état crû (non pasteurisé), il peut être dangereux . . . il
peut transporter des microbes qui provoquent différentes
maladies comme la fièvre typhoïde, la tuberculose
bovine, la fièvre ondulante, les maux de gorge
et la dysenterie.

Le lait pasteurisé est le seul lait garanti!

LA LIGUE CANADIENNE DE SANTÉ
914, édifice Sun Life, Montréal
publie ce bulletin dans l'intérêt de votre santé et celle
de votre famille

*(écrivez à la Ligue pour obtenir des renseignements au sujet des méthodes
de pasteurisation à domicile).*

Figure 7 Part of the Health League's pasteurization campaign, this poster encouraged
drinking pasteurized milk while on holiday. | LAC, MG28, I332, vol. 109, file 18.

Bates was obsessed with the dangers of consuming milk while vacation-
ing, a concern that developed after he purchased milk from a dairy in
Port Dover, where his family vacationed during the summer. The milk
soured quickly and Bates learned that the pasteurization process at the
dairy was flawed. He subsequently carried out a long campaign against

the milk supply in Port Dover, regularly sending missives to the editor of the *Port Dover Maple Leaf.*[150] This was perhaps an early sign of the crankiness that would emerge later in his life while campaigning for water fluoridation and the need for high moral standards, which we will discuss in Chapters 7 and 8.

In 1942, the Health League formed a National Committee on Milk to promote pasteurization. Dr. Alan Brown headed the committee, with A.E. Berry of Toronto's Department of Health as secretary. Berry was another important player in the public health community. He was a regular contributor to the *Canadian Public Health Journal* and had penned several articles for *Health* in the late 1930s. In 1943, the Quebec Health League launched an extensive campaign for pasteurization in that province. It released a series of fifteen-minute broadcasts by eminent physicians and professors over the Radio-Canada network. Several of these were reprinted in the journal *L'Union médicale*, which was sent to "all French-speaking physicians" in North America.[151] These talks were then distributed to parish priests, newspapers, and the presidents of Chambers of Commerce in all of the major cities and towns in Quebec. Nearly every newspaper in the province ran editorials in favour of pasteurized milk, while dozens of organizations, including women's clubs, chambers of commerce, and service clubs, sent resolutions to the government encouraging them to pass legislation for compulsory pasteurization.[152] A few victories were achieved: in Quebec City, the Catholic School Commission started providing milk to all children in their schools, and, as a result of the pasteurization campaign, the commission agreed that all milk would be pasteurized. The city of Hull also adopted pasteurization. Overall, however, the campaign failed to convince the provincial legislature.[153] In Vancouver, the Greater Vancouver Health League lobbied city council to pass legislation requiring that all milk be pasteurized. It also met with dairies to encourage them to voluntarily adopt pasteurization.[154]

In 1946, the Health League of Canada asked voluntary organizations across the country to sign resolutions in favour of mandatory pasteurization. It received signed resolutions from the Canadian Congress of Labour, the Canadian Order of Foresters, the Chief Constables Association of Canada, the Girl Guides Association, provincial teachers' associations, and the Canadian Nurses Association, among many others.[155] Throughout the decade, the league continued to produce a wide array of pamphlets and posters promoting pasteurized milk. It adopted the slogan "Pasteurized Milk Is the Only Safe Milk!" and circulated spot announcements on the dangers of raw milk and the value of pasteurization. It also prepared instructions on how to pasteurize milk at home.[156]

Bates often claimed that as many people had died from drinking raw milk as had died on the battlefield.[157] When questioned about the claim, he reasoned that "this is almost certainly true because human beings die from infected milk every day in all countries of the world, while serious wars are rare," making it clear that the claim was not based in actual data but on his own suppositions.[158] In any case, Bates never worried too much about playing fast and loose with the facts if he believed it would advance his cause. In addition, he had little patience with people who were unconvinced of the merits of pasteurization. In articles circulated to newspapers by the Health League in 1945–46, he condemned his opponents as "ill-informed and selfish."[159] He believed that pasteurization was opposed "by people who are either ignorant as to the necessity for such legislation or are financially interested in preventing its passage."[160] In one letter, he told a challenger that he was "unspeakably silly" and reprimanded him for not being more grateful to the doctors who were trying to help him, while in another he asserted that the opponents of pasteurization were selfish farmers who were willing to sell milk that crippled children.[161] On occasion, even his supporters urged him to tone down his rhetoric.[162]

The firmness of Bates' own opinions seemed to render him incapable of understanding the perspectives of those who disagreed with him. He himself had unwavering faith in the rightness of the medical profession and little understanding of why people might be suspicious of the claims of leading medical bodies. For him, it was enough that all leading health organizations had endorsed pasteurized milk, a fact that the league stressed in its pamphlets.[163] Bates' other problem was that he never seemed to realize that people in other parts of the country did not always take well to a Toronto-based organization telling them what they should do to improve health in their locality. He regularly promoted what Toronto and Ontario had done to reduce infant mortality, insinuating that other parts of the country were backwards or cared less about the health of their children.[164] A news release destined for Quebec in the 1950s highlighted that that province had the highest infant mortality rate in Canada and the highest rate of infant deaths from diseases that were attributed to consuming raw milk. It then pointed out the superior record of Ontario and Saskatchewan, which had passed mandatory pasteurization laws. It concluded on a nativist note, saying "it seems absurd to attempt to increase Canada's population by immigration at the same time thousands of native-born children are allowed to be poisoned by raw milk."[165]

Through the 1950s, the league continued to distribute pamphlets promoting pasteurization, and it published articles in *Health* in favour of the measure, but its Pasteurization Committee was largely inactive. It did conduct two surveys, which showed that the situation was improving, likely due to more communities mandating pasteurization as well as more milk distributors adopting it voluntarily (see Table 1). Despite the survey showing that most milk being consumed was pasteurized, the Health League continued to decry the fact that only two provinces had mandated pasteurization.[166] A 1964 pamphlet issued by the league to advertise National Health Week maintained that 45–50 percent of the milk consumed in Canada was unpasteurized – something that the league's own surveys had indicated was untrue.[167] This was typical of the Health League's tendency not only to sometimes bend the facts to suit its purposes but also to continue emphasizing the dangers even after a problem had largely been solved. Bates would be satisfied only by compulsion, regardless of whether pasteurization was actually taking place or not.

Table 1
Health League of Canada pasteurization surveys

Province	Percentage of pasteurized milk consumed	
	1951	1964
BC	85%	99% in urban areas; 97% in rural areas
AB	32%	90–95%
SK	35%	90%
MB	65–70%	Pasteurized milk available throughout province
ON	99%	100% except in a few settlements in the North
QC	85%	92% in cities and towns over 1,000
NB	88%	Mostly pasteurized
NS	55–60%	99%
PEI	Unknown	99%
NL	Unknown	75% but fluid milk consumption very low

Source: "Milk Pasteurization Survey of Canada According to Province," LAC, MG 28, I332, vol. 109, file 9; "Dairy Council Executive Praises League 'Impact' Progress Report," *Health News* 2, 1 (1964), 3 in LAC, MG 28 I332, vol. 109, file 1.

Evaluating the success of the pasteurization campaign is even more difficult than evaluating the success of Toxoid Week. In Ontario, as elsewhere, most people started drinking pasteurized milk not just because health authorities told them that it was safer, or because the law compelled it, but because this is what was increasingly available to them. Larger dairies had a strong incentive to pasteurize their milk – it was a safer product that also had a longer shelf life. As Canadians increasingly moved to larger centres, and fewer of them had their own cows or purchased their milk from a neighbouring farmer, they increasingly bought pasteurized milk. Pasteurization proceeded more quickly in Ontario than in the other provinces, but this at least partly reflected the fact that Ontario was more urban than the other provinces. That said, the campaign of the Canadian Social Hygiene Council/ Health League did help make many Canadians aware of the dangers of raw milk and perhaps pushed them in the direction of purchasing the pasteurized product.

***

During the 1930s, despite significant financial setbacks, the Canadian Social Hygiene Council/Health League of Canada transformed itself from an anti– venereal disease group to a much broader organization that took on a variety of public health issues, including, most notably, childhood immunization and milk pasteurization. Through its media program, the league became a source of valuable information for Canadians on a wide variety of health issues: Canadians learned about how to eat better, how to care for their children's teeth, what to feed an infant at various stages of life, and about chronic diseases like cancer, arthritis, and heart disease. The Health League, of course, was not the only source of information about these issues: federal, provincial, and municipal governments all provided health information to Canadians, as did businesses such as the Metropolitan Life Insurance Company. But the Health League, with its constant stream of press releases, its vigorous radio programs, and its magazine, *Health*, became one of the most important sources of health information in the country, although it must be noted that league materials were much more widely read in Ontario than in the other provinces. In all of its information, the league stressed the importance of health citizenship. It regarded toxoiding one's children, drinking pasteurized milk, and following other health recommendations as the responsibilities of citizenship in a democratic society. The league's disdain for those who did not follow these recommendations was palpable. While this may not have been the best way of encouraging Canadians to embrace its recommendations, the league had at least some positive impact. Torontonians *did* immunize their children, leading to significantly fewer childhood deaths from diphtheria in the city compared to other parts of Canada. People *did* drink more pasteurized milk, leading to fewer cases of bovine tuberculosis, septic sore throat, and undulant fever. They may not have enjoyed being hectored by the Health League, but they may have found some merit in its suggestions.

3

"Stamp Out VD!"
The Health League of Canada and Venereal Disease Education during the 1940s and 1950s

In 1942–43, half a million Canadians took a break from their busy wartime lives to see *No Greater Sin* (1941), an American anti–venereal disease film sponsored by the Health League of Canada. The film featured Betty and Bill, a young couple who fall in love while working at the same factory. In preparation for marriage, Bill takes a test for syphilis. The test is positive, but the doctor reassures Bill that the disease can be treated. He spends his savings to be cured, but the doctor is a quack. Unaware that he still has syphilis, Bill transmits the disease to Betty and their unborn child. When he learns of the situation through a test at the factory, Bill goes back to the doctor, who pulls a gun on him. In the ensuing struggle, the doctor is shot and killed, and Bill is put on trial. Bill is so ashamed that he refuses to tell the police what happened, but a kindly defence lawyer sees the truth and decides to take the case. On the stand, Bill refuses to cooperate until the lawyer suggests that he might have gotten syphilis from Betty. Bill attacks the lawyer, defending the honour of his wife, a response that underlined how much more shameful it was for a woman to be infected than for a man. The lawyer shows that the doctor had a false medical certificate, and the case is dismissed. Bill's father-in-law welcomes him back into the family. The film's central message is that syphilis is curable and that it is better to be tested and treated than to maintain secrecy about the disease. Bill is a sympathetic character whose premarital philandering is forgiven because he tried to do the right thing by getting tested and treated and because he was respectful of his wife's reputation.

Anti-Venereal Disease Campaigns during the Second World War

The Second World War brought renewed attention to health issues, as Canadians worried about the health of soldiers overseas and of the labour force at home. The Health League, which had been born out of wartime concerns about VD, alerted government authorities that venereal disease would increase once again and began an educational campaign to warn Canadians of the menace. During the 1940s, the Health League showed *No Greater Sin*, collaborated with the Canadian Junior Chamber of Commerce to promote National Social Hygiene Day, and produced educational materials to educate both teens and adults about venereal disease. After the war, it maintained its long-standing interest in health and morality by protesting against movies and books it considered to be immoral. During these years, there were signs that the Health League was growing increasingly out of sync with other organizations concerned with venereal disease. In part, the league was being squeezed out as provinces increased their activities in this area.[1] But the Health League's insistence that venereal disease should be seen as a moral problem also began to create a rift between it and other public health officials, who increasingly saw VD as something that could be easily treated and managed and who were less inclined to take a moralistic approach. Elizabeth Fee and Allan Brandt have noted similar tensions occurring over VD policy in the United States at this time: while Surgeon General Thomas Parran was more concerned with testing and treatment, organizations like the American Social Hygiene Association focused on vice and prostitution as the reasons behind the disease.[2]

During the 1940s, penicillin revolutionized venereal disease treatment, but other dramatic improvements predated that antibiotic. By the late 1930s, sulpha drugs provided an effective, safe, and quick treatment for gonorrhea.[3] In 1943, the Canadian Army adopted a shorter treatment for syphilis, reducing the average time of treatment from eighteen months to six.[4] During the war, penicillin was discovered to be effective against both diseases, although it would not be widely used in civilian treatment until the end of the conflict.[5] The very high rates of venereal disease seen in the First World War did not recur during the Second: the rate of infection remained well under 10 percent.[6] This may be because condoms, which had much improved in quality, were distributed to servicemen from the very beginning of the war. (At first, each man received just three condoms each month, but by 1944 they were unlimited.) Prophylaxis was also more readily available, although, as Ruth Roach Pierson revealed, women in the military did not receive the same protections as men.[7] The civilian population did not see a surge in cases either: a survey conducted by the Health League in 1943 showed that the incidence of syphilis in Toronto increased slightly during the war but the number of cases of gonorrhea fell.[8]

With more effective treatments available, VD education began to focus more heavily on testing and treatment than on prevention. The Health League heavily promoted premarital and prenatal blood testing and lobbied workplaces to provide periodic health exams that would include blood testing.[9] It also supported sex education, something that a growing number of Canadians were calling for, although the league promoted a fairly conservative version of sex education.[10] But the league began to worry that the moral side of the venereal disease question was being abandoned. The organization believed that many people got VD because they lacked discipline and character and that improved moral standards were vital. At the same time, it backed away from its earlier view that men were primarily responsible for spreading venereal disease. During the war, the Health League, like the armed forces and the federal government, warned men against "loose women" who would infect them and thus sabotage Canada's war efforts.[11] This approach marked a significant departure from the days of the Canadian National Council for Combatting Venereal Disease and the Canadian Social Hygiene Council (CSHC), when the organization had emphasized the "innocent" female victims of venereal disease.

When the Second World War broke out, the Health League urged that the federal government's booklet *The Diagnosis and Treatment of Venereal Disease* be reprinted and that a section on prophylaxis and new treatments for gonorrhea be added. It enjoined the government to do Wassermann tests for syphilis on all new recruits, and it recommended that prophylactic centres be established in military units and in major town and cities, to cope with soldiers who were on leave.[12] Although the league thought that "prophylactic packets" should be made available, it maintained that they should not be distributed too widely, for fear of sanctioning immorality. It recommended the use of social case sheets in military hospitals for the purposes of contact tracing, and it urged that pamphlets, posters, and films be enlisted in educating troops.[13] As the war continued, Bates became increasingly uneasy about the ready availability of prophylaxis and treatment. Although he himself had initially recommended prophylaxis, he soon complained that the military was relying far too heavily on prophylactic packets. In 1941, he warned that venereal disease could not be controlled by chemical means alone, as this would "damage the moral fiber of our people."[14] In keeping with his view that the medical profession played a vital role in educating people

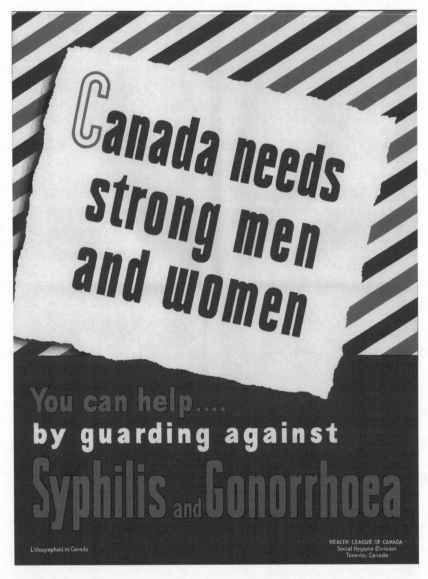

Figure 8 The Health League distributed this poster during the war as part of its campaign against VD. | LAC, MG28, I332, vol. 140, file 14.

about morality, Bates felt that prophylaxis should be given at doctors' offices rather than in the form of a packet available on military bases.[15] He worried that, as a result of prophylaxis and the newer treatments, "the public are likely to feel that illicit contact is quite without danger."[16] The Health League also never recommended the use of condoms as a venereal disease preventive, despite their widespread use in the military. Instead, Bates continued to harken back to the lessons that the CSHC had taught in the 1920s about self-control and self-respect and the importance of restricting sex to marriage. He argued that prophylactic packets might be acceptable in the army, "where all sorts of conditions of men are gathered together," but he still confessed "to some feeling of loathing to the whole idea."[17] Like many social hygienists, Bates was torn between his desires to uphold moral standards and to reduce disease.

Bates became convinced that venereal diseases were being spread by casual "pick-ups" and that many of these were fuelled by alcohol consumption.[18] While he had been aware of casual sex during the First World War, he tended to focus on men as the guilty party, although he believed that "feeble-minded girls" were a contributing factor. By the 1940s, it seemed to him that both genders were wantonly abandoning the moral codes that should guide their conduct. In 1943, Christian Smith, the social hygiene director of the Health League, complained that a recent league survey had shown that nine out of ten patients had been infected by casual pick-ups. He reported that girls as young as twelve were hanging out at railway stations or military camps, picking up soldiers and spending the night in hotels.[19] The Health League urged the Toronto medical officer of health to close eating or drinking establishments that appeared to be the source of an abnormally high number of VD infections.[20] As it had in the interwar years, it also encouraged churches and youth groups to provide wholesome recreation for young people in order to keep them away from roadhouses, hotels, and seedy restaurants.[21] At the same time, the league's literature took on an increasingly judgmental tone.

The Health League continued to distribute the pamphlets it had developed in the 1920s, but it also introduced some newer, more misogynistic material, including Gene Tunney's *The Bright Shield of Continence*, which the league reprinted from *Reader's Digest*. Tunney, a former boxer who was with the United States Naval Reserve, maintained that "sexual continence is the strongest weapon yet devised to combat venereal infection." He warned that syphilis and gonorrhea could lead to arthritis, invalidism, paralysis, and insanity, and argued that a "counter-army of prostitutes" threatened to reverse the gains that had been made on the venereal disease front before the war. Tunney claimed that "diseased classes of harlots" were plying their trade "in juke-box joints and red-light districts." He told men to be suspicious of "medical certificates" purporting to guarantee that a girl was free of disease and cautioned that "easy pick-ups" were likely to be infected. He lectured men that there was no physical need to engage in sex and warned that many men had lost the opportunity to distinguish themselves on the battlefield because "in an unguarded hour of weakness they succumbed to a more insidious enemy."[22] Given Bates' frequently voiced objections to the sexual double standard in the interwar years (and sometimes afterwards), it is hard to know why he found this pamphlet acceptable, but its adoption by the league seems to suggest that he was increasingly of the view that women were responsible for spreading venereal disease. *The Bright Shield of Continence* was widely taken up by military chaplains, and the Health League distributed tens of thousands of copies into their hands.[23] The league also produced a small pamphlet entitled *What Are the Venereal Diseases?* It warned that venereal disease "is damaging our war effort, bringing tragedy into home life and injuring children as yet unborn," the last point highlighting the league's ongoing concern with protecting "the race." The pamphlet threatened that the "person who indulges in sexual adventures" would sooner or later become infected.[24]

The Health League's material did not escape criticism. The Ontario government expressed concern that too much of the material produced by the league was American in origin.[25] In British Columbia, the acting director of venereal disease control, D.E.H. Cleveland, objected to the *Bright Shield of Continence*, saying that his division wanted to focus on the "medical aspects" of venereal disease and exclude "the moral aspect of the venereal disease problem." It did not want to preach about "chastity" and "sexual continence."[26] J.A. Leroux, who was involved in the leadership of the VD divisions in both Ontario and British Columbia over the course of the war, remarked that Health League materials had a certain "shallowness of interpretation."[27] At least one member of the public also complained: a widowed woman criticized the Health League pamphlets for taking a very negative view of sexuality. As she explained, "My husband and I were poor but we loved each other and weren't afraid to demonstrate it to each other. How can your husband know you love him if you don't show him? We felt it was all so very beautiful." Bates wrote back, "There surely should be some reticence about sex. How far would you propose to go?"[28]

The Health League continued to have considerable success showing anti-VD films, including *Fight Syphilis* (1942), *Plain Facts* (1941), *Health Is a Victory* (1942), and *With These Weapons* (1939). *Fight Syphilis*, a production of the US Public Health Service, began with soldiers marching off to war. A First World War veteran appeared on the screen. He would like to fight again but cannot because he was severely disabled by syphilis: we see him limping down the sidewalk. Next, an optimistic scene in a laboratory stressed that it was now possible to test for and treat syphilis. The film cautioned against dance halls, dark streets, and other places that "infect the people," while a melodramatic section warned against being treated by quacks. The film concluded with a vision of safe and comfortable homes across the nation.[29] The Health League urged high schools and churches across Toronto to show the film.[30] *With These Weapons*, produced by the American Social Hygiene Association (ASHA), emphasized that syphilis was curable, especially if it was caught early enough. It urged states to pass legislation mandating premarital and prenatal syphilis testing and recommended such testing in industry as well.[31] *Health Is a Victory*, another ASHA production, featured a lecture on gonorrhea in an industrial plant. It blamed prostitutes for the spread of the disease, and warned of dire consequences if the disease went untreated, but promised that new, highly effective treatments would bring an end to the suffering.[32] The ASHA's *Plain Facts* was a short film highlighting the dire consequences of syphilis and gonorrhea, showcasing syphilis sores, paralysis, and insanity, along with children blinded by gonorrhea.[33] The ASHA's films reflected the emphasis that the organization was putting on its industrial health program, an area that was also a growing interest of the Health League of Canada as well, as we will show in Chapter 4.

The Health League also showed feature-length films that focused on the subject of VD. *Damaged Lives*, a film that was a centrepiece of the league's educational campaign in the 1930s (see Chapter 1), was distributed to the armed forces, but it was not widely shown to civilian audiences, probably because new treatments had made some of the information obsolete.[34] Also, *Damaged Lives* had already been shown widely across the country, and people were eager for new material.[35] The league initially reverted back to the silent film *The End of the Road* (see Chapter 1), which it showed to three quarters of a million Canadians in the early 1940s.[36] (It is hard to know if people went to see the film for education or amusement. As early as 1927, a letter to the Saskatchewan Social Hygiene Council reported that the film had lost much of its educational value as a result of the old-fashioned dress and hairstyles. The writer reported that the protagonists' tennis clothes "produced howls of laughter and derisive screams.")[37]

The league had considerable success showing *No Greater Sin*, described at the beginning of this chapter.[38] The film received good reviews: these were often recycled from press releases sent out by the league, but even some independent reviewers praised the film. *Winnipeg Tribune* movie reviewer

Ben Lepkin asserted that most films dealing with "social diseases" were either "too sexy and risqué or scientific and dull" but that *No Greater Sin* was neither shocking nor didactic but "a serious portrayal of the human havoc these diseases play with human happiness."[39] The *Noranda Press* in Rouyn, Quebec, claimed, "It is a throbbing, vibrant document of human hopes and fears" (it's not clear if the sexual innuendo was intentional).[40] The jaundiced *Toronto Telegram*, on the other hand, asserted that "the audience yesterday was looking for thrills more than knowledge."[41] Major J.A. Leroux, then the acting director of British Columbia's VD Division, criticized *No Greater Sin* as a "third rate production with a not particularly strong story." He objected to the title, because he believed that it was important to reduce the stigma associated with venereal disease. He further claimed that the film *Plain Facts* (often shown before *No Greater Sin*) harkened back to an earlier era of venereal disease education when "we undertook to frighten people into cooperation by horrifying them with rare views of pathological lesions."[42] Even so, by March 1943, nearly half a million Canadians had seen *No Greater Sin*.[43]

While *No Greater Sin* emphasized that venereal disease could be treated, the Health League underlined the seriousness of such infections. In a press release for the film, the league claimed that syphilis "has been responsible for more deaths than any other infection" and warned that the disease could lead to insanity, infant death, and shortened life. It added that gonorrhea caused 80 percent of the blindness in babies and could have a "crippling effect" on women.[44] Such claims were a little exaggerated. It is unlikely that syphilis had caused more death than any other infection, and by the 1940s nearly all infants received silver nitrate drops at birth, preventing them from acquiring gonorrhea-related blindness.

No Greater Sin was remounted for a long showing in Toronto in 1944. The following week, venereal disease clinics at Toronto general hospitals achieved record attendance.[45] The film was also shown throughout Ontario and in Edmonton and Calgary.[46] Its message met with some criticism. Some people thought that the title perpetuated the idea of "sin, shame and prudery." Others objected to the common practice of showing the film to audiences segregated by gender, arguing that it was better that these issues be discussed between the sexes. The film was restricted to people over the age of sixteen, a fact that also led to criticism, as some people felt that it was adolescents who most needed such information. Finally, some observers objected to the advertising, which was somewhat lurid: a typical advertisement read, "SHOCKING ... because it is so true. DARING ... because it pulls no punches. EXCITING ... because it expresses facts ... A COURAGEOUS

SCREEN SHOWS the dire results of social evil in a love story, intimate and frank, of People Like You."[47]

Beyond using films and pamphlets to promote VD education, the Health League established a highly productive relationship with Junior Chambers of Commerce (Jaycees). In June 1943, at their national meeting, the Jaycees decided to focus their efforts on VD prevention and treatment for the duration of the war. They appointed Joe Lichstein, who had previously run a Junior Chamber of Commerce campaign against VD in Saskatchewan, to head their national campaign.[48] With the consent of the Jaycees, Lichstein moved to Toronto to work out of the Health League offices, with his time paid for by the league – another example of the league's effectiveness at building alliances.[49] The league put together an extensive volume of materials that was distributed to Junior Chambers of Commerce, health departments, and community groups across the country. It included literature, posters, background information, press releases, CBC-approved radio programs, a model sermon, advertising material, speakers' notes, a guide for panel discussions, and information on how to secure advertising.[50] The league also provided the Jaycees with films, pamphlets, and other publicity aids. By May 1944, forty-one different Jaycee groups had undertaken anti-VD campaigns, while another seventeen reported that they planned to do so.[51] These campaigns included public lectures, window displays, posters, pamphlets, newspaper advertisements, radio programs, and billboards. In some cities, Jaycee teams stenciled "Fight VD" on the sidewalks.[52] They distributed posters produced by the US Public Health Service, including "Know for Sure," promoting blood tests for syphilis, and "No Home Remedy Has Ever Cured Gonorrhea," as well as Canadian-produced posters including "Canada Needs Strong Men" and "Syphilis Strikes 1 out of 40." Pamphlets included league staples such as *Healthy Happy Womanhood, An Open Letter to Young Men,* and *Bright Shield of Continence*.[53] The Health League offered a prize for the best Jaycees campaign.[54]

Another area of close cooperation between the Jaycees and the Health League was National Social Hygiene Day.[55] The American Social Hygiene Association launched its Social Hygiene Day in the late 1930s. The Health League of Canada followed suit with Canadian Social Hygiene Day in 1943, marked with a few conferences in Toronto, Ottawa, and other cities.[56] The next year, the event broadened into National Social Hygiene Day.[57] The Canadian day was planned in coordination with the US event in order to take advantage of the American literature as well as American advertising that reached Canadian homes. In the week before Social Hygiene Day, the

Health League circulated a radio script that emphasized the importance of taking a blood test and urged healthy recreation for young people. Another script, to be read on Social Hygiene Day itself, emphasized that syphilis and gonorrhea were "responsible for much suffering and unhappiness, broken marriages, doomed children, sickness, chronic invalidism and early death."[58] By 1945, thanks to the combined efforts of the Health League and the Jaycees, National Social Hygiene Day had become a major event. That year, the Health League hosted a talk at Toronto's Massey Hall attended by 500 people. Percy Vivian, the minister of health in Ontario, spoke, followed by a panel discussion with representatives from labour, social work, medicine, and education.[59] Brooke Claxton, the federal minister of health and welfare, gave a radio address over the English language-network of the Canadian Broadcasting Corporation, saying "venereal diseases are among the greatest cause of disability and death!"[60] Spot announcements produced by the Health League ran on many local radio stations. There were also news releases, the use of a "Stamp Out VD" postal cancellation stamp, showings of *No Greater Sin*, and library displays. Many Junior Chambers of Commerce hosted panel discussions.[61] Similar events were held in 1946, although by that point the Jaycees had withdrawn from the campaign.[62] The Post Office used the "Stamp Out VD" cancellation stamp for several weeks; Claxton made another nation-wide broadcast, and the Health League sent out weekly news bulletins to Canadian newspapers over a ten-week period and provided radio spot announcements on most radio stations.[63] The National Film Board agreed to provide films and projectionists to community groups who wanted to show anti-VD films.[64] In spite of this success, by 1947 the Social Hygiene Division of the Health League was without a secretary, and National Social Hygiene Day was quietly folded into National Health Week.[65]

Another successful league initiative was the "Stamp Out VD" campaign of May 1945. The Health League convinced approximately 60 percent of drug stores across the country to put up a window display about venereal disease.[66] Provincial health departments provided the drug stores with more than 200,000 pamphlets on the subject. The league produced three advertisements and sought industry sponsorship to have them run in dailies across the country. Twenty-five newspapers ran at least one of these advertisements, including the *Montreal Gazette,* the *Montreal Star, Le Devoir,* the *Victoria Daily Colonist,* the *Regina Leader Post,* and the *Winnipeg Free Press.* The campaign stressed the importance of premartial and prenatal blood testing. During a radio address that was part of the campaign, H.C. Rhodes, assistant director of information services with the Department of

National Health and Welfare, said that such testing would "protect innocent victims." It would prevent marriages from breaking up as a result of one spouse learning that the other spouse had entered marriage infected with venereal disease and would prevent the suffering of innocent children.[67] In a press release, the Health League also emphasized that venereal diseases "arise from faulty human conduct and conduct is a personal responsibility," demonstrating that, despite the ostensible focus on testing, the league was still emphasizing the importance of individuals regulating and changing their moral behaviour.[68]

Throughout the war, the league attempted to coordinate its activities with various provincial and municipal governments and with the re-established Venereal Disease Division of the Department of National Health. The league saw itself as the clearing house for educational material and believed that it could provide a valuable service to governments. The league occasionally expressed frustration that provincial and municipal governments failed to recognize its contributions, one of several signs that government officials were increasingly wary of the league and of Bates.[69] When the Venereal Disease Division was re-established in Ottawa in 1943, there was no commensurate increase in federal grants to the Health League.[70] A memo in the files of the Department of Pensions and National Health suggested that the league dissipated its energies in too many directions, embarked on national campaigns without first testing them in local areas, failed to cooperate with other bodies, and had weak leadership.[71] In 1944, the Health League was excluded from a Dominion-Provincial conference of VD directors.[72] J.A. Leroux (then head of British Columbia's VD division) and D.H. Williams (the head of the Ottawa division) accused the Health League of spending too much money on salaries.[73] A few years later, Leroux, then back in Ontario, complained that the Health League acted too independently and that it should cooperate more fully with other health authorities. He scolded the league for starting projects it could not finish.[74] A number of provinces in western Canada complained that the league was too Ontario-centric, noting that they were not eager to cooperate with the organization until it established an office in western Canada or included western leaders in its activities.[75]

The Postwar Campaign for Premarital Syphilis Testing and Sex Education

The Health League continued its campaign in favour of premarital and prenatal testing for syphilis after the war. In 1946, it released a pamphlet warning that VD rates were increasing and urging premarital blood testing. In yet another example of the league's failure to adjust to changing times, this pamphlet cited the same case studies the league had been using for years, including that of the Brantford man who discovered that he and his wife and seven children were infected with syphilis.[76] The league lobbied the provinces, especially Ontario, to pass legislation requiring premarital testing. In February 1946, a national Gallup poll commissioned by the league indicated that 89 percent of Canadians were in favour of compulsory premarital testing. Support in Quebec, although lower, was a healthy 80 percent.[77] By 1946, five provinces (British Columbia, Alberta, Saskatchewan, Manitoba, and Prince Edward Island) had passed legislation making premarital blood tests mandatory, but only two (Alberta and Saskatchewan) followed through by having the laws proclaimed.[78] The zeal for premarital testing proved short lived. Despite five separate attempts to introduce legislation mandating premarital blood tests in Ontario in 1945–51, the bills all failed, largely because the ruling Conservatives felt that prenatal testing was sufficient and that the inaccuracy of the Wassermann test could create undue hardship for the people being tested.[79] Such reservations were not unfounded: in Alberta, during the first year of premarital syphilis testing, nearly 20 percent of the people initially given positive results were later deemed to not have syphilis. At the same time, only 1 percent of people tested proved to have syphilis.[80] Contemporary research suggests that perhaps 25 percent of the results of the Wassermann test might be false positives: one can only imagine the sense of betrayal, distrust, and distress created by these results.[81] By 1956, only four provinces – Alberta, Saskatchewan, Manitoba, and Prince Edward Island – had compulsory premarital testing.[82] British Columbia never proclaimed its legislation, because of the burden it would have imposed on provincial laboratories as well as unease about subjecting "deserving" women to compulsory blood tests.[83] This trend differed significantly from the United States, where the vast majority of states implemented compulsory premarital testing.[84]

During the postwar period, the league also continued to campaign for sex education, with a focus on morality. During the war, there had been considerable alarm in Canada about juvenile delinquency, especially female sexual delinquency.[85] At the time, many thought that better sex education could help counteract such behaviour. Numerous organizations passed resolutions in favour of sex education, including the Youth Labour Federation, the Ontario Educational Association, and the Winnipeg Council of Social Agencies. A Gallup poll released in June 1944 showed that 93 percent of Canadians favoured instruction about venereal disease in senior high schools.[86] The Health League wanted to ensure that this sex education would be taught in an appropriate manner, by which it meant that any discussion of sex per se would be secondary to a broader discussion of marriage and morality.[87] Students should be taught the value of continence: "Each lesson plan might even contain some information on the penalties nature exacts for deviations from the proper behavior patterns, i.e. illegitimacy and VD."[88] Bates argued that sex education "needed" to go beyond the "facts" and develop a "broad program needed to guide human beings in the matter of rational sex behavior."[89] After the war, the Health League passed a resolution recommending that any sex education be presented as part of the larger curriculum and not as a stand-alone course. It felt that the term "sex" should be avoided, and that "family-life education," "family relations," or "health and human relations" should be used instead.[90] Indeed, the league won this particular battle. As Christabelle Sethna outlines in her work on sex education in Ontario, an initial enthusiasm for sex education during the Second World War quickly disappeared. During the Cold War, family life education, with the goal of promoting marriage and parenthood, replaced any explicit discussion of sex and venereal disease.[91]

Yet, concerns with the behaviour of youth remained. In 1947, the Health League asked the Canadian Institute of Public Opinion to conduct a poll about whether or not teenagers were behaving better or worse than they had in the past. The poll reportedly discovered that "family life is deteriorating." Forty-five per cent of Canadians felt that teenagers were behaving worse than they had in the past, while only 11 percent thought that they were behaving in better ways.[92] As many historians have noted, attitudes like these reflected the heightened concern about delinquency, especially sex delinquency, in the postwar years.[93]

Regardless of perceptions of "sex delinquency," rates of infectious syphilis were plunging by the late 1940s. A league survey in Toronto in 1950 uncovered only 158 cases of early syphilis and 432 cases of later-stage syphilis, despite a high response rate from doctors. Rates of gonorrhea had also fallen, although not as substantially, but by this point gonorrhea could be easily treated and cured.[94] Statistics from the Department of National Health and Welfare bear out the trend found by the league (Figure 9). The issue of VD seemed less urgent, and as early as 1947, the Health League no longer had a paid director for its Social Hygiene Division. The division continued, but its major campaigns had come to an end.[95] Yet, in the pages of *Health*, and in Health League press releases, Bates continued to complain that the venereal disease problem was being poorly handled: "What is

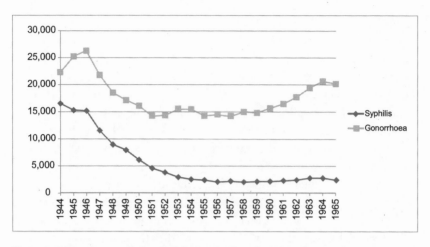

Figure 9 Rates of venereal disease infection in Canada, 1944–61
Source: Epidemiology Division, Department of National Health and Welfare, *Venereal Disease in Canada* (Ottawa: National Health and Welfare, 1965).

primarily a moral problem with a medical aspect is being treated as though it were a medical problem with a moral aspect."[96] Despite glaring evidence to the contrary, he believed that the introduction of penicillin was actually leading to an increase in venereal disease, as people's fear of the disease decreased. He concluded that "science has done just about all that science can do. There is now need for intense study of social action." In this, he had much in common with the American Social Hygiene Association, which also feared that penicillin would lead to promiscuity.[97] Bates returned to his critique of the sexual double standard, which he had muted during the war: "Isn't it time that we do away with the double standard of morals? There should be, as Mrs. Pankhurst once said, a single standards of morals and that is a high one." He complained about social hygiene posters that blamed women for the spread of venereal disease and claimed that venereal disease had disappeared in Russia because every woman had a job and women were paid the same as men.[98] He stressed that it was not enough to cure the disease with penicillin and move on. As an editorial in *Health* put it in 1948, "quick cures in the absence of social and moral controls" will increase disease rates. "Civilization," he railed, "has surely taught the value of monogamous marriage and pre-marital continence."[99]

This moralizing tone was also reflected in Health League campaigns against books and movies it felt were having a deleterious impact on the morals of youth. In 1949, Bates published an editorial in *Health* expressing concern about commercial films that played up the "salacious and sensational" with respect to venereal disease. He feared that such films were "subversive of the morals of the community." The Health League contacted all ministers of health in Canada offering to "assist in censorship."[100] In internal minutes, Bates expressed the view that censors should consult the Health League before all movie releases in Canada – an indication of the far-reaching role he felt that the league should play in Canadian life.[101] It was not just films that raised Bates' ire. In 1948, the league asked the federal government to ban the first Kinsey report, *Sexuality in the Human Male*, except for scientific purposes.[102] In an editorial, Bates expressed fears that the book would have dire consequences for the "innocents, adolescents and those of low mentality" who picked it up as pornography.[103] In 1950, the league urged the Ontario Censor Board to withdraw the sex education film *Bob and Sally* because it showed photographs of the sex organs.[104] Bates also published an editorial in favour of banning films in which Ingrid Bergman (not mentioned by name) appeared, because of her illegitimate pregnancy.[105] Five years later, Bates recommended banning the second Kinsey Report, *Sexuality in the Human Female*. He condemned Kinsey's methodology and claimed that the book libelled "womankind."[106] In 1958, he published an editorial complaining about the flood of obscene literature on the newsstands and blamed it for an alarming increase in venereal disease in New England.[107] The following year, Bates and the Health League supported new legislation, introduced by Justice Minister Davey Fulton, to control the publication of so-called obscene literature.[108] As Mary Louise Adams has shown, censorship campaigns against "indecency" reflected widespread concern about the corruptibility of youth in the postwar era.[109] Yet, many others felt uneasy about censorship and supported a more open discussion of sexuality.[110]

***

Although the Health League was able to garner significant support for its anti–venereal disease work during the Second World War and in the late 1940s, there were signs that this work was being taken over by provincial health units. Moreover, many experts in the field felt that the league's message was too focused on morality, sexual continence, and the dire consequences of venereal disease, and not enough on the basics of testing and treatment. In the years following the war, it became clear that penicillin was dramatically reducing the incidence of venereal disease in Canada. Bates believed that this was no cause for celebration: he feared that easy cures would create sexual licentiousness. By the late 1940s, the League had begun to back away from its work on VD prevention and to focus on other projects, as we will see in the following chapters. Yet, Bates would never lose interest in his first passion, and throughout the 1950s the league continued to editorialize against declining moral standards and in favour of censorship. In the 1950s, this raised few eyebrows, but as we will show in Chapter 8, by the 1960s, the Health League's views seemed increasingly dated.

4

Preventing Sickness and Absenteeism
The Health League and the Workplace

During the Second World War, the Health League began providing a series of posters and pamphlets to employers for their workers, covering a wide range of possible health hazards. One poster, "The Cold Facts," instructed workers to stay away from coughers and sneezers, to get lots of rest after work, to eat well, and to dress sensibly. The accompanying pamphlet instructed employees to take cod liver oil during the winter months, to avoid extremes of hot and cold, to prevent constipation, and to use their own cups and spoons. Another poster, "More Fresh Air Means Better Health," reminded workers that good health was a patriotic duty – a small flag proclaimed, "National Health Is Vital to Victory." The companion pamphlet instructed workers to keep their homes at 68–70 degrees Fahrenheit, to use a humidifier to clear and circulate the air, and to clean their furnaces regularly. A third poster, "Be Kind to Your Teeth," featured a large man with his head bandaged up against a toothache. It instructed workers to brush their teeth twice a day, to floss, to cut back on candy, and to eat green vegetables, raw fruits, whole wheat bread, and dairy products.[1] This campaign arose from the wartime desire to keep workers healthy and on the job, but it would continue in the postwar years as the Health League tried to develop its membership and promote the expansion of employer-delivered health services.

During the war, as many historians have detailed, the federal government and numerous voluntary organizations called on Canadians to change their ways of working, shopping, and living to help achieve victory.[2] As factories geared up production, employers and government officials were concerned with how to keep employees healthy and efficient.[3] Employers and bureaucrats were especially concerned about high employee turnover and days missed from work.[4] In response, the Health League created a Division of Industrial Health (also called the Industrial Division or Industrial Health Division) in 1940. This action reflected a long-standing interest among social hygienists in educating workers about health. In the United States, for example, as early as the First World War, social hygienists were warning employers about the costs of venereal disease, and the American Social Hygiene Association had an ongoing interest in industrial health.[5] In Canada, the Health League's Division of Industrial Health had strong support from the Industrial Hygiene Division of the Ontario Department of Health, the federal government's Industrial Hygiene Division of the Department of Pensions and National Health, and several corporations. The league's division had two goals: to keep workers healthy both physically and mentally, and to encourage employers to hire physicians and nurses and to recognize the improvements that they could bring to workplaces. The league took a paternalistic approach: it reached out to employers rather than to unions or workers and assumed that employers were generally acting in the best interest of their employees. The educational material directed at workers framed health problems as their own fault rather than the result of workplace conditions or low wages and poor living conditions.

The Health League felt that its contribution to industrial health could best be made through health education, and for a small fee it provided employers with posters and leaflets to be inserted into pay envelopes to teach proper health habits to workers. (The league was not alone in providing health education to workers; the federal government and provincial governments also produced educational material.)[6] For a time, the league provided employers with a newsletter, the *Industrial Health Bulletin*, which provided more detailed information geared towards factory physicians and management. From the 1940s to the 1960s, the league also ran regular articles in *Health* on workplace issues, focused mostly on how to avoid accidents and sickness and the subsequent absenteeism. By the 1950s, articles often focused on the mental health of workers.[7] The magazine took the side of management over employees; many articles celebrated what companies were doing to protect the health of their workers. This perspective is not surprising, given that *Health* was directed at a middle- or upper-class audience. And yet, the league also encouraged companies to employ disabled and older workers, emphasizing that they could be at least as valuable as able-bodied or younger workers. The league hoped that its Division of Industrial Health would help create a healthier and more stable workforce and citizenry, but, in entering the industrial health field, the league was also hoping to increase its revenues. Over the years, it developed several industrial membership schemes, although they achieved little success.

Related to its industrial health efforts was the league's Foodhandling Division, through which the league reached out to the Canadian Restaurant Association, offering to teach safe methods of storing, cooking, and serving food. The division hoped that restaurants, like industrial establishments, would enrol their employees as members of the Health League. As with many league efforts, funds for both the food safety and worker health programs were limited, and their ambitions exceeded the league's capacity. Consequently, the projects never came to full fruition.

Surprisingly little has been written about industrial health as a medical field or public health endeavour in Canada, in contrast to the more significant literature on the history of occupational health and safety.[8] Beginning in the late nineteenth century, labour organizations and middle-class reformers lobbied for legislation that would increase safety in the workplace, especially for women and children. The resulting Factory Acts introduced new rules and regulations around work hours, safety devices, ventilation, cleanliness, fire doors, and so on, and provided for factory inspectors to be appointed to enforce the regulations.[9] In the early twentieth century, most provinces passed workers' compensation legislation that allowed workers some (usually inadequate) cash payment in the case of industrial accidents. It was not until the 1970s that governments passed legislation mandating the establishment of health and safety committees that gave workers the opportunity to learn about and potentially combat the health risks they faced on the job. Even then, as Doug Smith reveals in *Consulted to Death*, these committees did not result in significant improvements to worker health.[10]

Canada lagged behind its more industrialized peers, Britain and the United States, in the adoption of industrial hygiene.[11] In Canada, as elsewhere, the initial focus was on workplace accidents and exposure to dangerous chemicals, but eventually it broadened to take in the well-being of workers more generally and especially the days lost to illness. Ontario was the first province to create a Division of Industrial Hygiene (as part of its Department of Health) in 1920.[12] Manitoba and Quebec established industrial hygiene divisions in the late 1930s.[13] These divisions carried out studies of the health hazards of various workplaces and engaged in health education. Running parallel to this activity was the expansion of industrial medicine (the provision of physician and nursing service in factories), which also occasionally went under the name industrial health or industrial hygiene.[14] After the Second World War broke out, the explosion of shift work and the employment of greater numbers of women and younger workers raised concerns about the special health needs that younger, inexperienced, and female workers might bring to the factory floor and encouraged a broader discussion about industrial health in the public health community. By the end of the war, the Health League indicated that somewhere between eight hundred and nine hundred firms in Canada operated an industrial health plan for their employees.[15] As industrial hygiene grew as a field, researchers increasingly pointed out that, because it was so common, illness was a much greater threat to efficiency than were industrial accidents.[16] While research continued on the environmental causes of disease, many people in the field of industrial health began to focus on the more mundane reasons behind absenteeism, such as colds, rheumatism, and other chronic conditions, as well as mental health.[17] This shift in focus was likely not accidental: as Claudia Clark points out in *Radium Girls*, university departments of industrial health were heavily dependent on corporate funding and tended to ally themselves with employers rather than workers.[18] Industrial physicians who worked in plants were beholden to the corporations that employed them. This bias in the field was also reflected in the Health League's approach, which paid relatively little attention to occupational hazards.

The league regularly stressed that an industrial health plan could save companies money by cutting down on absenteeism. It argued that studies had shown that the average worker in Ontario lost 9.5 days each year – nine of those days were lost through sickness and non-industrial accidents, while only half a day was lost to occupational accidents.[19] The league also contended that sick workers were more likely to have accidents and that they were more liable to exhibit "resentment" in the workplace. In other words, the healthy worker was a more compliant worker.[20] The league's emphasis on quelling labour unrest through better health habits was not surprising: during the war, union membership expanded, and the immediate postwar years were marked by growing labour unrest.[21] The idea that healthier workers would be less likely to strike or to protest workplace conditions was undoubtedly attractive to management.

The Industrial Health Division

Campaigns for Workers

The Health League formed its Industrial Health Division in 1940 under the leadership of honorary chairman J.S. McLean, the president of Canada Packers, one of Canada's leading industrialists.[22] Meat packing, of course, was an industry long associated with workplace accidents.[23] The division's chair was H.W. Weis, the president of Canada Glazed Papers, a mid-sized firm.[24] He was succeeded by F.D. Cruickshank, a medical doctor with deep roots in the industrial community of Weston (today a part of Toronto).[25] Other committee members included J.G. Cunningham, the director of the Industrial Hygiene Division of the Ontario Department of Health; several presidents of mid-sized corporations; and a number of factory physicians. People from Toronto dominated the division, and the league's efforts in this area were almost entirely confined to the province of Ontario.[26] (The Quebec Division of the Health League did produce a set of bilingual posters, but, unfortunately, no record of these remain in the files.)[27] The division started by circulating posters with captions like "Careless Coughers Are Dangerous People" and "Your Lunch Box May Be Your Worst Enemy."[28] These were followed by the three posters/pamphlets described at the beginning of this chapter.

Eventually, the league advertised a package of seventeen posters and pay envelope inserts on subjects ranging from foot care, summer health hazards, and correct posture to the importance of getting a good sleep and avoiding worry.[29] The topics chosen assumed that illness or poor health was the result of the worker's ignorance or apathy and was not caused by his or her working conditions. The poster program seems to have been fairly successful, with over three hundred corporations purchasing material from the league.[30] These posters were extremely attractive compared to most of the publicity material issued by the Health League. Brightly coloured and with large text, most featured a loose rhyme that could be easily remembered. Reflecting the wartime conditions under which they were originally produced, they highlighted the importance of keeping healthy for the nation. The majority of the posters featured male workers, reflecting the long-standing assumption that women's role was primarily in the home, although two featured male and female workers together, perhaps in recognition of the greater role that women were playing in the workforce during the war. A poster encouraging male workers to eat whole grains featured women in two-piece bathing suits, reflecting the growing presence of cheesecake images of women in the workplace.[31]

The poster "Watch Out for Summer Gremlins" focused on a theme dear to the Health League – the health hazards of summer. Every spring and summer, *Health* featured articles on the menace of sunburn, the possibility of drowning, and the dangers of drinking unpasteurized milk in rural locales. The poster featured a man lying in the grass while gremlins labelled sunburn, fatigue, and poison ivy tried to disturb his rest. A note explained that "summer gremlins are first cousins to the pesky little Air Gremlins who play tricks on our boys of the RCAF."[32] The accompanying pay envelope insert informed readers that it took sixteen days to safely suntan a child. It warned people against taking too much exercise all at once and recommended avoiding swimming for an hour after eating and taking plenty of salt. Reflecting the Health League's ongoing work on pasteurization, the material alerted readers to the dangers of unpasteurized milk in rural locations and cautioned vacationers to always purify their water.[33] The message assumed that workers were able to take their families on a summer holiday, a venture that was undoubtedly too expensive for most employees.

Several posters made the point that many workers worried unnecessarily about health problems that could easily be solved if only they sought a doctor's advice and treatment.[34] The "TB Is Dangerous" leaflet recommended that people set their minds at ease by getting an X-ray. It featured a grinning man and rhymed:

I really thought I had TB.
Hurray! I was mistaken;
I settled all my doubts and fears
By having an X-ray taken.

Notably, the leaflet said nothing about what would happen to the employee who discovered that he or she did have tuberculosis. It advised people to keep their hands away from their face, to ensure that they drank only pasteurized milk, to avoid drinking from a common cup, to exercise daily if they had a sedentary job, to sleep eight to nine hours each night, and to eat nutritious food.[35] The poster "Worry Causes Sickness" suggested that a "talk with the 'doc'" could easily put everything right (Figure 10). It featured two men in rocking chairs: a smiling doctor smoked a pipe and a relaxed worker who seemed to be in no rush to get back to the factory floor. The League assumed that workers worried more about possible illness than about financial or family troubles and anticipated that a "check-up" could reveal to the employee that she or he was not ill after all. It reassured workers that, even

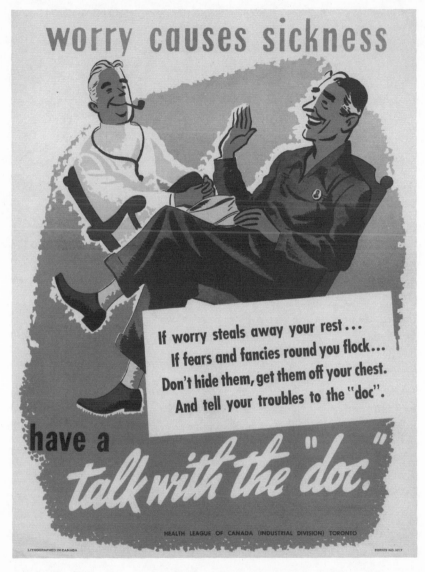

Figure 10 "Worry Causes Sickness" | LAC, MG28, I332, vol. 232.

if something was wrong with them, it was best to start treatment right away so that they could "start anticipating recovery instead of dreading conse-quences."[36] The message implied that modern medicine could solve nearly every health problem, and it underlined the Health League's position that doctors, dentists, and other health professionals were indispensable experts.

It also assumed that workers were taking no risk in confessing problems – whether emotional, financial, or medical – to the company doctor. Workers knew better. They were aware that doctors worked closely with management, making it potentially problematic to confide in the doctor.

Other posters recommended regular health habits. "Get 8 Hours of Sleep Every Night!" warned:

> You're behind the 8-ball when you're tired
> For everything goes wrong.
> So get your sleep, keep fit and well;
> "Canada wants you strong."

The related pay-stub insert instructed Canadians to sleep in a well-ventilated room, to rest before going to sleep, to read a "hard" book that will "bore you to sleep," to think about happy things, to sleep without heavy or oppressive covers, and to relax the muscles.[37] During the war, both provincial and federal industrial health divisions had heavily emphasized fatigue as an important contributing factor to sickness as well as to decreased wartime production.[38] Once again, this poster assumed that the cause of any troubles that the worker had in sleeping lay outside the workplace environment. Another poster warned against constipation. The pay-stub insert recommended exercising in the open air, drinking lots of water, and always using the bathroom when the urge arose. It suggested that "a good nourishing breakfast," flaxseed, and coarse vegetables would help with regularity and warned against constipating foods, including tea, large quantities of milk, potatoes, cheese, pork, veal, and spicy foods.[39] "Don't Sag: Stand Up for Canada" portrayed a young man and woman bent over and looking haggard. The information sheet told employees that "health depends on good posture" and warned that bad posture would prevent the lungs from filling and would cramp the stomach. It provided detailed instructions on how best to stand, sit, and sleep.[40] "Keep on Your Toes by Caring for Your Feet" highlighted foot care, another topic dear to the Health League, which regularly published articles on feet in *Health*.[41] The poster featured a row of women marching off to work in low heels, bandanas on their heads (à la Rosie the Riveter), and lunchboxes in their hands. They were shadowed by a group of men in the same formation.[42] It urged workers to wear well-fitting shoes and counselled that "sound active feet are vital to your work, your health, your happiness." The pay-stub insert suggested that daily footbaths would help remove corns and callouses, and stressed the importance of treating athlete's foot.[43]

Presumably, these baths were to take place on the workers' own time. All of these posters were notable for their patriotic appeal and their recommendation that workers regulate their eating, their leisure, and even their bodily movements to ensure better health and increased efficiency.

Several posters/flyers emphasized the importance of hygiene (usually at home). The poster "Health Depends on Cleanliness" had a dish-rack filled with soap and a scrubber and suggested that cleanliness was "The BEST defense against disease."[44] The pay envelope insert reminded employees to bathe regularly, suggesting that a warm bath would relax the muscles and promote sleep while a cold bath could stimulate the body in the morning.[45] The "Avoid Colds" poster featured a man violently sneezing and rhymed:

Don't mingle with coughers or sneezers;
Get plenty of slumber and rest;
Relax and keep fit – then you'll rarely
Have a cold in your head or your chest[46]

The insert warned: "The cold bug is more than a nuisance. He's a contagious menace. He's the greatest single cause of lost working time." It instructed workers to eat right, sleep in a well-ventilated room, avoid constipation, dress sensibly, and avoid using unwashed cups and spoons.[47] Again, these pamphlets urged workers to adopt new health behaviours on their own time in order to increase their productivity at work.

Several circulars urged employees to seek out regular medical care. The "Don't Be Shortsighted" poster instructed employees to have their eyes examined regularly and to read and work in proper light, and suggested that improved nutrition could help eyesight.[48] In yet another nod to the wartime environment, the eye chart read "VICTORY." The pay-stub insert reminded workers to wear safety goggles and to consult a first-aid attendant or nurse immediately if they got something in their eye, and recommended that workers give their eyes a rest by covering them during breaks or gazing at something green.[49] The poster "See Your Dentist Twice a Year" informed employees that a lot of their aches and pains might be due to an infected tooth. The pay insert stressed that oral health affected the whole body and that "a decayed tooth if neglected may lead to chronic serious or even fatal illness." It recommended avoiding refined sugar and eating green vegetables, raw fruits, and dairy products. It instructed people to brush their teeth after every meal and to use dental floss.[50] Notably, very few employees had benefits that would have covered dental visits; presumably, workers were to pay for dental visits themselves.

Many of the posters and flyers focused on the importance of good nutrition. The "Eat a Nourishing Breakfast" poster featured a giraffe and the tagline "It's a long way to lunchtime." The text suggested: "Start your day off with a nourishing meal; then the harder you work, the better you'll feel."[51] The emphasis on hard work no doubt appealed to employers. The corresponding insert provided a variety of breakfast menus. The poster "A Nourishing Snack" featured three stickmen in chef's caps. Each bore a snack on a tray labelled, respectively, milk and whole wheat sandwich; whole wheat doughnuts and fruit juice; and bran muffins and cocoa.[52] The pay-stub insert provided more detailed menu suggestions, including some unusual sandwiches – one of shredded spinach, ground liver, and sweet pickle, and another of cottage cheese, grated raw carrot, and chopped green peppers.[53] The pay-stub insert "Pack Power in Every Meal" listed six daily food rules, including drinking three glasses of milk and one of juice and eating four to six slices of whole wheat bread with butter, one serving of green or yellow vegetables, one serving of potatoes, one serving of oatmeal, and one serving of fish or poultry. It recommended liver, kidney, or heart at least once a week. Assuming that the worker was male and that he had someone to pack his lunchbox, it suggested "if you'd like a Health League booklet for your wife, girl friend, or mother, a booklet chock full of delicious and economical recipes and menu suggestions, send 5¢ to the Health League of Canada."[54] Another poster and insert urged workers to start a victory garden. It featured vegetables lined up in formation and rhymed:

> Grow these "fighting foods" at home
> It's a job we all can do
> The fresher food will do you good
> And you'll help your country too.

It provided instructions on how to plant beans, beets, cabbage, carrots, peas, and tomatoes.[55] "Keep Strong with Whole Grain Products" showcased a barrel-chested lifeguard striding past two women (Figure 11). The hearts radiating from their shapely bodies suggested how they felt about his physique. It told readers to "add whole grain products to your daily diet for Better Health" and reminded Canadians that "Canada grew great on grain."[56] All of these circulars urged workers to eat nutritiously in order to work harder and better, and promised that improved eating habits would strengthen the nation.

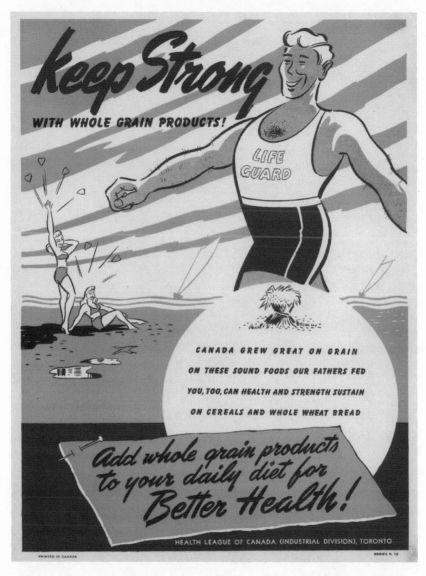

Figure 11 "Keep Strong with Whole Grain Products!" | LAC, MG28, I332, vol. 232.

A syphilis poster and pamphlet was not always included in the list of materials that employers could purchase. This gloomy poster featured a darkened sky and a lighting strike and warned "Syphilis Strikes One Out of Forty Canadians." It cautioned that many Canadians did not know that they were infected and that "about half of the victims are innocent of any wrong conduct" – they were infected by a wife or husband, a father or mother – a statement that perpetuated an understanding of the disease as a moral issue. The pamphlet warned that the consequences could be dire: "Syphilis is a crippling and killing disease. It unfits men and women for work. It fills many invalid chairs and sends many people to early graves. It provides a constant flow of patients to mental hospitals and other public institutions." It recommended that everyone get a blood test and reassured workers that plant physicians would keep the results confidential. While the front cover suggested that "Syphilis Can Be Cured if Treated Promptly," the main thrust of the pamphlet was to alarm and frighten.[57]

All of these materials aimed to cut absenteeism by reducing the number of colds, toothaches, and other ailments that regularly kept people away from work. Notably, they all assumed that it was home conditions or poor health habits that led to illness, and they proposed that workers, even while not on the job, should be engaging in health behaviours, like cleaning their furnace or flossing their teeth, that would keep them in good shape for their work. In keeping with the league's focus on white Canadians, none of the posters featured workers of colour; nor was there any attempt to reach out to immigrant workers by providing pamphlets in languages other than English.

It is hard to know how workers responded to this material. The Health League made at least one attempt to have a representative from labour on its Industrial Health Committee, but there is no indication in the records that he ever attended a meeting.[58] Several physicians in the Division of Industrial Health – including A.N. McKillop, who worked as an industrial physician for Goodyear in Toronto, and J.G. Cunningham – suggested that the posters were more useful than the pay inserts, as the latter often went unread.[59] By contrast, an employer on the committee suggested that workers did not pay much attention to posters, but that the circulars were helpful because wives and even children of the employees read them on occasion.[60] This, of course, is the problem with health education of any kind: it is hard to know how much people pay attention – even if they read the material provided – and it is even harder to know if it changes people's behaviour.

Promoting Industrial Health to Employers

In addition to the worker education materials, the Health League hosted regular conferences on industrial health, featuring high-profile speakers from government, industry, and labour. The major conferences were all held in Toronto. The first of these, held in 1943, attracted 500 people and included talks by L.B. Pett, the director of nutrition services, Department of Pensions and National Health; Eugene Forsey, the director of research with the Canadian Congress of Labour; and D.H. Williams, the chief of venereal disease control at the federal Department of Pensions and National Health.[61] In 1944, the keynote speaker was Brock Chisholm, then the deputy minister of national health in Ottawa, but soon to become the first director-general of the World Health Organization (Chisholm, like many people affiliated with the Health League over the years, was a supporter of the eugenics movement and had played a key role in the development of intelligence testing in the military).[62] In 1945, speakers included academics, government officials, and representatives of business and labour. Dr. C. Charles Burlingame, an expert consultant in psychiatry to the US Secretary of War, gave the keynote address on the reassimilation of war workers and veterans.[63] A final conference was held in 1946. The Health League also held industrial health conferences in smaller centres across Ontario including Niagara Falls, London, Kitchener, and Ottawa.[64] The conferences generated substantial material for the league to use in *Health* and other publications and demonstrated that in this field, as in others, it was well connected with leading professionals.

Near the end of the war, the division circulated a glossy pamphlet promoting its program. It encouraged corporations to implement industrial health plans that included employing a physician and/or nurse, depending on the size of the enterprise. It recommended that all potential employees be given a pre-employment medical examination that included a Wassermann test for syphilis. And it urged corporations to educate their workers about health. The pamphlet promised that such a plan would reduce absenteeism, "almost" eliminate serious illness, create "a kindlier feeling throughout the factory," and enable industry to do its part in employing veterans.[65] The league stressed that an industrial health plan could save companies money by cutting down on absenteeism.[66]

The league consistently emphasized the valuable role that the industrial physician could play in placing people in work environments that would best utilize their skills and talents and thus make them happier, more contented workers. Personnel placement was part of the wartime and postwar explosion of personnel planning, which has been described by Jennifer Stephen in *Pick One Intelligent Girl*. As she demonstrates, personal assessments, which purported to tell the "truth" about the worker, were grounded in racist, gendered, and classist assumptions about intelligence and vocational suitability.[67] The league argued that pre-employment and periodic health exams were for the benefit of the worker; for example, someone with allergies could be transferred to avoid having to work with chemicals and irritants. In one *Health* article, H.W. Urquhart, the chief medical officer of the Hydro-Electric Power Commission of Ontario, described the case of John J.: he had applied to operate a bulldozer, but his hearing and sight were below normal, and it would have been hazardous to allow him to handle heavy equipment. In another case, Bill W. applied to be an electrician, but he was partially colour blind, a characteristic that would have made it impossible for him to do complex jobs with multicoloured wires.[68] Notably, Urquhart did not mention what happened to these workers. At a dinner talk in Peterborough geared towards businessmen and voluntary organizations, Gordon Bates and J.G. Cunningham pointed out that some insurance companies requested medical exams before insuring employees, and there were instances where insuring unhealthy employees had bankrupted insurance companies. The takeaway message: the pre-placement exam would protect the company – and the insurer.[69] The league stressed that the industrial physician could place workers in jobs for which they were well suited: the less intelligent could be placed in repetitive work, while those who craved responsibility could be placed in more challenging positions.[70] The underlying assumption was that this type of screening would lead to a safer workplace environment as well as greater satisfaction among workers, but it also put enormous power into physician's hands.

Understandably, workers were often suspicious of industrial doctors, believing that medical examinations could be used to push out or punish workers who were regarded as activists or troublemakers, or that physicians would dismiss the seriousness of workers' illnesses in order to keep them on the job or deny them compensation.[71] Validating such fears, Jessica van Horssen has shown that in Asbestos, Quebec, company physicians seriously underplayed the risk posed by asbestos to workers at the Jeffrey mine.[72] Physical examinations could be used to regulate employees in other, more subtle, ways as well. For example, one league publication promoting the advantages of having a doctor on staff cited the case of a physically fit twenty-one-year-old woman who came to the doctor complaining of fatigue. Since the doctor "knew" the factory and the work that was done, he was aware that she did not have a heavy job. He examined the employee and found nothing wrong with her. He suggested that perhaps she was worried about something. She went back to work, apparently "reassured" that she was not ill. She returned to visit the nurse the next week and talked about her troubles. The league asked, what would have happened if the employer (in this case, George Weston Ltd.) had not employed a physician on staff? The publication suggested that, in such a case, the woman would have consulted an outside physician, who, knowing nothing of her work, would probably have given her a tonic and suggested that she apply to her foreperson for easier work. The news of the change in work would spread to fellow employees, and "the result would be a lowering of plant morale in her immediate group."[73] The story suggests that female workers were easily worried or troubled by small matters but that the authority of the doctor and nurse could easily put their minds at rest. It further assumes that company doctors could easily assess an individual's health to determine what kinds of work they were or were not capable of, and that the doctor could play a role in maintaining workplace morale.

The league predicted that physicians could bring about spectacular improvements in work performance through their understanding of psychology. This perspective was in keeping with the tremendous emphasis placed on psychology during the war and afterwards.[74] In an article in *Health*, the medical director of George Weston Ltd., Harold Harrison, described the case of John, a forty-five-year-old foreman in the shipping department. He had put in good work for twenty-five years and then suddenly began to suffer from fatigue and was often absent from work. The nurse learned that he had two brothers, one a doctor and the other a lawyer, and John, "doing his own hardworking, valuable, but not socially recognized job, felt himself to be a failure." The medical department recommended transferring John to a white-collar job, and "the exhaustion cleared up, as if by some miracle."[75] This article suggested that rectifying the proper class status of a worker could bring about substantial improvements in performance. Presumably, though, the same effect could not be achieved for a fatigued worker whose class background was not as privileged.

As the previous chapter showed, the league strongly supported pre-employment tests for syphilis, as it believed that many people with syphilis did not know they were infected. Not surprisingly, the league urged that Wassermann tests be part of any industrial health plan. It emphasized that the purpose was not to discriminate against those who were found to be infected, and especially not to fire employees with syphilis, but to ensure that they received treatment that would allow them to continue in their jobs. The league stressed the importance of confidentiality and emphasized that the syphilitic worker posed no danger to fellow employees.[76] But an article in *Health* makes it clear that the league valued the additional surveillance that an industrial physician could provide: if the worker was positive for syphilis, the factory doctor could ensure that "he receives adequate continuous care until such time as [he is] cured."[77] Presumably, workers would stay employed only if they agreed to treatment. The league also recommended that employers require X-ray examinations of all their employees for tuberculosis. This recommendation was in keeping with broader trends – X-rays of industrial workers were being taken across the nation both during and after the war.[78] The league did not mention what would happen to employees who were found to have the disease. Until the 1950s, infectious TB was still treated through long stays in sanatoria. While treatment was usually free and some provinces provided financial support to families, the confinement of a breadwinner could be devastating for the family economy. The league also recommended that the industrial physician ensure that all workers were vaccinated against smallpox. Again, there was no mention of what would happen to the worker who refused vaccination.[79]

As the poster program discussed above suggests, one of the inspirations of the League's Industrial Health Division was wartime excitement about how nutrition could contribute to the maintenance of efficient and healthy workers.[80] The division urged large corporations to establish cafeterias, assuring them that research had shown that "well-cooked meals" could improve the health of workers, reduce absenteeism, and increase efficiency.[81] If a cafeteria was impractical for a company, the division suggested providing workers with boxed lunches supplemented with milk, juice, and/or hot soup. It recommended that these meals be cheap enough that workers would want to buy them. Cafeterias were favoured, at least in part, because the division did not trust workers to put together nutritious lunches of their own accord. A cafeteria could rely on the expertise of dieticians, doctors, and other experts to provide meals that were based on "scientific knowledge of nutrition" and would help fight fatigue and illness.[82]

The Industrial Health Division was also concerned with the integration of veterans back into the workforce.[83] The league was not alone in this: there was widespread agreement in Canada that veterans needed to be compensated for their long service.[84] During the 1940s, *Health* devoted numerous columns to the topic of integrating the returned war veteran, most authored by Stanley Caldwell, the long-term secretary of the Industrial Health Division.[85] The league warned that the transition from military discipline to civilian life could be emotionally challenging for men, both at work and at home. The articles reflected the psychiatric language that had become so important in the military during the war and the growing emphasis on expert personnel placement.[86] One article explained that many veterans had had to struggle to adapt themselves to army life, but, now that the war was coming to an end, they would need to re-adapt themselves to civilian life. Many in the military had learned to take orders rather than taking initiative; civilian life would require a different set of skills.[87] Veterans would also need to adapt to families that had changed while they were overseas: women had become more independent, and children had grown up, with some barely remembering their fathers. There had been infidelities on both sides.[88] Adjustments in the workplace could help veterans adapt to these more personal challenges. Veterans, one author argued, should be treated with leniency at first. Every effort should be made to integrate them into their departments, in an attempt to emulate the sense of belonging that many had felt in the military, and a warm relationship should be established between office executives and the new workers.[89] In another article, Caldwell argued that veterans were "torn between a need for discipline and resentment towards it. Many seek adventure but also long for security."[90] He raised the example of Pete, a man who had suffered a head injury while fighting overseas and had been in a coma for three weeks. When he returned to work, he was restless and had difficulty concentrating. The plant physician explained that "he needed a lot of assistance, a lot of guidance, a lot of co-operative effort between management and supervisor and medical department."[91] Eventually, he adjusted. The story of Pete again highlights the league's assumption that the industrial physician would have psychological insight into the workers under their supervision and that this insight would improve workplace relations. In fact, in Canada at this time, most plant physicians had no specialized training in industrial hygiene, nor had their medical degrees provided them with much education in psychology or psychiatry.[92] Nonetheless, proponents of industrial health seemed to assume that a medical degree guaranteed expertise in such areas.

The league stressed that employers had a duty to employ men who had been injured overseas. The league, through its magazine, appears to have been a particularly forceful voice on this issue: the *Canadian Medical Association Journal*, by contrast, ran few articles on the needs of the disabled soldier.[93] *Health* insisted that disabled workers could be excellent employees. It argued that people with disabilities often had higher powers of concentration and were often more productive, less likely to be absent from work, and less likely to leave their place of employment.[94] The league also emphasized all that modern medicine could accomplish, noting that "physical and mental disabilities can be corrected by modern techniques."[95] It believed that industrial physicians played a vital role in the integration of disabled veterans, as the plant physician could determine the "physical and mental condition of the applicant" and place him in the most appropriate job.[96] Such recommendations speak to the league's faith in experts, as they gave enormous power to physicians to determine potential employees' capacity for certain tasks, which also determined their wages and working conditions.

Over the next fifteen years, the league would continue to argue for the value of disabled employees. It maintained that "handicapped" workers could "usually compete favourably with [their] fellow workers, and exceed them in loyalty and attention to the job if placed in the right occupation." This condescendingly assumed that disabled workers would be better people purely as a result of their condition, a common trope in the treatment of the disabled.[97] The league stressed that disabled workers worked as efficiently as, and with less absenteeism than, able-bodied workers. It began to argue that all workers were "handicapped" in one way or another and that the role of an industrial health program was to build on an employee's strengths.[98] One article in *Health* attested that only 1 percent of workers were in perfect health and that "handicapped persons can actually perform many skilled and delicate jobs as well as or even better than able-bodied workers." The author argued that, as long as the person was emotionally adjusted to his or her disability, there was usually no problem finding a job that was suitable: she suggested that deaf-mutes could be employed as sheet metal hand formers, people with leg amputations could work as drafters, and blind people could work as telephone dispatchers.[99] While such attitudes were condescending and assumed that disabled people would have to adjust to society more than society adjusting to accommodating them, at least they acknowledged the ubiquity of disability, and offered hope of empowering disabled people through gainful employment.

From the late 1950s onwards, the league used similar arguments to support the employment of older workers. It frequently celebrated the contributions of older workers and argued that they, like the disabled, had lower rates of absenteeism than younger or able-bodied workers. In taking this position, the league was confronting significant discrimination that existed against older workers in the post–Second World War period. As one writer in *Health* put it, "We are all aware these days that workers over the age of 40 have, in many industries, little hope of finding a job."[100] The Health League maintained that people had very different capacities at different ages and that it was important to determine a person's capacity and employ that individual accordingly. As one article put it, "The mature or elderly worker is no job-hopper, has a 20% better attendance record and a better safety score than his younger shop mate." The league celebrated workers like a ninety-year-old janitor in San Diego "who has been with the company nearly

20 years with an excellent attendance record" and the sixty-six-year-old auto service station owner who found himself bored after retirement, sought employment as a stock clerk, and redesigned the shop's inventory system.[101] While the league acknowledged that not everyone would want to work into their nineties, its focus on the value of older workers helped to counter the pervasive ageism of the era.[102]

The league's concern with older workers was reflected in its campaign against mandatory retirement. Bates himself was determined to never retire. In 1971, journalist Sidney Katz reported that the then eighty-five-year-old Bates exclaimed, "Retire? Never! A person can keep going as long as he wants to. I'll never quit. I'm working 15 hours a day. Look at all the things I have to do!"[103] Bates believed that it was "perfectly ridiculous to develop a society in which there is nothing to do for people over 65 many of whom are much more capable than their younger associates."[104] On more than one occasion he claimed that retirement drove men to suicide.[105] In *Health*, several articles pointed out that retirement at sixty-five was arbitrary, as many Canadians could be ill before or healthy long after that age, and argued that Canada was losing a vital cohort of potential workers and incurring unnecessarily high pension costs.[106] The personnel director at Consolidated Edison in the United States, Dwight Sargent, testified that his company had seen the harm done by forcing their workers to retire at sixty-five and had improved the company's financial situation by extending the age of retirement.[107] In 1962, the Gerontology Committee of the Health League submitted a brief to the Royal Commission on Health Services, complaining that many retired people were "perfectly capable" of continuing at work. The Gerontology Committee contended that as lifespans increased, Canada would soon be "confronted with an intolerable tax burden" and "millions" of people who were capable of working would "deteriorate" because they were not working.[108] At the same time, *Health* acknowledged that retirement, whether voluntary or mandatory, was a reality for many Canadians, and the magazine included articles on how to prepare for this transition.[109] It urged retirees to continue to contribute to society in different ways and find new forms of work that they could enjoy.[110]

In the late 1940s, *Health* ran a series called "Industry Protects the Workers," celebrating what various companies were doing to protect the health of their employees. An article on the Robert Simpson Company raved that the department store employed two doctors and two nurses in its Toronto location. The company provided all its employees and their dependants with a Blue Cross plan for hospital expenses (the company paid half the cost of the plan, and the employee the other half). Realizing that workers often returned to work too early after a serious illness or operation, Simpson's provided a convalescent hospital for those recuperating employees who lived in boarding houses rather than with their families. The hospital included a swimming pool, tennis courts, and gardens.[111] The Bell Telephone Company provided doctors and nurses at its head office in Montreal, as well as in its Toronto offices. It gave workers pre-placement examinations (to place workers in jobs for which they were physically suited) and promoted health through education. It also carried out periodic exams on "absentee repeaters, sickness prone individuals and those recently returned to work after any prolonged illness." Bell hoped to extend this program towards early detection of illness. The company covered assessment and exams, but, if medical needs were discovered, employees were expected to undertake treatment at their own expense.[112] An article on Bristol-Meyers enthused, "It is apparent ... that private enterprise has taken tremendous strides in providing for and protecting its workers." At that company, every employee who had worked for at least ten months was entitled to two weeks' paid vacation each year, and workers with ten years received three weeks. The company offered yearly medical exams to all its employees. It provided tea, coffee, and snacks at rest periods and lunch at cost in the cafeteria. It also provided a variety of insurance and medical plans at no cost to its employees, including disability insurance and coverage for hospital expenses and doctors' visits.[113] By praising what some employers were doing, this feature many have encouraged other companies to adopt similar plans. Certainly, some of the programs described were advantageous for workers. At the same time, the series created the impression that employers were doing all that they could for workers and that workers should be grateful for the attention that they were receiving, when, in fact, the programs were usually limited and often entailed increased surveillance over workers' lives outside of work.

The league's Division of Industrial Health produced a monthly bulletin called *Industrial Health*, which was sent free of charge to the employee welfare and medical departments of businesses. The Division of Industrial Hygiene within the Department of National Health and Welfare already produced a similar publication – it is unclear why the Health League felt a second publication was necessary.[114] From its inception during the war, the newsletter was a very basic typewritten publication of ten to twelve pages, with a circulation of approximately three thousand. In 1949, it became a twenty-page digest-style periodical, a format that the Health League claimed increased circulation. Just two years later, the league (temporarily) discontinued publication, hoping that employers and/or their employees would subscribe to *Health*. Such new subscriptions apparently did not materialize, as *Industrial Health* resumed publication in the mid-1950s and continued until the mid-1960s, albeit with a fairly small circulation.[115] Compared to *Health* or the poster program, *Industrial Health* included more information about occupational diseases, suggesting that the league felt comfortable addressing workplace hazards only with an audience of employers, management, and/or company doctors. Presumably only the "experts" could be trusted to manage this information, which might lead to anger or distrust among workers.

The league hoped that its industrial division could help increase the circulation of *Health*. In the summer of 1942, it devoted an issue of that magazine to the subject of industrial health. It circulated copies of the periodical to industrial plants in Canada and offered bulk discounts in instances where more than twenty members of a firm subscribed to *Health* or where the employer subscribed to *Health* on their behalf. Bates suggested to potential subscribers that "one article alone might save months of illness and perhaps death in any one of our homes."[116] But the offer apparently had little impact, as subscriptions to *Health* did not noticeably increase.[117]

Employer Membership Schemes
In 1952, the Health League initiated an industrial health membership scheme. The idea was that companies would enrol their employees at the rate of $2 per person. For that fee, each employee would receive *Health* at home, the idea being that the entire family – especially wives/mothers – could read the magazine. In addition, the company would be provided with the now-resurrected *Industrial Health Bulletin*, posters for the bulletin board, and general information on absenteeism.[118] One pamphlet promoting the scheme, *Absenteeism ... Is It Stealing Your Profits?*, promised that the Health League would help control absenteeism by bring knowledge of advances in medicine to workers. Inside were endorsements, including ones from the presidents of Dominion Stores, O'Keefe Brewing, and the Toronto-Dominion Bank. More surprisingly, the president of the Canadian Labour Congress (CLC), Claude Jodoin, also provided an endorsement.[119] Employees received a pamphlet explaining why their company had enrolled them. They were told that "a great deal of sickness never need occur – when we know how to prevent it." Specifically, they were instructed to lose weight, to immunize their children against whooping cough, to drink pasteurized milk, and to get tested for diabetes.[120] As was the case with the posters and

pay envelope inserts discussed earlier in this chapter, these publications assumed that health was the responsibility of the worker, not the employer, and most of the health behaviours being promoted involved the employee's own time and expense.

This was not the first time that the league had attempted to develop a membership scheme out of the Industrial Health Division. In 1947, the division had tried to persuade restaurant owners who were members of the Canadian Restaurant Association to enrol their staff as members of the Health League. Employee members would receive issues of *Health News* (a short-lived bulletin produced by the Health League from 1945 to 1947, which updated members on activities) and a copy of the Department of National Health and Welfare publication *If You Serve Food*. The employer would receive a set of the league's industrial health posters, and the league would offer a course on food handling to employees and management.[121]

Such membership schemes were driven at least partially by financial considerations. Beginning in 1944, the league received funding from the United Welfare Chest, more than doubling its revenue. But, as a member of the Welfare Chest, the league was unable to fundraise independently.[122] The membership plan provided a way of circumventing these restrictions.[123] The Health League had high hopes for its membership plan: an April 1958 brief suggested that the scheme might provide $1 million in income every year.[124] This was not to be. The league was initially able to enrol some large companies, including George Weston Limited (300 employees enrolled), the Robert Simpson Company (100 employees), Canadian Breweries (567 employees), and the Dominion Bank (60 employees). However, for some companies, the number of workers enrolled represented only a fraction of their actual employees.[125] Moreover, growth was slow. In the end, the plan was never a notable success. The league indicated in its annual report for 1953–54 that fifty companies had enrolled in the scheme. By 1956–57, apparently only 2,500 employees from twenty-two companies were enrolled. Subsequent reports indicate that the scheme never expanded beyond these numbers.

The scheme faced some significant criticism. J.G. Cunningham of the Ontario Department of Health feared that companies would purchase the Health League scheme instead of developing a proper industrial health plan that included medical care, which, of course, would be much more expensive. In interviews with a league staffer, most companies indicated that the magazine did not provide enough value to justify their enrolment. Several suggested that they were already supporting the Health League through their donations to the United Community Fund (the latest incarnation of the Welfare Chest).[126] In 1957, the league decided to expand its campaign by selling industrial memberships to service clubs. The league hired Colonel R.J. Williams to give speeches to service clubs to try to induce them to enrol. The hope was that Rotary members would become interested in enrolling their own employees.[127] As with earlier membership drives, this campaign met with little success, as only six service clubs enrolled.[128] The various attempts to raise money through memberships led to significant conflict with staff, three of whom were fired because they failed to make a success of the industrial membership scheme. Ironically, the industrial health membership scheme was hindered by the fact that Health League staff members were poorly paid and often left after only a short period of time in service.

The Foodhandling Division

The Foodhandling Division began in 1946 as part of the Industrial Health Division of the Health League. Its goal was to enrol members of the Canadian Restaurant Association in the league and to promote courses in food safety. The first such course was held for workers at the Chateau Laurier in Ottawa, one of Canada's most prestigious hotels. Similar courses were then offered in the Maritimes, parts of southern Ontario, and Vancouver. The courses involved a combination of films, quizzes, lectures, and posters. They informed workers about how fast bacteria multiplied but reassured them that they could be killed by heat, soap, water, and sunlight. The courses instructed employees to always wash their hands after going to the toilet, to avoid putting their fingers inside clean glasses and cups, to avoid picking up utensils at the eating end, and to stay home when they had a cold. (They said nothing about the loss of income this might entail.) They provided instruction on how to keep food safe, recommended cleaning dishes with chlorine bleach, and urged restaurants to serve only pasteurized milk. While the main focus was on customer safety, the courses warned workers that they too were at risk: "Think of the customers you served to-day. Were they all healthy? You can't tell."[129] The courses, although offered long after the widespread acceptance of germ theory, were part of the hygienic revolution that Nancy Tomes has described as the "Gospel of Germs."[130] League courses encouraged restaurant workers to imagine germs spreading from food handler to utensil to customer. Workers were told that the health of the nation rested in their hands, and that healthy citizenship involved their taking pride in their work.[131] Unlike the industrial health program, which usually focused on the male worker, the food-handling course put significant emphasis on female workers. The lessons reflected the gender norms of the time. Waitresses were told that they should look attractive, with "neat clothes and cheery smile." Instructions highlighted stereotypically female talents for cleanliness and artistry, urging workers to display food attractively and to ensure that their workplaces were scrupulously clean.[132]

The energetic league secretary, H.C. Rhodes, initially ran the Foodhandling Division, but in 1949 he left the league to work for the Canadian Restaurant Association. The league continued to offer classes to the army of food service staff at the Canadian National Exhibition (CNE) every year and offered films and literature on request, but its food-related activities shrivelled after Rhodes left. Even so, the CNE program remained significant. Classes were offered to every food handler at the CNE, attracting somewhere between 800 and 1,500 workers.[133] The CNE had long been an important locale for the league: it had hosted exhibits on the exhibition grounds since the 1920s, and it saw the event as an important showcase for the city and – as befitted the league's Toronto-centrism – the nation.

***

The health messages delivered by the Industrial Health Division and the Foodhandling Division were fairly typical for their time and place: they urged people to avoid germs, to seek out medical care on a regular basis, to eat nutritiously, to exercise, to relax and avoid stress, and to take care of their bodies for the good of the nation. The Health League seems to have sought out workers, not necessarily because they thought that they were in special need of health education (it was just as assiduous in trying to form links with women's groups, churches, and men's service clubs), but because workplaces provided a potential audience. Its message was designed to appeal more to employers than to workers themselves, likely because it knew that employers had the resources to support the league. It was employers, not workers, who would purchase posters and pay-stub inserts and subscribe to *Health*. As a result, the Industrial Health Division celebrated all that employers did for the health of their workers while counselling employees to adopt new health behaviours that would enable them to stay hard at work. The division was apparently oblivious to the ways in which industrial physicians could be used to keep a workforce in line, and it was remarkably silent on the consequences that medical examinations could have on workers deemed to be unfit. It not only trusted that industrial physicians had the best interests of the workers in mind, it also believed that the power of modern medicine and psychology would allow physicians and management to devise fair solutions for any employee who felt unwell. In short, the division envisaged a world remarkably free of class conflict, in which everyone (owners, management, health professionals, and workers) worked together for the benefit of their health and that of the nation. This vision assumed an economy characterized by rising salaries and opportunities, and a society marked more by consensus than conflict. It reflected the elite orientation of the Health League, which paid little attention to workers' voices while devoting considerable space to the voices of physicians, capitalists, and other "experts" in the emerging postwar world.

5

"The Human Factory"
Nutrition, Efficiency, and Longevity

The cover of the January/February 1954 issue of *Health* magazine featured a grinning girl on her toboggan (Figure 12). Below the photograph, a banner promoted National Health Week, which would begin at the end of January. The cover also promised that interested readers could learn why "Too Many Executives Die Young." While *Health* often focused on issues of children's health, it also evinced a strong interest in the health of the middle aged, especially men. Such concerns reflected a recognition that the leading cause of death was changing from infectious diseases to so-called chronic diseases, like cancer, heart disease, and diabetes, and that women were outliving men by ever-larger margins.[1] This particular issue of *Health* had several articles on male health, including one entitled "Memo to Fathers: Why You Can't Sleep" that stressed how difficult a man's business life could be. Other articles focused on nutrition, another long-standing interest of the Health League of Canada, including one on salads, another on nutrition for teens, and a third on food for the elderly. The magazine also always stressed the importance of physical exercise, and one article in this issue instructed parents on how to teach their children to cycle safely.

In the middle decades of the twentieth century, public health workers became interested in how to prolong life and ensure good health over the life course. While the Health League focused much of its effort on infectious disease, its leaders were mindful of the mortality transition that was taking place. They attempted to address this change by stressing the importance

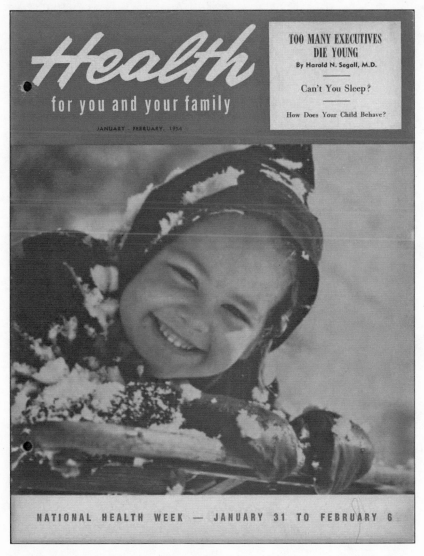

Figure 12 The cover of the January/February 1954 issue of *Health* promoted National Health Week. | LAC, MG 28, I332.

of periodic medical exams (which, they promised, could lead to the early diagnosis and treatment of chronic conditions) and, especially, of good nutrition, which many authorities agreed could help prevent both chronic and infectious disease by enabling children to grow up healthy and strong, while helping their elders lead lives free of heart disease, diabetes, and other

diseases common to old age. The league also advocated exercise and stress
reduction as ways of improving quality of life and longevity. The league's
chronic disease program often compared the body to a machine, one that
would wear out more quickly than necessary without regular inspection and
proper care.[2] At other times, especially in the nutritional material, the body
was compared to a factory, whose many systems required different inputs
to keep them in working order. As was the case in most of its programs,
the league urged people to take personal responsibility for their health by
adopting health habits that would keep them well and on the job and would
thereby help strengthen the Canadian nation. Such programs, especially
the nutrition program, took on special force during the Second World War,
when Canadians worried about the health of enlistees and of workers on the
home front, but they were a key part of the league's activities throughout
its existence. While the Health League did have programs directed towards
workers, as discussed in Chapter 4, its more general health education advice
tended to assume a middle- or upper-middle-class audience who had time
for exercise and leisure and could afford regular visits to the doctor and
dentist. Many of its articles on chronic disease were geared towards the
"executive," whom the league assumed to have special health needs because
of the stressful conditions of his work. Indeed, the "human factory" envisaged by the league was male: *Health* and other league initiatives paid relatively little attention to the health needs of adult and aging women.[3] This,
too, was in keeping with larger trends: North American periodicals in the
1950 and 1960s emphasized how the "organization man's" stressful working
conditions were leading to an epidemic of heart disease.[4] The preoccupation
with men's health reflected the privileging of men over women in society
more generally, but it was also connected to the fact that the gap in life
expectancy for men and women was widening: in the early 1920s, women
could expect to live two years longer than men, but by the early 1960s that
gap had widened to six years.[5]

Periodic Health Examinations

By the late 1920s, the Canadian Social Hygiene Council (CSHC) had established a Committee on Periodic Health Examination, which publicized the
value of such exams.[6] In this advocacy, the CSHC was following contemporary trends: from the second decade of the twentieth century, insurance
companies, public health authorities, and physicians all promoted the value
of annual physical examinations, with the goal of early detection of chronic
diseases such as cancer and of educating patients about how to care for

themselves.[7] The theory behind periodic examinations assumed that a doctor could determine the state of a patient's health through a physical exam and that the examination and counselling process could improve that patient's health. Because the movement underlined the authority and expertise of physicians, it was a perfect fit for the Health League, which wanted Canadians to follow doctors' guidance as one of the duties of health citizenship. In 1930, the CSHC released a pamphlet recommending periodic medical exams, which promised "Your Death Might Be Postponed."[8] The pamphlet explained that many diseases were preventable and that many others once thought to be incurable could be treated. Reflecting the enthusiasm of the preceding decade for radiation treatment, the pamphlet went so far as to claim, "If most types of cancer are treated in the early stages, there is nowadays every chance of effecting a permanent cure."[9] The pamphlet featured a skeleton mounting the stairs outside a comfortable-looking home. It wore a black cape of death bearing the words "communicable diseases," "cancer," "tuberculosis," and "heart disease." At the door, a doctor with "periodic health examination" written on his jacket held up his hand, preventing the skeleton from entering.[10] To promote periodic health exams, the CSHC mounted an exhibit in the summer of 1930 at the Canadian National Exhibition in Toronto and at fall fairs in Leamington, Meaford, Beaverton, St. Catharines, and Niagara Falls, using the slogan "Don't wait until you're sick. Get examined while you're well."[11]

After *Health* began publishing in 1933, it regularly promoted the value of annual exams. In 1936, articles by F.C. Middleton (former president of the Canadian Public Health Association and director of the Division of Communicable Disease of the Department of Health in Saskatchewan) and J.H. MacDermot (the president of the Greater Vancouver Health League and editor of the Vancouver Medical Association *Bulletin*) argued that periodic health exams would boost efficiency, earning power, and national prosperity. MacDermot claimed that annual exams could save 35,000 Canadian lives annually by detecting disease in its early stages.[12] In 1937, the league established a Periodic Health Examination Committee. The committee, which was chaired by Dr. A.J. Mackenzie (a former president of the Toronto Academy of Medicine), had eighteen other members, all physicians, including Gordon Bates.[13] The committee hoped that the promise of annual medical examinations would encourage people to become members of the Health League.

The committee created a standardized form for periodic health examinations and distributed it to doctors. Patients who were league members would go to their own physician, who would undertake the examination and send the completed form to the league. The league would then store the form at its head office and provide a summary of the findings to the patient.[14] The form appears to have been modelled on a sample created by the Canadian Medical Institute, which was a consortium formed by three of the leading insurance companies in Canada.[15] It included sections on patients' demographic information and on the health background of their parents, siblings, spouse, and children. Patients were asked about their dental habits, urination and bowel movements, sleep patterns, and exercise.[16] Once the responses to these questions had been recorded, the physician used the reverse side of the form for the results of the physical examination. Physicians were expected to record height, weight, and temperature, and then log their findings with respect to the patients' eyes, nose, sinuses, ears, mouth, throat, general appearance, glandular system, back and spine, chest, cardiovascular system, hernias, rectal examination, legs and arms, nervous system, blood, and urine. Once this extensive examination had been completed, physicians were asked to summarize any "defects noted" and to record any advice they provided to the patient.[17] An additional form was created for female patients, which recorded their marital status, menstrual and obstetrical history, and pelvic health, and provided for a breast and pelvic examination.[18] Prior to launching its plan, the Health League had it reviewed by the Toronto Academy of Medicine's Committee on Ethics. The committee found nothing unethical about the scheme, but pointed out the great amount of work involved in the exams and expressed the opinion that the fee for the physician was inadequate.[19]

The scheme of tying membership to health exams was motivated in large part by the league's belief in the value of periodical medical examinations in improving health. Yet, it was also designed to raise money for the league. Indeed, this scheme, like the industrial health membership plans discussed in the preceding chapter, illustrates how the need for revenue influenced the league's decision to emphasize certain health issues. While the membership plan cost $10, the Health League paid examining physicians only $5, with an additional $1 for completing a pelvic examination or Wassermann test.[20] Despite the paltry fees, physicians were eager to join the league's roster of doctors who could carry out these examinations, and the organization quickly recruited 400 such physicians within Toronto.[21] The league seems to have had less success recruiting potential patients. There is no clear record of how many signed up as members at the $10 rate and followed through with a health examination. Only four receipts for payment are apparent in the archival record.[22] The Health League's report back to one of these patients showed that she was generally healthy but suggested that she pay attention to her weight and blood pressure, and it encouraged her to be examined again the following year.[23] While a dismal failure as a membership scheme, the league's promotion of periodic health examinations may have played a role in encouraging people to seek out yearly visits to their family physician or to sign up for the increasing number of private insurance programs that were beginning to offer similar services.[24] In any case, the Health League continued to emphasize the value of visiting one's doctor and dentist regularly.[25] In keeping with the league's tendency to regard the body as a machine, at least one article promoting regular dental visits chided Canadians for having their cars checked every 5,000 miles, while their children's mouths went without care.[26]

Nutrition

From the 1930s onwards, the Health League had a strong interest in nutrition: nearly every issue of *Health* had an article about how to eat better. Such content may have been to meet the demands of the readers and appeal to the food advertisers who dominated *Health*. As Valerie Korinek shows for *Chatelaine*, articles about food and health, especially those with recipes, were popular with both readers and advertisers.[27] But such themes also had to do with the growing recognition that nutrition played a vital role in health. Researchers believed that good nutrition would help children grow stronger and be more able to fight disease, would make workers more efficient and less likely to be absent from work, and could stave off many of the degenerative conditions of old age, especially heart disease and diabetes. The Health League began its work at a propitious time for nutrition education: during the 1920s and 1930s, nutritional researchers had isolated many vitamins, greatly complicating nutritionists' view of what constituted a healthful diet. During these years, many nutritionists came to believe that there was an epidemic of "hidden hunger" caused by the inadequate intake of vitamins and minerals. Over the course of the Second World War, interest in nutrition spiked, as many researchers, bureaucrats, and members of the public believed that better nutrition could improve the health of military recruits and reduce the fatigue of those working long hours on the home front.[28] At the same time, the introduction of rationing provoked concern among many housewives as to how they could feed their families healthily under new restrictions.[29] Consequently, a variety of different groups, including the league, launched nutrition classes. As Ian Mosby has shown, learning about nutrition became a way for women to make a patriotic contribution to the war effort.[30] In short, healthy eating, like other health duties, became part of citizenship.

During the war, the league tried to keep a full-time nutritionist on staff, but turnover in the position was high. Near the end of the war, the league hired Margaret E. Smith, who remained in the position for the next decade. The Canadian-born Smith had an MSc in nutrition from the University of Wisconsin and had been an assistant professor of nutrition and biochemistry at the University of Arkansas before becoming the director of the league's Nutrition Division.[31] Throughout her tenure, she wrote articles for *Health*, produced press releases, answered public queries, gave talks, and conducted surveys. When she left in 1955, the league did not replace her, although it continued to publish regularly on the importance of nutrition. In the years after the Second World War, the league, like many other organizations, became less worried about the possibility of mass malnutrition, at least in Canada. Yet, it continued to emphasize the importance of a balanced diet, especially for children, teenagers, the elderly, and workers. It informed Canadians about the strengths and weaknesses of fortified foods like margarine and enriched bread, and warned about the dangers of obesity. By the 1960s, *Health* was drawing on the federal government for its food-related materials, and its focus shifted away from nutrition and towards promoting Canadian food products.

The Health League held that eating properly (although still inexpensively) would prevent illness, create more efficient workers, and build a stronger nation. Its belief that eating should be "scientific" left little room for taste, cultural preferences, or pleasure. In this, the league was not alone, as numerous food scholars have shown.[32] At the end of the nineteenth century, nutritionists began analysing foods according to the various components, including water, protein, fat, carbohydrate, and "ash," and determining their caloric content. They began measuring what subjects ate, and what they produced in waste. They used these measurements to show that cheaper foods could be as valuable nutritionally as more expensive luxury foods. Under Wilbur O. Atwater, Russell Henry Chittenden, and other physiologists, food became something that could be broken down and measured, and nutritionists and domestic scientists stressed the value of teaching people how to eat properly and inexpensively. The science of eating became even more complicated in the interwar years, when the discovery of numerous vitamins led to the realization that healthy eating involved more than just protein, fat, and carbohydrates. It became even more intricate in the postwar years, as experts warned that overeating could shorten life and that excessive fat consumption would lead to heart disease.

The tendency of nutrition professionals to regard the body as a machine that required careful feeding to avoid premature breakdowns and or slowdowns was in keeping with most of the Health League's material. The league's nutritional lectures, which were called "The Human Factory," urged people to think of their bodies not as temples but as "work shops or factories." To work properly, the league explained, the human factory needed fuel in the form of food: the body builders were proteins, the body protectors were vitamins, and the body regulators were water, minerals, and roughage. As time went on, the league's materials would emphasize other issues, like the threat of obesity, but the mechanistic idea that what went in the body would affect how well it worked remained strong. In addition, Health League material drew extensively on the language of home economics, which emphasized Taylorist principles of scientific management to stress that housekeeping could be improved through maximizing efficiency and reducing costs.[33]

The Health League's nutritional efforts reflected what was happening more broadly in Canadian public health. Until the Second World War, nutritional education at the provincial level was usually folded into child and maternal health activities, and it focused primarily on infant feeding.[34] In 1938, the Canadian Council on Nutrition (CCN) was created, on the Department of Pensions and National Health's recommendation. The council included dieticians, nutritionists, home economists, doctors, biochemists, economists, and social workers. Its goal was to consolidate expert knowledge about nutrition and provide guidelines on how Canadians should eat.[35] In 1941, the Department of Pensions and National Health added a Nutritional Services Division, headed by influential CCN member Lionel B. Pett.[36] At the same time, provinces and municipalities began their own nutrition programs, while voluntary groups such as the Red Cross, the Women's Institutes, the National Council of Women, and the Health League also began providing nutrition education. By 1943, there were eighty community nutrition campaigns operating in Canada. These programs, as Ian Mosby has shown in *Food Will Win the War,* drew on a common set of beliefs about the nutritional status and needs of Canadians that was highly influenced by the CCN.[37]

In 1939, the CCN established the Canadian Dietary Standard (CDS). The CDS was adapted from American researcher Hazel Steibeling's set of nutritional recommendations, which defined an ideal diet rather than a simply adequate one, in the process significantly overestimating dietary needs. The CCN pared down Steibeling's caloric suggestions for women but directly appropriated the rest of her recommendations.[38] The extremely generous nutritional criteria enshrined in the CDS practically ensured that most people would fall short.[39] Indeed, when several influential dietary studies sponsored by the CCN in Halifax, Toronto, Edmonton, and Quebec City compared Canadians' actual diets to the nutritional requirements set out in the standard, the findings suggested that Canadians were significantly malnourished. Such surveys helped create concern about "hidden hunger" and subclinical malnutrition.[40]

As Mosby has shown, there were different responses to the discovery of apparently widespread malnutrition among Canadians. Some, like E.W. McHenry, a nutritionist based at the University of Toronto who would head the Health League's Nutrition Committee during the war, believed that the biggest problem was ignorance: Canadian women needed to be educated on what to eat and how to make better use of their food dollar. In contrast, the Toronto Welfare Council, which had planned the initial survey in Toronto, believed that the results of the surveys showed that Canadians lacked sufficient income to pay for the foods they required, and used the survey to call for more generous income supports. The Health League, following McHenry's lead, tended to emphasize the need for better education about nutrition and home economics: thus, its wartime materials provided economical menus and often berated Canadians for eating poorly out of choice rather than necessity.

Initially, the league drew attention to the crisis of malnutrition. For example, in *Health* in 1939, Elizabeth Chant Robertson, a nutritional researcher at the Hospital for Sick Children, wrote that, even though most Canadians would never suffer from a full-blown deficiency disease, "the absence of actual disease is quite a different thing from active energetic health."[41] Other educational material emphasized what could befall Canadians who took in insufficient vitamins. In a series of classes offered by the league in 1943, the instructors explained the symptoms of various subclinical deficiencies. One lecture described "sub-scurvy" as characterized by "tiredness, pains in the limbs and joints, irritability and headache." That lecture concluded that Canadians "are probably getting enough to prevent any specific symptoms of deficiency but not enough to keep them at their best as regards to vitamin C nutrition." Sub-optimal vitamin A intake was blamed for night blindness, poor light adjustment, susceptibility to infection, thin tooth enamel, and skin irritation. As regards vitamin B, "If the diet is low in thiamin," the lecture read, "poor appetite, intestinal disorders including constipation, [and] nervous depression may result."[42]

Much of the league's material promised that the nutritional crisis could be averted through knowledge of nutrition and careful planning. It treated the body as a machine that needed refuelling and maintenance. A 1941 *Health* article on lunches for businessmen began, "Have you a car? Does your company operate trucks? There is no mystery as to the amount of gas and oil needed for motor vehicles in business. Today, there should be

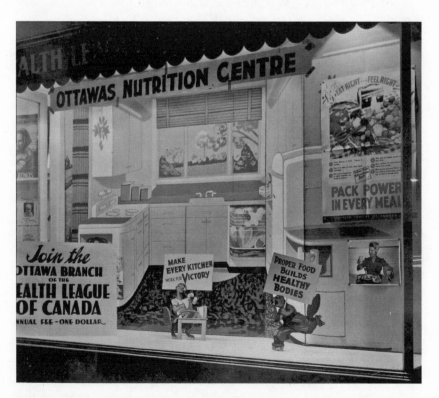

Figure 13 The Health League ran nutrition classes at nutrition centres like the one featured in this display. | LAC, MG 28, I332, vol. 202.

a greater interest in the fuel needed for the body. The foods necessary can be estimated in terms of protein, fat, and carbohydrate, also the important vitamins and minerals."[43] A 1941 pamphlet, *Eat Correctly for Health and Victory*, claimed that in some countries malnutrition was due to food shortages, but in Canada "it comes more often from an unwise choice of foods." It claimed that one could spend a lot of money and be undernourished, while inexpensive foods could provide a highly nutritious diet. It instructed Canadians on what they should be paying for food, according to their income, and encouraged them to eat a broad range of foods, including meat, fish, and eggs, fresh fruit and fresh vegetables, bread and cereals, milk and cheese, and small amounts of sugar and fats. It provided a weekly menu that featured daily porridge for breakfast, a roast beef dinner on Sunday, cold roast beef on Monday, and some extremely minimal suppers (Monday's supper consisted of cold tomato soup and apple sauce).[44] The league also provided a menu with recipes and a shopping list for a typical week.[45] In addition to providing these materials to the public on request, the league used them as material for its very popular nutrition classes in Toronto, which would run from 1939 until at least 1944.[46] The classes were taught by graduates of the household science program at the University Toronto and attracted thousands of students every year.[47] In 1945, the league reached out to other parts of Ontario when Edith Elliot, a federal Department of Agriculture home economist, gave lectures on home canning and preserving to branches in Toronto, Stratford, Simcoe, Weston, Niagara Falls, Welland, Port Colbourne, Port Erie, Midland, Peterborough, and Lindsay. This initiative, the league hoped, would contribute to the war effort as well as encourage thrift.[48]

The league's wartime nutrition program centred on Anglo-Canadian food choices. As in many of its educational campaigns, the league was largely blind to the fact that not all Canadians were of British background, although its suggestion of fish on Fridays suggests that it were prepared to make some concessions to Catholics. The diets recommended by the league were based primarily on Canada's Food Rules, another initiative of the CCN. The Food Rules were introduced in 1942, with minor revisions in 1944 and 1949. In 1961, the title was changed to Canada's Food Guide.[49] The Food Rules, which were based on Steibeling's 1933 optimal nutrition standards, grouped foods into several categories: milk, eggs, whole wheat bread and cereals, vegetables, fruit, and meat or fish.[50] As Mosby has shown, although their creators claimed that the rules reflected Canadian preferences, they drew on foods from a limited cultural repertoire.[51] The rules were practically impossible to follow in the North, and suggestions as to milk consumption would have been extremely difficult for Indigenous people and Asian Canadians, who are often lactose intolerant.[52] Although lists of vitamin recommendations and broader lists of food choices would have been more culturally neutral, the rules were intended for public use, so they focused on foods that were commonly available in Canada.[53] Such an approach was easier for the public to understand, but it implied that only these specific foods were healthy and others were not. The league, basing its educational efforts on the rules, conformed to this process in its menus, shopping lists, and recipes. In *The 1941 Menu Shopping List Recipes for a Week* pamphlet, the most exotic meal suggestion was macaroni with tomato sauce. Although, as Franca Iacovetta has explained, Canadian investigators valued pasta as a thrifty way to extend meat and vegetables, the league's recipe was a travesty of Italian cooking: the sauce was made from salted, tinned tomato soup.[54]

The league also used the rules to promote Canadian agricultural produce, and its material linked Canadian farm goods to food security, patriotism, and good citizenship. The CCN had intentionally based the rules on Canadian goods, aside from citrus, and projected that, if everyone in Canada followed them, farmers' earnings would dramatically increase.[55] At one 1940 lesson, E.W. McHenry instructed listeners to base their diet on milk, eggs, meat, whole grains, fruit, and vegetables. As a newspaper reported, "Dr. McHenry stressed the fact that all these foods are produced in Canada and that concentration upon them would be a help to the country by cutting down the necessity for importation of foods." McHenry, in this case, was referring to the problems of wartime shipping as well as the need to support Canadian farmers.[56] Along similar lines, the league's 1941 pamphlet of menus, shopping lists, and recipes, upon which the year's nutrition classes were based, included an "adequate week's meals, Using Canadian and Empire Goods Only."[57]

In addition to specifying what Canadians should eat, the league's nutrition materials stipulated how they should cook these foods. Like other nutritionists and cookbook writers at the time, the league continually urged Canadians to cook for vitamin preservation.[58] One quite comprehensive guide explained that leafy vegetables should be cooked without a cover, while beets, carrots, corn, parsnips, peas, potatoes, squash, and string beans should be cooked with one. Ideally, vegetables were to be eaten raw. If one insisted on cooking them, they should be baked or steamed rather than boiled. Furthermore, if one did boil vegetables, then the water should be conserved and turned into soup, gravy, or even a beverage. Cooked vegetables, the guide concluded, were to be served immediately: they lost vitamins with every moment they were left to sit.[59] Clearly, homemakers had to follow numerous guidelines if they were to fulfil their duties as health citizens.

The league framed these multitudinous responsibilities of health citizenship as contributions to the war effort. In a 1940 *Health* article, Minster of Pensions and National Health Ian Mackenzie argued that all Canadians needed to be fit for war work or battle, writing, "The field of nutrition ... is above all the one [in] which we, as individuals, can learn the most with the greatest benefit to ourselves. We need health in our armed forces. We need health in the nation – and we can achieve it only by having health in the home."[60] In that vein, the league's Industrial Health Division, which, during the war, worked closely with the federal government's Nutrition Division of the Department of Pensions and National Health, created pamphlets with titles such as *Foods for Health* and *Economical Health Menus for Every Day of the Week* for distribution to industrial workers. The latter included shopping lists, menus, recipes, a lunch box guide, and a vitamin chart.[61] The goal, as in all of the league's industrial programs, was to combat absenteeism.

From Malnutrition to Obesity

By the late 1940s, most nutritionists, McHenry included, began to revise their earlier claims about mass malnutrition. After the war, images of true want and starvation were emerging from Europe; it was abundantly clear that Canadians' playing at malnutrition was offensively privileged.[62] Also, as Ian Mosby argues, McHenry, Pett, and other architects of nutritional guidelines in Canada were no longer convinced that the "optimum standards" that had guided food policy during the war were necessary. In 1945, the CCN advised researchers and nutritionists to disregard the 1942 Canadian Dietary Standard and de-emphasized subclinical malnutrition as a health problem.[63] Even so, the league continued to emphasize that it was possible to be malnourished even if one's caloric intake was sufficient. The head of the league's Nutrition Division, Margaret E. Smith, was particularly concerned that children were getting insufficient vitamin D to prevent rickets, but she also warned that modern foods lacked vitamins and minerals because of modern food-processing methods and soil depletion.[64] Practising what it preached, the National Nutrition Committee of the league frequently concluded its evening meetings in the early 1950s with a snack of whole wheat bread, raw fruit, and tea (the league was a stalwart supporter of whole wheat bread).[65] During this same period, Smith carried out a number of nutritional surveys in schools and found that the diets of Canadian children were woefully inadequate. She complained that the majority of children drank only the minimum amount of milk required, half of them had fruit juices only three times each week instead of daily, many ate no green or yellow vegetables, few ate whole wheat bread, and only a small percentage were getting an adequate amount of vitamin D.[66]

As during the war, the league tended to blame nutritional inadequacies on ignorance or on the refusal of Canadians to eat what they should. One league pamphlet, *The Best Kinds of Meals*, lectured that "malnutrition has been found among the wealthiest people in the richest country in the world – a product of ignorance, indifference and neglect." It provided a number of suggestions for eating nutritiously on a budget: consuming skim milk instead of whole milk, mild cheddar in preference to other types of cheese, small thin-skinned oranges to get better nutritional value for cost, raisins and medium-sized prunes over other types of dried fruits, cheap lean meats, and rolled oats rather than more heavily processed cereals.[67] While this material suggested that there was little excuse for poor nutrition, even if one's income was low, the league also condemned the rising cost of food in its yearly food budgets in *Health*. Even here, though, the individual came in for scolding, as Smith critiqued Canadians for continuing to consume tea and coffee despite their high cost, an antagonistic approach that implied that the poor did not deserve even small pleasures.[68] At the same time, Smith believed that modern food-processing and agriculture techniques were contributing to the problem of inadequate nutrition, indicating that consumer ignorance was not entirely to blame.[69]

The league continued to heavily emphasize the Food Rules. During National Health Week (to be discussed in Chapter 6), it routinely distributed paper placemats printed with the Food Rules (and later the Canada Food Guide). In 1961, it sent out 180,000 placemats to restaurants throughout British Columbia, Alberta, Saskatchewan, Ontario, New Brunswick, and Nova Scotia; in 1963, it distributed 350,000.[70] After the Food Rules became Canada's Food Guide in 1961, the league worked both to publicize the new name and to show that, in essentials, the rules remained unchanged. *Health* explained that the word "rules" was thought too inflexible. The diet recommended by the new Food Guide was almost exactly the same as that under the Food Rules; it included substantial amounts of milk, fruit juice, vegetables (including one serving of potatoes), breads and cereals, meat, and fish, as well as recommendations for vitamin D.[71]

At the same time as it was promoting these nutritional guidelines, the league began to emphasize the dangers posed by obesity. As several scholars have noted, thinness was held up as an ideal from the beginning of the twentieth century, and this trend intensified as the century continued. And, as new research demonstrated the links between overweight and the risk of early death, both men and women were told that they needed to be slim for the sake of their health, and not just because it was considered to be more attractive.[72] In 1948, *Health* published an article by McHenry that lauded the Canadian food supply but complained "that many Canadians use too much food, or too many food constituents." He argued that Canadians needed to be "as much concerned with the excessive use of food as with deficiencies, even though the consideration of deficiencies is more fashionable these days." He pointed out that people who were overweight put a strain on their organs and had lower life expectancies.[73] An article two years later warned that, for children, being overweight was probably more dangerous than being underweight. It emphasized that overweight adults had often been overweight children and that just twenty-five pounds of excess weight at forty-five years of age decreased life expectancy by 25 percent. The author stated that, while many parents claimed that their obese child hardly ate anything, "this is very unlikely." This unwillingness to believe obese patients and their parents suggested a lack of sympathy for those who found it difficult to control their eating.[74] Margaret Smith warned her readers that "overweight is dangerous, particularly for people over 40 years of age, and it is generally brought about by eating too much." She said that very few people who were overweight suffered from glandular disorders; they just ate too much. She told them that they would need to cut down on fats and sugars while eating nutrient-rich foods, noting that obesity led to hardening of the arteries, heart attacks, and gallstone attacks.[75] Another article on obesity, entitled "NO! – It May Be Fattening," featured an obese man being fed tea and pastries by two attractive young women (Figure 14), suggesting that being fat was not only unhealthy, it could also make a person a laughing stock. It exclaimed that 2 million overweight Canadians "will have more illness and die earlier than the rest of the population!

To consider yourself big-boned, pleasingly plump, stylishly stout, chubby, well-rounded or just of heavier build is pure fancy. If you are 10 per cent heavier than your ideal weight you are obese!"[76] The title of an article by Louis Dublin, the influential statistician at Metropolitan Life Insurance, promised that "Reducing May Save Your Life." He warned that the company's insured clients who were overweight were 50 percent more likely to die than clients who were not overweight. They died of cardiovascular and renal diseases, diabetes, and gall-bladder disease. A separate study showed that those who lost weight significantly reduced their risk of dying.[77] This emphasis on the dangers of obesity shows that the league,

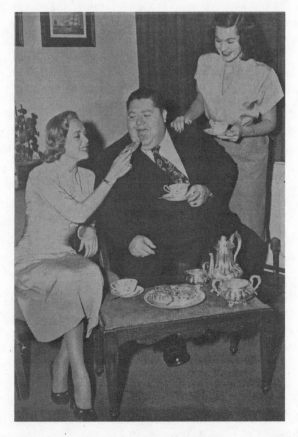

Figure 14 Photograph accompanying an article entitled "NO! – It May Be Fattening." | *Health*, March/April 1953, 8. LAC, MG 28, I332, vol. 181.

like the medical profession more generally, was gradually thinking more about problems of chronic disease.

The Nutrition Division withered after Smith left in 1955; it no longer conducted surveys or held public talks. But the league continued to commission articles on nutrition for *Health*, often from people with a close relationship with the league, including McHenry, Pett, and Chant Robertson. It also ran a series of articles by Corinne Trerice, who was the director of nutrition at the Bakery Foods Foundation of Canada. Not surprisingly, most of these focused on recipes for bread or cookies, indicating that the league, like most Canadians at the time, still had a significant sweet tooth despite its rhetoric around the need to cut back on sugar consumption.[78] Indeed, *Health* accepted advertisements for Coca-Cola, Orange Crush, and Crown Brand Corn Syrup. In 1959, the Health League was able to hire another nutritionist, Catherine Mahoney, although her tenure was short, as the league decided that her salary was too expensive to justify the cost of keeping her. After she was hired, *Health* introduced a new series entitled "Foods for Health." It covered topics such as preparing salads, holiday meals, and food safety. It continually referred to the Food Rules/Canada Food Guide and usually included at least one recipe.[79] Like the rules, the "Foods for Health" segment promoted the nutritional values of specific foods but took the extra step of linking good nutrition to proper cooking. The series usually focused on Canadian produce, since those goods were prominent in the Food Rules. After Mahoney left, the series continued to appear, but without a byline.[80] It drew recipes from the Department of Agriculture's Consumer Section and the Department of Fisheries, and it seems likely that the copy was also drawn from these same sources.[81] These articles praised Canadian goods, including cheddar cheese, milk, cream, peaches, tomatoes, apples, strawberries, and pork (fresh and cured). They explained Department of Agriculture grades when they existed for the specific food, and how to buy for quality when they did not.[82] The Department of Fisheries provided similar information on fish salads and cooking canned and frozen fish and explained Canada's frozen fish grades.[83] Sometimes the articles veered away from the strictly healthy to discuss goods like ice cream. One instalment noted that ice cream was "a delicious dessert and between-meal treat," adding that "the important nutrients of cream and milk are retained in its manufacture." Consumer Section recipes for strawberry, honey nut, and apple butterscotch sundae sauces followed this copy.[84] Another article, "Maple: Canada's Unique Sweet," included recipes for maple syrup pie and maple chiffon pie.[85] Some of the articles abandoned healthy nutrition almost entirely, suggesting that *Health* had become a vehicle for Department of Agriculture initiatives.

Indeed, in 1963, 1965, and 1966 *Health* included "food forecasts" that explicitly discussed agricultural yields and urged Canadians to eat foods that were in surplus. A 1963 issue began by stating that it "should be no problem at all to eat well in Canada in 1963 for we are fortunate in having an abundant supply of all the foods necessary for good nutrition and good health produced right here in our own country." The article then instructed Canadians to drink more fluid milk, as production had increased but consumption was decreasing. It suggested that if Canadians all drank the amount of milk recommended in the Food Guide, "there would be no surplus of milk in Canada." It also noted that canned pears would be particularly plentiful that year, and that Canada's Food Guide recommended two servings of fruit each day.[86] The next page recommended that Canadians use poultry as well as beef to fulfil their protein needs, as beef would be expensive for the rest of the year. Similarly, a "bumper crop of tomatoes last fall" meant that canned tomato products were plentiful. It further noted that tinned tomatoes "are a relatively inexpensive way to get colour, flavour and Vitamin C (ascorbic acid) into our meals." Should readers want more information about food grades, the author directed them to send away for the Department of Agriculture's "handy, purse-sized booklet 'Buy by Grade.'"[87] The food forecasts for 1965 and 1966 paid even less attention to nutrition and more to getting Canadians to eat Canadian produce, especially items deemed to be in surplus.[88] Culinary citizenship was not just a matter of optimum nutrition for energy, efficiency, and longevity, but it also involved doing the best for the Canadian economy.

Exercise and Leisure

From its beginnings, the Health League had stressed the value of exercise. As the Canadian Social Hygiene Council, it had encouraged young men and especially young women to exercise to help build their bodies for parenthood, thus ensuring the health of future generations. *Health* drew attention to the link between heart disease and inadequate exercise as early as the 1930s. The magazine encouraged people to be active, although it cautioned that too-vigorous exercise for those over forty could be dangerous (in this case, too vigorous meant playing singles games of tennis and badminton).[89] *Health* also ran numerous articles on the value of physical education in schools, stressing that it was just as important to have a healthy body as a healthy mind and that, indeed, the two things often went together. One author, A.S. Lambe, the director of the Department of Health and Physical Recreation at McGill University, promised that physical education would correct "remediable defects" and promote "the harmonious development and functioning of the body."[90] In the late 1930s, the magazine lauded what other countries, including the USSR, were doing to promote physical fitness and warned that Canadians were falling behind.[91] Surprisingly, given the attention that it paid to the issue in the pages of *Health,* the league never established a committee devoted to physical fitness. Perhaps it felt that the field was already too crowded or that the issue was not "medical" enough.

Health's attention to exercise intensified in the early 1960s, after the Diefenbaker government decided to devote more attention to amateur sport and fitness. In 1961, Bates editorialized that a healthy nation "must be composed of citizens who are physically fit and healthy."[92] From 1961 to 1963, *Health* devoted its May/June issue to physical fitness. These articles stopped warning about the danger of over-exercise, emphasizing instead that people's capacity for vigorous exercise differed and that it was wise to consult a physician before undertaking a new exercise program. During these years, the league also commissioned several articles by Dr. Paul Dudley White, the cardiologist who gained international fame as Dwight Eisenhower's physician after the American president had suffered a heart attack while in office.[93] White believed that heart attacks could be prevented through regular exercise and improved nutrition. He advised that it was wise to consult a physician before beginning any exercise program, but he strongly recommended that middle-aged Canadians exercise more. He promised that toning the large muscles would help the heart maintain good circulation, that physical activity would reduce tension, and that exercise could help combat excess weight (a significant risk factor for heart disease) and slow up the process of "arterial rusting" (atherosclerosis).[94] In another article, White advised readers that exercise could keep the heart healthy, benefit digestion and prevent obesity, help the psyche, improve the lungs, and serve as an antidote for "nervous tension and strains."[95] In the late 1960s and early 1970s, frequent contributions by Rex Wilson, the medical director of the BF Goodrich Company, underlined the links between exercise and cardiovascular health.[96]

Throughout *Health's* existence, the magazine ran articles promoting particular sports, with titles such as "Canoeing for Health and Pleasure," "Gymnastics for Health," and "Learn How to Swim."[97] Covers of the magazine often depicted people engaged in outdoor sports, including skiing (at least twelve covers of the magazine were devoted to this pursuit), canoeing, and fishing. In articles, the sports most commonly referenced were skiing, swimming, tennis, and golf – not coincidentally, the sports most often played by middle- or upper-class Canadians, who could afford skiing trips and country club fees. As Catherine Gidney has pointed out, swimming, golf, and tennis were all promoted by university-based physical education programs in this period.[98] A focus on these activities reflected the magazine's class bias, although, to be fair, *Health* also promoted calisthenics, rhythmic gymnastics, and walking, all activities that could be undertaken in the home or the local neighbourhood.[99] Compared to today, when we are bombarded with very specific instructions about how much exercise we should do, and what our heart rate should be while doing it, *Health*'s instructions around exercise were vague. While its writers believed that a healthy body could prevent illness, they were not terribly specific (with the exception of heart disease) about the mechanisms by which this would happen. *Health* urged its readers to think of the body as an automobile, but in the case of exercise, the instruction manuals provided by the magazine lacked detailed instructions. Moreover, the magazine valued exercise as much for its effect on the mind and the emotions as for its specific disease-fighting properties.

A survey of photographs and illustrations in the magazine reveals that the bodies portrayed by *Health* were usually young and toned and were always white. There were no pot bellies, but neither were there voluptuous, skinny, or overly muscular bodies. They were "regular" bodies, clearly in line with the often-used Metropolitan Life height and weight tables. Women were frequently featured with babies or toddlers. Children were involved in outdoor sports or nature activities, or were shown at school or, occasionally, reading or playing the piano. Younger women frequently appeared on the cover of the magazine, often doing calisthenics, swimming, or skating. Men were often engaged in outdoors activities: camping, fishing, family picnics. Such images reveal the legacy of social hygiene, with its emphasis on building a healthy race. As historian Dorothy Porter notes, ideals about the healthy body were rooted in "eugenically inspired pre–Second World War movements"; the images in *Health* show that these ideals persisted long after the end of the war.[100]

In addition to advocating exercise, the league promoted the idea that taking regular holidays and having hobbies was an important aspect of good health. Summer issues of *Health* were often devoted to holiday health. Not surprisingly, the articles assumed that people would have the funds to send their children to camp, to spend time at a cottage or a "holiday" resort, or to travel across the country by automobile.[101] In addition to summer holidays, the league encouraged Canadians to incorporate leisure pursuits into their daily life. Articles recommended hobbies like reading, travelling, painting, gardening, and bookbinding, among other activities.[102] The league believed that meaningful recreation would improve mental as well as physical health.[103] Enjoyable and productive leisure activities were important, it argued, not just because they provided relaxation in the present but also because they would give people something to do in their later years, helping to alleviate the boredom, loneliness, and feelings of uselessness that could arise in old age.[104]

Executive Health

Throughout the 1950s, *Health* carried a number of articles on the health of executives. These focused on topics such as heart disease, nervous breakdowns, and digestive complaints, characterized as the suffering of men who, though they did not do physical labour, were contributing their all to the betterment of their companies. Portraying executives as overburdened cast them as selfless health-citizens, sacrificing their own well-being for the betterment of their families and industries. These articles reminded executives to take care of their own health and promoted measures such as periodic health examinations.[105] Such attention to executive health, the league argued, benefited both the individual and the company. According to the subtitle of one such article, "modern preventive methods protect [the] health of executive[s] and prevent industry's loss."[106] Dr. Harold Segall, who was, fittingly, involved with both the National Heart Foundation and the Canadian National Railway Company, advocated in *Health* for the periodic health examination as the best avenue to protect both the physical and mental health of the nation's executives.[107] Even the educated executive needed the guidance of his physician if he was to live a long, healthy, and productive life. Furthermore, he needed to protect his health and stay fit in both body and mind by monitoring his diet, exercising, and getting adequate sleep.[108] The message was clear: despite the demands of his job, the executive had the responsibility to remain in good health so as to continue his contributions to industry. Only by following the advice of *Health*'s physicians, undergoing periodic health examinations, keeping his weight down, exercising appropriately, and adopting healthy hobbies would he be fulfilling the obligations of health citizenship.[109]

By contrast, the executive's wife – the presumed reader – received little attention in *Health*. While women were urged to pay careful attention to the health of their husbands and children, the magazine offered little information about women's health, especially for the middle-aged women who were the most likely readers of the magazine. For example, *Health* seems to have run only two articles on menopause in almost fifty years of publication. Perhaps this was because the trend of women living longer than men was already well-established by this point, so there seemed to be less need to educate women on how to increase their lifespan. It probably also had to do with the fact that women, at least once their children left home, were not generally seen to be productive members of society, and therefore women's health was less important.

***

By the time the Health League came into existence, it was clear that the rate of death from infectious disease was declining, while the number of people dying from diseases of old age (such as cancer and heart disease) was increasing. As we have seen in earlier chapters and will show again in Chapter 6, the league continued to devote much effort to combatting infectious diseases. That said, as this chapter shows, it also attempted to address chronic disease. It did so through its nutritional program, its support for periodic medical examinations, and its general health education program, which urged people to eat well, get enough rest, exercise moderately, and adopt hobbies as ways of increasing longevity and improving the quality of life. The league was very concerned about healthy aging, which was consistent with its respect for the contribution that older people could make to society. Consequently, the league provided considerable advice on how to live healthily and happily into old age. With the exception of some of the nutritional materials, the league's advice tended to be blind to the constraints of poverty. It never addressed how people could follow the league's expensive advice to take summer holidays, adopt hobbies, or take up sporting activities like tennis and skiing. The focus on the middle and upper classes likely reflected the actual readership of *Health*, but it was also indicative of the Health League's chronic inattention to the inequalities of class, ethnicity, and race in Canadian society.

6

Fighting Apathy and Ignorance
National Campaigns

In the late 1940s and early 1950s, a Health League advertisement showed a mother holding a pair of baby shoes to her face, with the caption "He Was Just Beginning to Walk."[1] A banner blared "Whooping Cough! Diphtheria! Smallpox!" Accompanying text warned parents that whooping cough and diphtheria could prove fatal, especially for children under the age of five, and urged them to have their children vaccinated. The advertisement's message – that parents (and more specifically mothers) who failed to have their children vaccinated were endangering their lives – was typical of the league's guilt-inducing approach to public health education.

In the postwar years, the Health League bombarded Canadians with messages about how to keep themselves healthy: they were to immunize their children, visit their doctor and dentist regularly, eat according to Canada's Food Rules, support water fluoridation, drink pasteurized milk, and protect themselves against chronic disease. Two of the league's most successful projects were National Immunization Week (1943–71) and National Health Week (1944–80). Both campaigns started during the heady wartime years, when the Health League was undergoing a rapid expansion. In the first quarter decade that followed the war, most Canadians were probably aware of these national campaigns: schoolchildren received information in the classroom; newspapers, radio, and television covered the events; pharmacies put up posters and streamers; and service clubs hosted speakers and events. The two initiatives reflected the league's national aspirations, its skill at garnering publicity, and its ability to work with a wide range of organizations, including public health agencies, schools, churches, service clubs, unions, and businesses. While the two events had slightly different goals, both used a combination of information, criticism, and guilt to induce Canadians to meet their health responsibilities, as defined by the league. Surprisingly, given extensive immigration to Canada during these years, and the long history of public health agencies regarding immigrants as a source of contagion, these initiatives made relatively little effort to reach out to "New Canadians." Instead, the message focused on a Canadian nation that was presumed to be white and Christian.

National Immunization Week built on Toxoid Week, which the league had run in conjunction with Toronto's Department of Public Health. As shown in Chapter 2, the use of diphtheria toxoid had dramatically reduced the rates of disease and death caused by diphtheria in Toronto, and the league wished to spread this success across the country.[2] By the time it launched National Immunization Week, new vaccines were making promising inroads against many childhood diseases. The new name reflected an expansion beyond diphtheria, and its preventive toxoid, to a broader range of diseases for which vaccines (not necessarily toxoids) had been developed.[3] A vaccine against whooping cough (pertussis) had been introduced in Canada in 1936–37, and by 1943 it was available in combination with diphtheria toxoid. In 1947, tetanus toxoid was added, and the DPT (diphtheria, pertussis, and tetanus) vaccine became the agent of choice in most provinces.[4] At first, Immunization Week emphasized protecting children against smallpox, diphtheria, and whooping cough. In some provinces, the week also targeted scarlet fever; however, because it was unclear if the scarlet fever vaccine was effective and the vaccine required many doses, Immunization Week campaigns did not always include it as a focus.[5] (Scarlet fever came to be effectively treated with penicillin and eventually the vaccine was abandoned.)[6] After the Salk vaccine became available in 1955, polio was added to the list.

National Immunization Week

National Immunization Week reflected the league's long-held interest in child and maternal health. This, of course, was not just the league's focus – until the 1970s, most health agencies and government health departments emphasized child and maternal health. In the early years of the twentieth century, few families were untouched by serious childhood diseases. Communicable diseases killed at least one in six children under the age of fourteen, and rates of infection were even greater.[7] During the interwar years, childhood mortality dropped significantly. While progress in combatting childhood illness slowed in the years after the Second World War, death rates for children continued to decrease in the 1940s and through the 1960s. Sulpha drugs and penicillin played a role in decreasing the mortality of children, but so did rising immunization rates. When the Health League began National Immunization Week, it was clear that many children were still not immunized. For example, in Montreal in 1943, only 55 percent of children aged four and under had been immunized against diphtheria.[8] Over the years that National Immunization Week operated, immunization became increasingly widespread, and death and morbidity rates from infectious diseases such as whooping cough, diphtheria, and polio underwent a remarkable decline (see Figure 15). Of course, this trend was not entirely, or even mostly, due to National Immunization Week. During these years, provinces across Canada operated extensive immunization programs, which likely played a far more important role both in publicizing the availability of immunizations and getting children immunized. Even so, National Immunization Week helped to remind parents of the importance of immunization.

Immunization undoubtedly reduced childhood deaths and suffering, but it also had unintended effects. Mona Gleason has pointed out that the

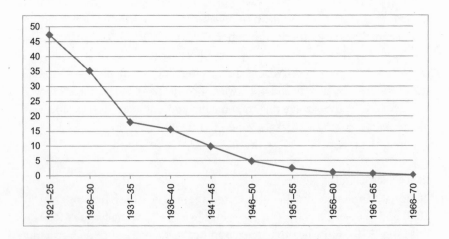

Figure 15 Death rates from communicable disease (including diphtheria, whooping cough, measles, scarlet fever, and typhoid fever) in Canada, 1921–70
Source: Death Rates from Communicable Disease (All Ages, per 100 000 population) (Historical Statistics of Canada http://www.statcan.gc.ca/pub/11-516-x/sectionb/4147437-eng.htm).

focus on childhood health in the first four decades of the twentieth century encouraged parents to think of children's bodies in new ways. She argues that the idea of children's bodies as inherently vulnerable was replaced by the idea that children were under threat from a variety of outside conditions and diseases.[9] Such a perspective may have slowly fed into the idea that children needed to be protected from all threats, and helped create the cosseted childhood that many observers have critiqued in the late twentieth and early twenty-first centuries.

National Immunization Week was organized by the Health League's National Immunization Committee, chaired first by Dr. Nelles Silverthorne (1944–49) of the Hospital for Sick Children and later by Dr. F.O. Wishart (1950–66) of the School of Hygiene at the University of Toronto.[10] Silverthorne, one of the most important specialists in infectious disease in Canada, had helped to develop the whooping cough vaccine in the 1930s and researched polio vaccines in the 1940s and 1950s.[11] Wishart was also a researcher, who published on the diphtheria toxoid and the tetanus vaccine. Both men were actively involved in the organization of National Immunization Week, with the support of other committee members (primarily male Toronto-based physicians) and the Health League's paid staff. The fact that such well-known and respected physicians led National Immunization Week helped to ensure its success. Moreover, it testifies to the success of the Health League in building relationships with important medical allies in the period during and after the Second World War.

National Immunization Week had high-level support from other quarters as well. From the beginning, it received yearly endorsements from the governor general, the minister of national health and welfare, and the Canadian Medical Association.[12] During the event's first decade, the Health League cooperated with the National Film Board to show pro-immunization shorts before movies in commercial theatres.[13] In the first of these, the minister of pensions and national health, Ian Mackenzie, emphasized that government departments were doing all that they could to develop vaccines and eradicate disease by funding scientists and clinics, and that it was the duty of Canadians to take the available measures to protect themselves and their families.[14]

When the league first established National Immunization Week, it sought the support and assistance of provincial ministers of health. Generally, the ministers' responses were positive – they found the publicity useful. However, some criticized the event for competing for advertising space with other campaigns, including a Victory Loan campaign during

the war. Others objected to the autumn timing of the week: some officials claimed that parents more commonly vaccinated their children in
the summer months, while the health officer in Prince Edward Island complained that the campaign coincided with potato-picking season, during
which time the province's schools were closed.[15] British Columbia believed
that National Immunization Week made little difference because the province was carrying out immunization activities continuously throughout
the year.[16]

The level of support for the initiative varied across the provinces, based
in part on individual ministers' engagement with the campaign and on the
alignment between the Health League's promotional materials and the vaccines available in each province. However, most ministers of health expressed
their support, approved of the Health League's literature, and assisted in
distributing league materials to physicians and through schools.[17] Saskatchewan's director of health education, Christian Smith, who had previously
directed the Health League's Social Hygiene Division, was particularly
enthusiastic in supporting the league's work and providing opinions on its
initiatives. As a result, campaigns such as National Immunization Week
appear to have been implemented more extensively in Saskatchewan than
in other provinces, with the exception of Ontario and Quebec, where the
Health League was most securely established. Of course, Saskatchewan had
long been a leader in public health and the provision of medical services, so
it is not surprising that it provided active support to Health League campaigns.[18] By the end of the 1950s, the provinces' interest in National Immunization Week had waned. By then, most children were immunized, and the
provinces came to feel that the program had served its purpose and that
other public health issues had greater priority.[19]

As the organization's first national campaign, National Immunization
Week allowed the Health League to establish mechanisms for national
publicity campaigns. With the support of the Health League's Publicity and
Promotion Division, the National Immunization Week Committee made
extensive use of the media to reach as many Canadians as possible, particularly those interacting most frequently with young children. In this, they
were in keeping with major trends in public health: in both Great Britain and the United States, public health organizations were taking advantage of advertising and the mass media to promote immunization.[20] The
Health League placed articles on vaccination in national magazines and
journals, and encouraged newspapers across the country to run sponsored

advertisements. For example, in 1943, *Chatelaine* and the *Canadian Home Journal* both ran articles on immunization, while *Maclean's, Liberty,* and the *Canadian Public Health Journal* all ran editorials endorsing the work.[21] National Immunization Week editorials and advertisements often appeared in women's magazines or in the women's sections of newspapers, highlighting the particular responsibility of mothers to ensure that their children were vaccinated. The league also circulated spot announcements to radio stations (and later television networks), which ran them for free as part of their public service time. These concise announcements reminded Canadians that it was National Immunization Week and that children were still dying unnecessarily from diseases such as diphtheria and whooping cough.[22] In addition to these mass media sources, the league promoted Immunization Week on billboards, in window displays, on streetcars, on family allowance cheques, in doctors' offices and laboratories, and through life insurance companies. It broadcast its message through short films and radio plays and numerous press releases. It created catchy slogans to promote its work, such as the concise call to "Be Wise – Immunize!"[23] Each year, the National Immunization Week Committee repeated the publicity efforts of past campaigns while seeking to expand its promotional reach. All in all, National Immunization Week was likely successful in reaching many Canadian families.

During the first National Immunization Week in 1943, the league built on wartime anxieties, including fear of epidemics – a significant concern for those who remembered the Spanish flu pandemic that had followed the First World War.[24] A poster (also reproduced as the cover of a pamphlet) titled "War Brings Epidemics" featured a young boy sitting peacefully in a field of flowers while soldiers and storm clouds gathered in the distance (Figure 16).[25] The pamphlet raised fear that soldiers returning home would bring new diseases to North America, which would then spread among the civilian population, and it underlined the vulnerability of children. In a news bulletin, the Health League also made use of war rhetoric to justify the need for an immunization campaign: "Casualties from preventable diseases in Canada since the beginning of the war have far outnumbered the casualties among the country's armed forces."[26] This bulletin provides another example of the tendency of the Health League to exaggerate the extent of the problems it was addressing: although Canadian children were dying of preventable diseases, these numbers were far smaller than the number of men and women who were dying overseas.

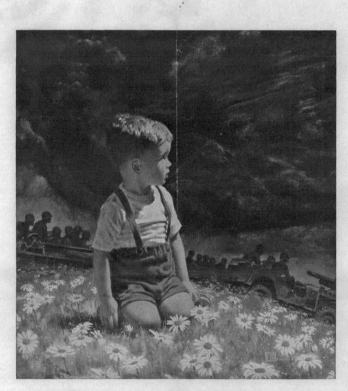

Figure 16 "War Brings Epidemics" | LAC, MG28, I332, vol. 94, file 4.

Another common theme was the notion that diseases were invisible threats to children's health that parents should fear. This approach was most evident in a 1950s advertisement picturing an alert infant nestled under a blanket, with the banner asking the question "Safe and Snug?" (Figure 17). The text responded, "Well, snug maybe ... But not safe. A warm blanket in a cozy home will keep out the cold and the wet ... But disease can enter the coziest home and pass through the warmest blanket ... If your child has not been immunized, he is an easy mark for diseases that lurk just around

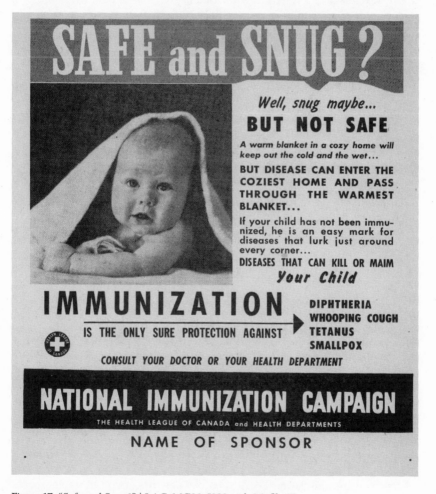

Figure 17 "Safe and Snug?" | LAC, MG28, I332, vol. 96, file 17.

every corner."[27] As conscientious parents and health citizens, mothers and fathers had the responsibility to adequately protect their children. If they failed in this regard and their children became sick, the league did not hesitate to exploit parental guilt, reminding them that their child could have avoided the illness if they had taken the proper measures. For example, a National Immunization Week advertisement that first appeared in 1945 portrayed worried parents leaning over a child's crib as a doctor stood in the doorway. The text read, "'Yes ... You have a *very* sick baby' – And that baby should have been protected by immunization" (Figure 18).[28] Visually, the Health League's advertisements often depicted both parents, suggesting that the duty for immunization and blame for illness was shared. However, the league's general approach to family dynamics reflected the contemporary social consensus that the primary responsibility for childcare lay with mothers. As a result, it was they who were most to blame if a child were ill. These advertisements also communicated to parents that appropriate child-rearing involved the expert advice of physicians. At times, the league conveyed this message in a fairly positive way, as in the advertisement "Partners – your Doctor and your family," which portrays a mother, a child, and a physician: the child smiles at the doctor, who is about to vaccinate him, while the mother offers her support. But others, including "You have a *very* sick baby," suggested that parents who did not follow expert medical advice were inadequate and irresponsible.

Together, the messages contained in National Immunization Week advertisements taught parents about the most fundamental roles of the Health League's ideal health citizen: they must listen to, accept, and act on the advice of experts, including those associated with public health organizations, to ensure their own well-being and that of their families. Certainly, parents and the Health League had valid reasons to be concerned with immunization. Rates of childhood disease and mortality were higher than they needed to be. Some of the vaccines had only just emerged on the market, and education was required to let people know what was available and when children needed to be vaccinated.[29] In such a context, the Health League was justified in its convictions about the need to promote immunization. Even so, their materials demonstrated that there was a hierarchy to health citizenship – parents needed to listen to the advice of doctors and perform appropriately.

National Immunization Week was relatively pragmatic in its approach. The league allowed provinces a great deal of autonomy in implementing the campaign. It made changes to promotional material at the provinces'

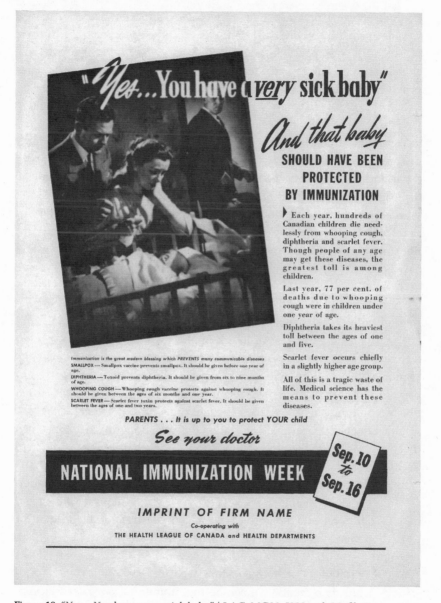

Figure 18 "Yes ... You have a *very* sick baby" | LAC, MG28, I332, vol. 94, file 9.

request, such as altering the list of diseases to be featured, based on the opinions of ministers of health and the feasibility of administering particular vaccines.[30] The provinces also disagreed about vaccine schedules, and the Health League was willing to work around these differences.[31] Another example of league pragmatism involved the BCG (bacilli Calmette-Guérin) vaccine against tuberculosis. Despite the vaccine's widespread use in parts of Europe, it was not widely adopted in Canada, except for high-risk individuals such as nurses and medical students. Few contemporary studies convincingly established the efficacy of the vaccine, and concerns regarding its safety and utility were raised in the international medical community.[32] Despite these findings, the league advocated for the vaccine in *Health*.[33] Yet, its communication with the provinces revealed that only Newfoundland was undertaking a widespread BCG vaccination program.[34] Likely in response to the scientific uncertainty and the limited use of the BCG vaccine in Canada, the league never included tuberculosis in its National Immunization Week promotional material. This flexibility likely improved the initiative's success, as the provinces frequently ordered pamphlets, posters, and other promotional material from the league by the thousands – something they would have been unlikely to do had the materials been inconsistent with provincial preferences.

Nevertheless, behind the scenes, observers expressed concern that the Immunization Week materials were too Toronto-centric. In 1952, J.S. Robertson, the deputy minister of health in Nova Scotia, penned a sharp letter complaining that the Health League's materials suggested beginning immunization at six to nine months of age, when many provinces recommended that they begin at three to four months of age. He complained that this was an example of "so-called Toronto thinking." He grumbled that the Health League was not really a "national association" and recommended that branches be established in Nova Scotia. The league eventually agreed to alter the wording around the commencement of vaccination.[35]

Interestingly, the Health League did not lobby for compulsory immunization. This stood in significant contrast to its campaign for compulsory pasteurization and its support for mandated water fluoridation and for legislation mandating premarital blood-testing. But it was in keeping with the approach of other public health agencies and doctors at the time.[36] In a 1964 policy statement on immunization, the Canadian Public Health Association included no mention of compulsory immunization.[37] In Ontario, it was mandatory for children to have a smallpox vaccination before attending school, but this legislation dated back to 1914. It was not until 1982 that Ontario and New Brunswick passed laws requiring schoolchildren to be vaccinated; even then, there were exemptions if parents objected on the grounds of "conscience or religious belief."[38] This emphasis on mandatory immunization paralleled what happened in the United States, where mandatory immunization programs gathered strength in the 1970s.[39] The fact that the Health League chose to promote immunization rather than urging provinces to pass laws mandating it undoubtedly contributed to the success of National Immunization Week. There is a long history of resistance to vaccination in Canada, as historians such as Katherine Arnup and Paul Bator have shown, although their work does not focus on the middle decades of the twentieth century.[40] Yet, the Health League's files reveal few instances of resistance, and those primarily by people who were concerned about the impact of vaccine production on animal welfare or who believed that vaccination was driven by pharmaceutical companies seeking profits.[41] Indeed, as Denyse Baillargeon showed in *Babies for the Nation*, most mothers believed that vaccination contributed to the significant decline in infant mortality and were eager to have their children vaccinated.[42]

National Immunization Week was, in many ways, a crucial initiative for the Health League. As its first national campaign, it allowed the league to expand and solidify its relationships with the media and provincial governments, which would facilitate the promotion of future campaigns such as National Health Week. In both practical and symbolic ways, National Immunization Week revealed the Health League's belief in the importance of protecting children and ensuring their health as the future of the nation. In this respect, it was a natural extension of the social hygiene principles that had animated the organization from the beginning. Also, through this work, the Health League reinforced the notion that if Canadian parents would adhere to the health behaviours advocated by the league, both they and their children could prevent illness. The league's expectation that good citizens would accept the guidance of voluntary health organizations, schools, churches, and other social institutions is also revealed in its second national campaign, National Health Week.

National Health Week

National Health Week originated in 1944 as a project in some of the Ontario branches of the league and grew to become a national event by 1946. It may have been inspired by New Brunswick's Health Week, an initiative of William F. Roberts, who, in 1918, became the first provincial minister of health in Canada.[43] Health Week came to be the league's most important event and was described by Gordon Bates (never shy about self-promotion) as "the greatest annual publicity event in Canada, and ... the biggest annual health week in any country in the world."[44] Like National Immunization Week, National Health Week obtained endorsement from the governor general of Canada, the federal minister of national health and welfare, and the Canadian Medical Association. Health Week had a particularly strong presence in schools, as will be discussed below, and the Canadian Education Association and a number of teachers' associations and boards of education across the country also endorsed it.[45] The league's Clergy Committee actively promoted Health Week in churches and synagogues, while the Publicity Committee distributed free streamers and posters and bombarded the press with news releases. The initiative received support from the Canadian Labour Congress and the Canadian Manufacturers' Association, both of which distributed material to their members. The Canadian Pharmaceutical Association and the Canadian Restaurant Association were also valued patrons and prominently featured Health Week material. As with several of the programs discussed in preceding chapters, the strong support National Health Week received from broad sectors of Canadian society shows that, in the first few decades following the Second World War, the Health League had many important allies and significant social and cultural capital.

National Health Week stressed the importance of preventive medicine. Publicity urged Canadians to visit their doctor and dentist regularly, drink pasteurized milk, immunize their children, engage in safe behaviours to prevent accidents, promote water fluoridation, and educate themselves about chronic disease. Most Health Week slogans emphasized personal responsibility: "It is better to *stay well* than to have to *get well*"; "Prevention is better than cure"; "Healthy Ways mean Happy Days"; and "Health is YOUR business!"[46] Like other league materials, Health Week publicity often took a righteous tone, berating Canadians for failing to pay sufficient attention to their health. In a 1953 news release, Bates complained that some communities in Canada still failed to pasteurize their milk, provide safe water, and vaccinate their children. He argued that these services should be available across the country and that "in these days of general prosperity only public apathy and ignorance stand in the way" of such measures.[47] Another press release that year fumed that "ignorant and gullible Canadians" were still purchasing "quack remedies and nostrums." Bates urged citizens to become better informed about the services available from governments and from their own physicians.[48] In an editorial in *Health* celebrating Health Week in 1961 (which was also circulated to the media), he pronounced:

> Most sick people shouldn't be sick, but they are. Most people who are overweight should be thin, but they are not. Most of the millions of people with

defective and decayed teeth should have good teeth, but they haven't. A multitude of different ailments fill the hospital beds and cut short the lives of people who should be, instead, contributing to the national economy because they are healthy.[49]

In 1971, the announcement for Health Week proclaimed that, "every individual must assume responsibility for maintaining his own health and that of his family at the highest possible level."[50] Such pronouncements were in keeping with Bates' view that much illness was preventable and that Canadians needed to assume the duties of health citizenship to protect themselves, their families, and the economy. Other material was less judgmental and more informative: press releases on arthritis, epilepsy, muscular dystrophy, heart disease, cancer, and mental health were a common feature of Health Week.

In its first few years, Health Week was planned to correspond with Social Hygiene Day, which was itself organized to align with American Social Hygiene Day.[51] Early advertisements for National Health Week reflected this social hygiene influence: one featured a young couple walking arm-in-arm, with the text challenging parents, teachers, churches, and youth leaders to prepare young people for the responsibilities of marriage and parenthood and emphasizing that three-quarters of venereal disease infections occurred among people under the age of thirty.[52] Before the end of the 1940s, Social Hygiene Day had been abandoned, and Health Week rarely made mention of venereal disease until the 1970s, when the league returned to the topic.

While Bates exerted strong control over most aspects of the Health League's programming, Health Week was the brainchild of the league's secretary, Dr. E.A. Hardy, a dedicated educator and activist, who started Health Week when he was in his late seventies. Hardy was a teacher, writer, and editor who played a key role in the establishment of public libraries in Ontario. He also served as chair of the Toronto Board of Education and president of the Canadian School Trustees Association. He compiled several books of poetry and was active in the Canadian Authors Association.[53] Hardy passed away in 1952, and the league went through a number of secretaries until Murdoch McIver, a former headmaster, took the reins in the mid-1950s. As a result of Hardy's and McIver's leadership, National Health Week had a substantial presence in schools. Bates' connections lay more in the fields of medicine, public health, and business, and he was occasionally frustrated by National Health Week's operations, fearing that there was too much focus on schools and not enough cooperation with public health authorities.[54]

It may have been undervalued by Bates, but the success of Health League in schools should not be underestimated. In 1949, over 40,000 students heard a health talk at assembly during Health Week, over 27,000 students made health posters, more than 25,000 sang health songs or recited health poetry, over 14,000 witnessed physical training demonstrations, and over 20,000 took a written or oral quiz on health.[55] In 1953, the Department of Education for Alberta indicated that about half of the province's schools made some effort around Health Week. Some brought in a visiting speaker, while others had the children listen to the Health League's radio broadcasts.[56]

Much of the early educational material associated with National Health Week was intended for students. *Heroes of Health,* first produced in 1946, provided engaging biographies of key figures in the history of medicine, such as Edward Jenner (who discovered the smallpox vaccine), Marie Curie (who discovered radium), Louis Pasteur (who developed pasteurization), and Frederick Banting (the Canadian who co-discovered insulin), which stressed that they had made their discoveries through extensive study and hard work.[57] The booklet compared health heroes to the missionaries who had come to Canada to "claim this country for the service of God." Canada was "destined" to become one of the leading countries of the world, it said, but the country needed Canadian children to become "missionaries for health," a phrase that reflected both the league's emphasis on health citizenship and its Christian bias. It urged young Canadians to improve their health habits and to talk about health at home and in their communities.[58] These booklets received positive feedback from teachers and other educators in Canada.[59] In 1946, 50,000 English booklets and 30,000 French booklets were circulated to departments of education in the nine provinces.[60] Yet, by 1953, overall circulation had declined to about 30,000, and by 1955 it was down to just over 4,000.[61]

In 1950, the league compiled a second school booklet, entitled *Guardians of Our Health,* which was distributed to schools until the mid-1960s. This volume, geared to Grade 8 students, identified promising careers in medicine, including that of doctor, dentist, druggist, nurse, and laboratory technician. Doctors were heroes – the doctor in the booklet had recently saved two toddlers from poisoning by speeding in a jeep through heavy mud to reach the children and hurrying them to the hospital, while taking "emergency measures" that saved their lives. This, and other scenarios in the booklet, presented a very masculine version of what doctoring could be. It glamorized the northern doctor who got around almost entirely by aircraft. It told "young men" how to prepare for the profession, stressing that it was physically demanding. Only at the end did the writer admit, "all this applies to women doctors also." The dentist was a less heroic figure – the pamphlet merely emphasized the importance of regular dental care. Strangely, though, compared to its section on physicians, it provided much more detailed information on how to become a dentist. The booklet also made it clear that that career was open to both men and women: this suggests that the booklet may have been influenced by the Canadian Dental Association, which had produced its own pamphlet encouraging both men and women to become dentists.[62] The booklet portrayed the other health professions – including nursing and pharmacy and lab work – as less challenging, less exciting, and less prestigious. The writer assumed that nurses were female, highlighting the nurturing and caring aspects of the job. The booklet stressed that there was a vast need for nurses in Canada, while acknowledging that the wages were low, suggesting that anyone who went into nursing did so to help "suffering humanity." By contrast, it depicted the druggist as male. It described the profession as requiring diligence, courtesy, and an interest in scientific issues. Salaries were "fair." The career of laboratory technician was described as open to both men and women. The booklet described it as a practical profession that did not pay well but had its rewards in saving lives.

Following these professional profiles, the booklet provided nutritional information, promoted pasteurization and immunization, and listed great names in the history of medicine, including Vesalius, Florence Nightingale, and Health Week favourites Jenner and Banting. It concluded with a few suggestions to teachers for discussion and further research.[63] The Health League's linkage of nation and citizenship with health was evident in the words that opened the booklet – "Our Goal: Canada to Lead the World in Health" – which was followed by an article discussing what made Canada a "great nation."

Despite the attention dedicated to schools, National Health Week went far beyond the education system. The league ran an extensive publicity campaign, with sponsored advertising in sixty-eight newspapers across the country in 1946.[64] In 1953, at least nine newspapers, including the *London Free Press*, the *St. Catharines Standard*, the *Guelph Daily Mercury*, and the *Saint John Times-Globe*, devoted an entire page to Health Week activities.[65] In 1961, the league noted that newspapers across the country had run at least 248 articles on Health Week.[66] The league also relied on the increasingly popular medium of television. In 1957, a short film about the Health League was broadcast during airings of popular programs such as *The Lone Ranger*, *The George Burns and Gracie Allen Show*, *Cavalcade of Sports*, and

The Adventures of Robin Hood.[67] In 1960, Health Week was featured on *Gillette Cavalcade of Sports,* the Ontario showings of *Sky King, The Perry Como Show, Tabloid,* and the *Imperial Esso Hockey Broadcast.*[68]

The league also promoted the campaign through churches and, eventually, through synagogues. This may say something about how the league envisioned the ideal Canadian health citizen – presumably someone who attended church, or possibly synagogue. When the league first established its Clergy Committee in 1950, it included representatives of the Anglican, Roman Catholic, Baptist, Presbyterian, and United churches, as well as the Salvation Army.[69] The committee eventually branched out to include other Christian groups as well. Early letters from the committee indicate that it was thinking about only Christian churches as a venue for health messages. By 1950, members expressed interest in having a Jewish representative on the committee, although the files indicate that a rabbi did not join the board until 1957.[70] From the Clergy Committee's perspective, the question of Jewish representation was complicated by the fact that Jewish congregations were not linked to a single Canadian body, making it harder to find a national representative.

The league solicited endorsements for National Health Week from the leaders of Christian denominations in Canada, which were generally granted enthusiastically.[71] Each year, the Clergy Committee sent a letter, co-signed by representatives of several denominations, to all churches, asking them to promote Health Week.[72] These letters used religious rhetoric and scripture to remind clergy of God's gift of health and the example set by Jesus in healing and caring for the sick. For example, the first clergy letter argued that God bestowed good health and expected people to take care of it. It reminded clergy that "St. Matthew Ch. 14:14 tells us that Jesus healed the sick."[73] These letters urged clergy to promote Health Week in their sermons, announcements, and local press and by arranging for speakers on health-related topics. The committee often followed with a survey asking what had been done to promote the campaign in the churches. Survey responses reveal that churches often announced the week in bulletins and mentioned it from the pulpit, but they did not usually devote sermons to health.[74]

Christian rhetoric pervaded Health Week material. For example, from the mid-1950s onwards, the Health League used the slogan "Crusade for Health." Booklets and newsletters entitled "Join the Crusade for Health" featured a medieval crusader bearing the Health League's symbol (a cross enclosed in a circle with the Health League's name around the circumference) as his emblem. Presumably the active involvement of the Clergy Committee in Health Week had something to do with the rhetoric. But it also reflected Canadian society at the time: in 1957, a Gallup poll indicated that 87 percent of Roman Catholics and 43 percent of Protestants reported having attended church in the past seven days.[75] Moreover, the vast majority of Canadians at this time identified themselves as Catholic, Anglican, or United Church in the census.[76] The Christian rhetoric, while not as apparent elsewhere in the Health League's materials, also reflected the organization's belief that health and morality were intimately connected.

While the league attempted to include Jewish congregations in its messaging, there is no indication that it reached out to other non-Christian denominations; indeed, even its efforts to involve Jews were half-hearted. In 1963, the league received a letter from Samuel Lewin of the Canadian Jewish Congress pointing out that "the circular letter [sent to clergy each year regarding National Health Week] is not inter-denominational but Christian only" and that the league's approach "would have to be broadened if it were to be directed also to synagogues and rabbis."[77] Although, the Canadian Jewish Congress endorsed National Health Week in 1958, and, by that time, the Clergy Committee had a Jewish representative (the well-known Toronto rabbi Stuart Rosenberg), there are indications as far back as 1957 that the secretary of National Health Week was aware that its material was not particularly well suited for distribution to synagogues.[78] Still, it took until 1960 for the Clergy Committee to devise a letter that would be acceptable to both Christians and Jews.[79] The Health League's interaction with Jewish clergy in National Health Week planning demonstrates that the organization was not necessarily hostile to those outside its assumed audience, but its efforts to be inclusive were often ineffectual or limited. The league was pleased to have a prominent rabbi on its Clergy Committee, but it was in no rush to make its material more palatable to Jewish congregations.

Nor did the league make much effort to address immigrants. There was a long history in Canada of regarding immigrants as a public health threat.[80] While this specific concern had diminished by the post–Second World War period, public officials were often dubious about immigrants' ability to assume the roles and responsibilities of Canadian citizenship, particularly its moral dimensions.[81] At a 1964 meeting, the National Health Week Committee explained its reasoning for not involving representatives of the Eastern Orthodox Church in its activities: "They are an important group," the committee acknowledged, but concluded that "we must give them time to adapt to Canadian ways."[82] Despite the fact that there was an extensive conversation in Canada about "New Canadians" in the 1950s, the Health League made little attempt to include them in National Health Week programming. In 1951, the league specifically reached out to new Canadians to inform them about free health services, such as chest X-rays, childhood immunization, and venereal disease treatment, by distributing pamphlets to teachers of citizenship classes in Ontario, but this appears to have been a one-time effort.[83] It may be that, because the Health League emphasized public education – as opposed to on-the-ground public health work – it thought that the specific needs of new immigrants would be better left to local public health units. More likely, however, given its unthinking focus on middle-class, white Canadians, it probably did not spare much thought for the wave of immigrants who were reshaping Canadian society during these decades.

The Health League did make a special effort to include women during National Health Week. Beginning in 1946, E.A. Hardy collaborated with the Federated Women's Institutes of Canada to distribute National Health Week material.[84] At the same time, he requested that Women's Institutes ask their members to write to government representatives in support of compulsory testing for venereal disease.[85] Additionally, the league distributed National Health Week materials through women's groups, including the Catholic Women's League, the National Council of Women of Canada, homemakers' clubs, and the Young Women's Christian Association.[86] In addition to these women's organizations, the league corresponded annually with Home and School Associations and Parent Teacher Associations, using them as additional channels for the dissemination of educational materials for Health Week.[87] The league urged local branches of women's organizations to "observe Health Week during the month of February, either by arranging for a special health meeting with a Health speaker, or the showing of a Health film, posters, pamphlets, etc."[88] National Health Week's correspondence with women's organizations was in keeping with the league's goal of educating women, whom it saw as the gateway to the Canadian family and therefore of vital importance in raising the future generation of health citizens.

The Health League had considerable success generating support among male-dominated service clubs as well. In 1960, for example, it sent mailings to over 1,750 service clubs seeking their participation in National Health Week.[89] Organizations such as the Rotary, Kinsmen, Gyro, Lions, Kiwanis, and the Optimists often hosted health speakers during National Health Week. Not surprisingly, these talks frequently focused on diseases affecting middle-aged men, such as cancer and heart disease, although dental care and problems affecting children were also popular topics.[90] The league encouraged every service club to form a health committee, although this initiative met with limited success, as many organizations felt that that they were already involved in health issues through their work with more specialized organizations, that they had more pressing commitments, or that there was no need for more health work in their communities.[91]

In addition to support from the voluntary sector, Health Week received significant corporate support. To mark the week, the Royal Bank of Canada devoted an issue of its monthly newsletter to health. In some years, the bank printed up to 150,000 extra copies for circulation by the league to schools and businesses.[92] The league prepared sponsored advertisements for newspapers across the country, ads frequently paid for by drug stores.[93] Beginning in 1959, the league printed Health Week placemats and sold them at cost to restaurants and lunchrooms across the country. The production of the placemats, which was supported by the Sun Life Insurance Company, was a highly successful endeavour. In 1960, some 332,000 placemats were distributed, with the slogan "Every Week Is Health Week."[94] Organized labour provided additional support for Health Week. From the late 1950s to the mid-1960s, the Canadian Labour Congress (CLC) distributed thousands of promotion folders and pamphlets to its member organizations.[95]

Along with these placemats, pamphlets, and folders, the league distributed *Health Facts*, its annual publication of statistics and information regarding the status of various diseases in Canada. It suggested that individuals and organizations could use the booklet both as a personal source of information and as a reference for speakers. *Health Facts* was an extensive booklet: in addition to mortality and morbidity statistics, it contained sections on the importance of pasteurized milk; nutrition (which included a set of guidelines on how to eat, based on the Canadian Food Rules); industrial health and the need to prevent sickness at work; mental health; and information on cancer, heart disease, arthritis, dental health, diabetes, alcoholism, and the problems of aging. It included information on public health activities in Canada at the federal, provincial, and municipal levels, and descriptions of the leading voluntary health groups in Canada, including the Health League, the Red Cross, the Canadian National Institute for the Blind, the Canadian Mental Health Association, and the Canadian Arthritis and Rheumatism Society. The front page provided advice to speakers using the booklet as a resource: they should celebrate the decline in mortality in many diseases and the progress that had been made in nutrition, medicine, and mental health, but emphasize that there was still much to do in the fields of cancer, tuberculosis, venereal disease, arthritis, pasteurization, and proper care for old age.[96] By its very existence, the booklet testified to the importance of facts and figures in understanding health. It valorized medical progress while mobilizing citizens to continue to act in ways that kept them healthy. Readers as well as lecturers and their audiences were encouraged to follow proper nutrition, to keep themselves healthy at work, to get themselves immunized, to drink pasteurized milk, to brush their teeth, and to visit a dentist regularly.

Health Week seems to have been most prominent in Ontario. In 1960, the government of Saskatchewan, experiencing growing frustration with the Health League's unwillingness to work in cooperation with provincial health authorities, announced that it would not be endorsing the initiative. The same year, the government of Manitoba decided to provide only "passive support."[97] As the league's funding dwindled from the mid-1960s onwards, National Health Week declined. At least in some years, the league continued to send out press releases, short radio announcements, and slides for television, but there is little indication the campaign achieved the reach that it once had. One of the last Health Weeks occurred in 1978, when Mabel Ferris was executive director of the Health League. In an article promoting the event, she told journalist Zena Cherry that "in our lifestyle we overeat and eat the wrong kinds of food. We smoke when we know we shouldn't. Many drink to excess. We under-exercise."[98] Ferris' words revealed that, while the magnitude of the week had changed, the messaging apparently had not: through National Health Week, the league continued to scold Canadians for failing to take better care of themselves.

***

National Immunization Week and National Health Week became major media events in Canada in the 1940s, 1950s, and early 1960s. They helped to inform Canadians about the importance of immunization, milk pasteurization, dental health, chronic disease, and accident prevention, among other topics. They took root in a Canada where the vast majority of people went to church (at least occasionally) and many, especially members of the middle and upper classes, belonged to service clubs and women's organizations.[99] These two initiatives were powerful during the baby boom years, when Canadians were particularly focused on the health and well-being of their offspring.[100] The messaging perhaps appealed to a citizenry that had considerable faith in experts such as doctors and believed that modern medicine could protect their children and themselves from disease. The message of personal responsibility likely also resonated with a generation that believed in active citizenship, as evidenced through their involvement in service clubs and other associations. But the league's failure to consult sufficiently with provincial health departments, its declining financial situation, and its failure to renew its leadership and networks eventually led National Immunization Week and National Health Week to fade away.

7

"A Malicious, Mendacious Minority"
Fighting for Water Fluoridation

In 1958, the head of the Health League's Fluoridation Committee, the young dentist Wesley Dunn, appeared as the mystery guest on CBC's famed *Front Page Challenge*, a show on which panelists tried to guess the news story associated with the guest. One of the panelists, the radio broadcaster Gordon Sinclair, was well known for his opposition to fluoridation, which he decried as "shoveling rat poison into the drinking water." For his part, Dunn counselled the television viewers that all medical and dental organizations agreed on the merits of water fluoridation, that it would greatly benefit children's teeth, and that it was best for citizens to take the advice of experts on this issue. Dunn emphasized the importance of Canadians deferring to experts by saying that it would be inappropriate for him to vote on what his child was learning at school, and that fluoridation, too, was a matter best left to the most knowledgeable individuals.[1] The Health League's belief that citizens should listen to experts came out strongly in the fluoridation debate, which would prove to be the most controversial public health issue of the postwar era.

Water fluoridation involves adding approximately one part per million (ppm) of fluoride to municipal water supplies. Studies completed in the immediate postwar era indicated that this could cut tooth decay by as much as 60–70 percent. But opposition to water fluoridation arose quickly. Some opponents believed that adding fluoride to municipal water supplies medicated people against their will, and argued that it was a violation of civil liberties. Others thought that the measure had been insufficiently studied and that fluoride, which was an active ingredient in pesticides, could have harmful effects on overall health that were not yet known. Still others believed that the measure was too expensive, and was wasteful because most municipal water was used for irrigating lawns and washing dishes, clothes, and cars. A few believed that fluoridation was a communist plot. They claimed that it could be used to "weaken people's wills" or for sabotage – the argument being that it would be easy to add this colourless, tasteless product to water supplies, thereby poisoning an entire population. The debate quickly became highly fractious: anti-fluoridationists circulated pamphlets, posters, and newspapers condemning fluoride as a dangerous poison, while pro-fluoridationists touted the benefits of better dental health. Pro-fluoridationists, who were appalled by how much misinformation circulated, failed to understand how anyone could oppose a measure that would improve the health of children. The Health League, in close cooperation with the Canadian Dental Association, became a leading force in the fight for fluoridation, especially in Toronto, which finally fluoridated its water in 1963 after years of debate. Gordon Bates became one of the most prominent supporters of fluoridation, best known for his claim that the anti-fluoridationists were a "malicious, mendacious minority."[2]

The league's support for water fluoridation may ultimately have helped children's teeth, but it was costly for the organization. Compared to childhood immunization, better nutrition education, or even testing and treatment for venereal disease, fluoridation was not a popular measure. Moreover, the league's unwavering support for fluoridation in Toronto highlighted that the organization was never really a national body – it was a Toronto group whose campaigns often extended across Canada. Its campaign for water fluoridation lost the league friends and supporters, and it significantly hurt the organization's bottom line. Due in part to the league's support for the measure, the United Community Fund of Toronto (which provided more than half of the league's revenues) decided to stop funding the organization, a move that resulted in financial devastation.[3]

The idea of fluoridating municipal water supplies originated in the United States. In 1931, two separate studies concluded that excessive amounts of naturally occurring fluoride in local water supplies had caused a distinctive mottling of white spots on teeth. Trendley H. Dean, a dentist with the US Public Health Service, subsequently demonstrated that mottled teeth were particularly resistant to decay. Over the next six years, a series of epidemiological studies showed that 1 ppm of fluoride in water significantly reduced dental decay without causing unsightly mottling. The US Public Health Service undertook a series of studies on fluoride excretion and the impact of fluoride on bones to ensure that there would be no health risk to adding fluorides to the water supply. In January 1945, the first controlled experiment began in Grand Rapids, Michigan, with another in Newburgh, New York, a few months later. In Canada, the first city to add fluoride to its water was Brantford, Ontario. In 1946, the Dental Health Division of the Department of National Health and Welfare commenced a long-term study comparing Brantford with Stratford, which had 1.3 ppm naturally occurring fluoride, and Sarnia, whose water was free of fluorides.[4]

In the meantime, dental researchers studied whether or not the benefits of fluoride could be delivered through other means. One option was fluoride tablets or drops, but studies of their effectiveness were inconclusive. Another option was "painting the teeth" with aqueous solutions of sodium fluoride and, later, stannous fluoride. Given the severe shortage of staffing in dentistry, this time-consuming process was not practical. Finally, manufacturers began to produce fluoridated toothpastes, but it was not until the mid-1950s that studies began to show their value.[5] Today, the growing consensus is that the effects of fluoride are topical and not systemic, and that fluoridated toothpastes may have played an important role in the enormous decline of dental caries in North America in the second half of the twentieth century.[6] But, in the 1950s and 1960s, dental researchers were convinced that fluoridated water was a better solution to the problem of dental decay. In part – and somewhat ironically, given that much of the opposition came from people who felt that adding this substance to the water was "unnatural" – pro-fluoridation dentists and scientists believed that it made the most sense to emulate the benefits of fluoride as they had first been discovered, and adding fluorides to water replicated how they existed in nature.

The three initial studies of artificial water fluoridation, in Grand Rapids, Newburgh, and Brantford, were scheduled to run for ten to fifteen years, but activist dentists in the United States believed that Dean had already demonstrated that fluoride could lead to dramatic improvements and urged the US Public Health Service to act quickly. In 1950, the Health Service and the American Dental Association endorsed water fluoridation.[7] The following year, the American Medical Association followed suit. There was reason for optimism. The three trials were showing that fluoridated water could cut tooth decay in children by as much as half.[8] But in Canada, the dental and medical communities feared that not enough was known about the long-term effects of fluoride.[9] Still, the evidence in favour of fluoridation was mounting, and, in April 1953, the *Journal of the Canadian Dental Association* published its first editorial endorsing fluoridation. Soon afterwards, the Canadian Dental Association's tone became much more strident, accusing fluoride's opponents of sensationalism and misusing evidence. In October 1953, the Canadian Dental Association endorsed the fluoridation of Canadian water supplies, and, eight months later, the Canadian Medical Association also gave its unqualified approval.

The Health League first endorsed water fluoridation in 1954. That same year, the Canadian Federation of Mayors and Municipalities asked the league to produce a report on the opinions of experts on the issue. The league surveyed professors of preventive medicine at ninety-two North American universities for their opinions. Well before the report was completed, Bates sent a letter to every deputy minister of health in the country, informing them that, of the thirty-two responses received so far, none were negative. Eventually, the Heath League received replies from seventy-one departments of preventive medicine: sixty-four were in favour of fluoridation, six claimed that they were not sufficiently educated about the subject and declined to give an opinion, and the one expressed a desire for caution and further study.[10] The Life Insurance Officers Association gave the Health League a grant of $500 to print 10,000 copies of the report, although the association did so only after considerable debate and a request to the Health League not to give the association any credit for the funding, an indication of how controversial this subject already was.[11]

At the same time, Bates gave an important address to the annual conference of the Canadian Dental Association. He started with one of his favourite quotes, "Sickness is the greatest cause of poverty." Then, drawing on cold war rhetoric, he emphasized that communism "thrives in poverty stricken countries." Thus, promoting health could defeat communism. He proclaimed that the World Health Organization did more to deter the expansion of communism than an international police force could ever do. Having established the crucial role of health, he turned to the fluoridation issue, attacking those who opposed fluoridation on the grounds that "it's only teeth." He asserted that, "I have a sneaking idea that normal dentition has much more to do with good health and long life than most of us imagine." He argued that people needed teeth to properly digest food, and that improperly digested food could lead to irritation, which was a major cause of cancer. Worse yet, "the toothaches which seem to be the lot of average man" were a sign of infection, which could cause problems in other parts of the body. In alluding to such concerns, he urged dentists to revisit the theory of focal infection.[12]

The theory of focal infection held that problems such as rheumatism and heart disease were the result of infected teeth. The first person to expound the theory was E.C. Rosenow, head of experimental bacteriology at the Mayo Clinic, who described it as a general or local infection caused by bacteria travelling through the bloodstream from another point of infection in the body. In 1910, the British physician William Hunter gave a lecture at McGill University in which he criticized dentists for focusing on restoration instead of extraction. He argued that restorations were a "veritable mausoleum of gold over a mass of sepsis." He believed that infected teeth were the cause of many illnesses, including anemia, dyspepsia, and nervous complaint. Weston Price, an American dental researcher, subsequently began a two-decade study of focal infection. His publications on the topic in the 1920s led many dentists to become "100 percenters," who recommended extracting all pulpless and endontically treated teeth. Dental journals touted the cures that had been achieved through this method, and many dentists jumped on the extraction bandwagon. But, by the 1930s, dental researchers began calling the theory of focal infection into question. They criticized Rosenow and Price for not using controls and called for a return to restorative treatment.[13] By the 1950s, most dentists had rejected the theory of focal infection.

But Bates, who had been trained at a time when the theory had first been articulated, remained a firm convert. He believed that the removal of several infected teeth had cured his bursitis.[14] Later in life, he wrote that a number of his friends had suffered strokes that had been caused by the removal of teeth, which had led to infection circulating in the blood.[15] Throughout his pro-fluoridation career, he stressed the dangers of focal infection, and such a belief would clearly have affected his view of the importance of the measure. Thus, in a letter to the *Globe and Mail*, Bates claimed that tooth decay had led to deaths from septicemia and other causes and that it might be the cause of arthritis.[16] In an editorial in *Health* in 1962, he asserted that "thousands of people have died of infection caused by tooth decay." He claimed that the theory of focal infection, as expounded by Price and Rosenow, had once been "looked on as gospel" but had fallen out of favour when the widespread availability of penicillin reduced the dangers of such infection. But, Bates argued, "it is the opinion of many authorities that the pendulum has swung too far at the moment and that there is a fatal tendency to treat dental focal infection too lightly."[17] This was not true: when dental journals addressed the question of focal infection in the 1950s and 1960s, it was mostly to dismiss it as a mistaken idea that had led to much unnecessary tooth loss.[18]

By the end of his life, Bates was making fairly outrageous claims about the dangers of focal infection: in 1975, when thousands of people were still dying of smallpox in India, he wrote the mayor of Los Angeles to say that "more lives are lost through focal infection arising from infected teeth than are killed by smallpox."[19] As we have seen in other Health League campaigns, Bates was willing to misrepresent the medical literature if it served his polemical purposes. From the Health League's perspective, one advantage of promoting the idea of focal infection was that it made fluoridation seem beneficial to all people, not just children. The league used this argument to counter anti-fluoridationists, who argued that even if fluoridation benefitted children, it could harm others, especially the elderly. If preventing tooth decay reduced arthritis and strokes, then its pro-fluoridation campaign showed that the Health League was committed not just to the health of children, but also to that of all Canadians over the life course.

The emphasis on focal infection was not the only peculiar feature of the Health League's fluoride promotion, as Bates expounded the idea that sugar was not the cause of caries and that it was a vital food. In an editorial in *Health*, Bates wrote, "One of the pet arguments of the recalcitrant uninformed is that if only children would eat or drink less sweet things all would be well. They ignore the fact that this love of children for sweets is the result of a physiological tissue demand. To deny children sweets would be to deprive them of an essential element in child nutrition."[20] This prompted a sarcastic letter from Canada's best-known expert in the field of nutrition, long-time league ally E.W. McHenry, who retorted, "This is such an interesting new concept in the field of nutrition that I would not like to ignore it in teaching the subject," and requested that Bates send him the references supporting his claims.[21] Bates responded that his opinions were merely a matter of "common sense" and suggested that he (Bates) could provide evidence in the form of letters from pediatricians.[22] Throughout his years of fluoride activism, Bates continued to blithely defend the consumption of sugar. In a letter to fellow fluoride promoter Ron Haggart of the *Toronto Star*, he wrote that "sugar does not cause caries" and that advising against the consumption of candy, ice cream, pop, and white sugar was "pure prejudice."[23] In a letter to an opponent, Bates claimed "sugar is also essential in the human diet and is the origin of energy."[24] His defence of sugar was surprising at a time when most mainstream nutritionists believed that obesity posed a greater threat to the health of North Americans than hunger or malnutrition and when dentists consistently warned about the dangers of refined carbohydrate consumption. Indeed, as Chapter 5 shows, the Health League itself regularly warned readers about the dangers of obesity. It may be that Bates was reluctant to condemn sugar when Coca-Cola and 7-Up were major advertisers in *Health*, or perhaps he genuinely believed fluoride would magically reduce decay to such a degree that cutting back on refined carbohydrates would be unnecessary.

Like many fluoride proponents, Bates believed that opponents were acting in bad faith. He accused the best-known anti-fluoridationist in Toronto, Gordon Sinclair, of only pretending to oppose fluoridation because it increased the ratings of his radio show. He believed that George Macmillan, a health food store owner who organized the anti-fluoridation campaign in Toronto, was against fluoride because the publicity brought more people to his store.[25] He insisted that anti-fluoridationists made large sums of money from selling pamphlets.[26] The claim that anti-fluoridationists were making money from their efforts seems hard to believe, as anti-fluoridation campaigns in most cities were led by just a few dedicated opponents, and there is little evidence that they possessed much in the way of financial resources. The literature was produced by small-scale publishers and was sold cheaply – it seems far more likely that these people were driven by their beliefs rather than by the hope of financial gain.

Bates' ad hominem barbs and his disdain for his opponents distinguished the Health League's approach to the fluoridation campaign from that of its allies. Never one to mince words, Bates told Roy Farran, the publisher of the *North Hill News* (a Calgary newspaper), "If you really believe the nonsensical views to which you have given expression then I believe you should resign your position as editor and publisher of your two newspapers and seek another position which requires less intelligence."[27] In an editorial in *Health* criticizing the citizens of North Battleford, Saskatchewan, for rejecting fluoridation, he wrote, "The efforts of the health authorities were defeated by the fanaticism of a misguided group which waged a battle against the health of children. This was silly enough, but the real tragedy is that there should be people so gullible to believe nonsense foisted on the public by uninformed people."[28] Such arrogance did little to promote reasoned debate on the issue.

The Fluoridation Committee and the Politics of Health Citizenship

By the mid-1950s, the Health League had formed a Fluoridation Committee under the leadership of Wesley Dunn.[29] Dunn was a young, forward-thinking dentist, who was already making a name for himself as registrar-secretary of the Royal College of Dental Surgeons and editor of the *Journal of the Canadian Dental Association*. Although Dunn headed the committee, it soon took the view that fluoridation should be promoted by "citizens" and not by dentists or medical professionals. The dentists on the committee believed that fluoridation was primarily a political problem, not a scientific one.[30] The need for citizen involvement in pro-fluoridation campaigns was becoming an increasingly common view in pro-fluoridation circles and was the opinion of Bates himself, who believed that a campaign for fluoridation in Calgary in 1957 had failed because it was led by dentists and not by citizens. As a result, when the league's Fluoridation Committee began to discuss plans to form a new committee to promote fluoridation in Toronto, it decided that it should be called the Citizens' Committee for Fluoridation, in the hopes of creating the impression that the local committee expressed the "spontaneous desire of citizens to obtain fluoridation."[31] The league hoped to find a leading citizen, and one not currently affiliated with the Health League, to chair the Toronto committee. Recruiting such an individual proved difficult, and a vice-president of the Health League board of directors and a former city councillor, E.C. Roelofson, finally stepped in as chair of the Citizens' Committee for Fluoridation in June 1962. That month, the committee was renamed the Metro Committee for Fluoridation, on the recommendation of several campaign consultants who felt that shorter name was better.[32]

In terms of strategies, Bates was particularly impressed by a pro-fluoridation campaign led by dentist Aberdeen McCabe in Montreal in the late 1950s. McCabe had delivered letters and fluoridation pamphlets to dentists throughout the city. He had asked the dentists to explain fluoridation to their patients and to leave pro-fluoridation pamphlets in their waiting rooms. On a subsequent visit, the patient was asked to sign and date a form letter promoting fluoridation, which was then sent to the appropriate city councillor. As a result of McCabe's efforts, Montreal dentists, their patients, and their friends sent more than 60,000 letters to municipal officials. While a number of the outer suburbs of Montreal fluoridated as a result of this campaign, it did not lead to fluoridation in Montreal proper. Even so, McCabe and Bates concurred that political pressure from citizens was key to achieving success in the fluoridation struggle.

Bates' efforts to engage citizens was part of the Health League's larger strategy of reaching out to service clubs and other organizations, including women's groups, in the hopes of mobilizing them in pursuit of health. The Health League had taken a similar approach in its campaigns against venereal disease, in favour of milk pasteurization, and to promote National Health Week. But citizen engagement only went so far. Bates still felt that medical professionals were the most authoritative voice on any medical question: citizens needed to take the advice of doctors and dentists and mobilize accordingly. Part of the reason why the anti-fluoridationists infuriated him was because they were expounding opinions on issues that Bates believed were well beyond their expertise. Thus, in a letter to the *Montreal Star*, he complained that anti-fluoridation letter-writers had been "influenced by people who pose as authorities but who are not. They have been led down the garden path by false prophets who rely on the too frequent gullibility of mankind to exploit their prejudiced ideas."[33] Bates' ideal health citizens never questioned medical authorities but leapt to put medical knowledge into political and personal practice.

In Bates' view, not everyone was an equally valued member of the Canadian public: he saw some citizens as more trustworthy than others. First on the list of less desirable citizens were those who were unlikely to embrace the health instructions of groups like the Health League. In an editorial in *Health* that condemned the "stupendous ignorance" of the citizens of Regina for rejecting fluoridation, Bates indicated that the goal of *Health* was to "carry light into dark places – in other words, instruct the intelligent un-informed."[34] (The metaphor of bringing light into dark places was commonly used in the battle against venereal disease. As Mariana Valverde makes clear, the metaphor of light pervaded moral reform in early twentieth-century Canada.[35] Bates' use of this language is demonstrative of the ways in which the league was failing to adapt to changing times.) When it came to fluoridation, he was opposed to referendums, believing that only the "informed citizenry" should make the decision as to whether or not a community fluoridated its water supply – and, presumably, one measure of "informed citizenry" was whether such citizens subscribed to the views of the Health League in such matters. In one press release, also printed as an editorial in *Health*, Bates thundered, "A referendum on a subject such as fluoridation is just about as ridiculous as asking for a referendum as to whether a dangerous tiger should be disposed of when it is already killing women and children."[36] In 1961, when the Ontario government introduced legislation allowing municipalities to add fluoride to their water, Bates wrote to Premier Leslie Frost to complain that the bill made it too easy for groups to force a referendum. He added the "vast number of foreign-born people in Toronto" made it likely that any referendum would be defeated: "There are some 150,000 Italians in Toronto and a large proportion of them cannot even read English. It would only be logical to expect that they would vote against anything which they could not understand."[37] In Bates' view, such people should not have the right to engage in the democratic process because they could not be trusted to listen to the appropriate experts and put health first. Bates, of course, was not alone in questioning the ability of "New Canadians" to become good citizens in this period; as Franca Iacovetta outlines in *Gatekeepers*, a wide network of social workers and bureaucrats was devoted to turning new Canadians into citizens, often in extremely patronizing ways.[38]

As we have seen, for the Health League, part of citizenship meant taking care of one's health for the good of the nation. Bates could be strikingly dismissive of those whom he felt paid insufficient attention to their health, and he believed that working-class people, immigrants, and the poorly educated were less likely to look after themselves. One of the arguments put forward by anti-fluoridationists was that people who wanted fluoridation for themselves or their children could get it by using tablets and adding them to their water supply at home. Bates opposed this solution on the grounds that many parents could not be trusted to faithfully use the tablets. In one letter, he wrote that, "If tablets were used as a substitute it is quite likely that that section of a population which needed fluorine the most would be neglected. People who are indolent or ignorant, especially among the group with less education, would certainly neglect to see that their children got fluorine in some form."[39]

For Bates, citizenship sometimes entailed giving up one's personal liberty for the greater good. However, the Health League preferred to avoid this issue, arguing instead that fluoridation did not interfere with people's civil liberties. It frequently compared fluoridation to the addition of chlorine to water. Both made the water safe and healthy, and neither required people to give up their rights. In an editorial in *Health* entitled "What Is Wholesome Water?" Bates explained that ordinary water was not just H_2O – it was "H_2O mixed with a great many chemicals coming from the beds of rivers and lakes which make it palatable." Since it had been discovered that fluoride protected teeth from decay, "competent scientists" believed that water was "pure" only if it had sufficient amounts of fluoride to counteract tooth decay. In the view of the Health League, municipalities were failing in their obligations to provide "pure and wholesome water" if they refused to add enough fluoride "to ensure healthy teeth."[40] Such an argument put Bates outside the mainstream of fluoride activists, who generally argued that adding fluoride would be beneficial for oral health, not that it would make the water more pure.[41]

The Health League represented fluoridation as risk free. Although, in scientific circles, it was well known that fluoridation might increase the possibility of tooth mottling, the league refused to acknowledge this as a potentially negative side effect. Similarly, while a small minority of doctors and scientists cautioned that fluoridation might accumulate in the bones, or that further study was needed, the league insisted that fluoridation had been proven to be safe. Thus, in a press release issued during the Toronto campaign, it quoted Toronto medical officer of health A.J.R. Boyd as saying "fluoridation is safe. There isn't a scrap of authentic evidence of risk to the health of anyone ... There is no risk for either the old or the young, the sick or the well, the feeble or the robust."[42] But even if the league had acknowledged possible risks to fluoridation, it likely would have pushed ahead, as it believed that sometimes citizens needed to make sacrifices for the overall health of the body politic.

Campaigning for Fluoridation in Toronto

The Health League was always a Toronto-centric organization. Not surprisingly, then, it became more heavily involved in the fight for fluoridation in Toronto than in any other city. The fluoridation battle in Toronto was a long and fractious one. Metro Council approved the principle of water fluoridation in 1955. (Two years earlier, Metropolitan Toronto had been created out of the City of Toronto, Etobicoke, North York, Scarborough, and other smaller municipalities, including Forest Hill.) The Health League was one of several groups, including the Academy of Medicine and the Academy of Dentistry, that gave presentations to Metro Council urging it to take this measure. Dr. Alan Brown, the physician-in-chief at Sick Children's Hospital, who was then serving as chair of the Health League's Fluoridation Committee, presented the league's brief. The league left it to others to promote the scientific merit and health benefits of fluoridation; its brief focused on why the arguments of the antis were wrong. Drawing on a document produced by the Fluoridation Committee of the Vancouver Dental Society, it defined the anti-fluoridationists as fitting into several categories, none of them positive. The first were the "uninformed," who did not take the time to study the evidence. The second were the "misinformed," who had been "misled by baseless allegations." The third were people "who have something to sell or promote," such as faddish foods and pamphlets. Finally, there were "the crackpots," who were probably in search of notoriety. The rest of the brief refuted the specific claims of the anti-fluoridationists. It concluded that opposition to fluoridation was similar to the opposition to chlorination, pasteurization, and vaccination, and instructed that all people "interested in the health of the children of this country should procure authentic literature originating in health departments or from recognized medical or dental authorities."[43] The brief was indicative of the league's disdain for the anti-fluoridationists and their position as well as of its own strong belief that political decisions needed to be guided by expert medical knowledge.

Several weeks after Metro Council approved fluoridation, the Forest Hill Council announced that it would take Metro Toronto to court to prevent enactment of the measure. The reeve of Forest Hill, Charles O. Bick, believed that fluoridation violated people's individual rights and that it might increase gum disease.[44] In March 1956, the Ontario Court of Appeal prohibited Toronto from proceeding with fluoridation. Chief Justice Pickup argued that existing municipal legislation did not allow the city to add a medicine to the water supply.[45] Metro Toronto appealed, but the Supreme Court of Canada agreed that water fluoridation exceeded the powers of the existing Municipal Act.[46]

As a result of the campaign originating in the wealthy, well-educated community of Forest Hill, the Health League decided to do a survey of the neighbourhood – the idea was to prove that the residents of Forest Hill wanted fluoridation but were being denied it by their reeve. The league sent out approximately two thousand cards soliciting opinions on water fluoridation. Only 11 percent of recipients responded, although 66 percent of those who did said that they were in favour of fluoridation. Only 17 percent said that they were against the measure.[47] Bates was frustrated by the progress of the survey and decided to shelve it because the response rate was so low.[48] At the same time, the league asked every member agency of the United Community Fund to pass a resolution urging the provincial government to enact special legislation that would allow Toronto to fluoridate its water supply.[49]

The Health League drew on strategies and connections from its earlier initiatives to generate support for fluoridation, both municipally and nationally. It corresponded with Home and School Associations in Toronto with the goal of gaining support for fluoridation.[50] It investigated the possibility of organizing of exhibition of goldfish swimming in fluoridated water to counter the opposition from stores selling tropical fish.[51] At a Canadian Restaurant Association convention, it sponsored a booth with a full-sized replica of Sherlock Holmes and a banner reading "Sherlock can't tell the difference! CAN YOU?" People were asked to try water from two large bottles and guess which one contained the fluoridated water. Answers were evenly split: 87 people chose incorrectly; 85 chose correctly; and 80 said that they couldn't taste the difference.[52] The league also kept up a regular stream of articles and editorials in favour of fluoridation in *Health*. In 1959, it hired Lloyd Bowen as executive secretary for the Fluoridation Committee. Bowen put out press releases, wrote letters to the editor, and sent fluoridation literature to provincial health units, members of provincial legislatures, radio stations, and newspapers.[53]

That same year, the Ontario government appointed a royal commission to investigate water fluoridation. After a year of study and public hearings, the commission came out in favour of the measure. In the spring of 1961, the Ontario government passed legislation that permitted municipalities to fluoridate their water, unless 10 percent of the electorate signed a petition requesting a referendum. In Metropolitan Toronto, the law stated that a referendum had to be held if it were requested by 10 percent of the electorate in a majority (i.e., seven of thirteen) of municipalities. On March 14, 1961, Toronto City Council voted in favour of immediate fluoridation. That vote galvanized the antis and, by the end of the month, anti-fluoridationists had formed the Ontario Citizens' Rights Association. Spearheaded by A.H. Woods, a business school administrator, and George Macmillan, a health food store owner and long-time anti-fluoridation activist, members of the association campaigned door to door in the seven smallest municipalities in Toronto and easily obtained the required number of signatures to request a referendum.[54] On his daily talk show on CFRB, the influential Toronto broadcaster Gordon Sinclair objected to being medicated against his will.[55] The *Globe and Mail* opposed fluoridation because it violated "freedom of choice."[56] In contrast, the *Toronto Star* and *Toronto Telegram* supported it, and columnists Ron Haggart and Frank Tumpane produced a regular stream of columns on its merits.[57]

The Health League organized a Citizens' Committee for Fluoridation, later renamed the Metro Committee for Fluoridation. The Metro Committee had to function at arm's length from the league: the league received a significant grant from the United Community Fund of Greater Toronto, but the fund had specified that this money was not to be used to promote fluoridation. (That requirement may have resulted from the fact that, in 1958, the fund reported that several people had withdrawn their contributions because of the league's support for fluoridation.)[58] Moreover, the terms of its agreement with the United Fund prohibited the Health League from raising money on its own.[59] And so the Metro Committee for Fluoridation – ostensibly independent of the league – did its own fundraising, although much less successfully than it had hoped. It began with the goal of raising $100,000, but succeeded in raising only $3,800, mostly in $5 and $10 increments from dentists after circulating a letter to them pleading for funds.[60] In the end, the committee overspent its budget on newspaper advertising (which was supposed to be covered by an outside donor), and the Health League covered an outstanding debt of $400.[61] Despite the supposedly arm's-length nature of the Metro Committee, it used the services of the Health League secretarial staff. The executive secretary of the league's own Fluoridation Committee, Lloyd Bowen, was heavily involved in daily operations of the Metro Committee, whose members included Gordon Bates and Mabel Ferris. Clearly, attempts to separate the Metro Committee from the Health League were less than thorough.

The Metro Committee was extremely active, especially in the months preceding the referendum. It hired a public relations officer to work full time for eight weeks before the day of the referendum. Two insurance companies agreed to hand out literature to their employees, and the Women's Electors Association handed out material at political meetings in Toronto. The Salvation Army and a number of other churches agreed to distribute literature to their members. University of Toronto dental students delivered pro-fluoridation material door to door in their local communities. Two days before the vote, the committee ran a large newspaper advertisement announcing the measure's endorsement by the local medical officers of health. It sent press kits to eighty-three newspaper editors, columnists, radio announcers, and other local press personalities. These kits included fillers for the newspapers and spot announcements for radio and television. The radio announcement featured local dentists on the theme "why I support fluoridation."[62] The kits included the front cover of that month's issue of *Health*, which featured a young girl drinking from a water fountain and the command "Vote for Fluoridation" (Figure 19).[63]

The Metro Committee followed up with additional press releases over the next three weeks. It also sent four feature articles on fluoridation at weekly intervals to thirty-four foreign-language newspapers. It purchased two thousand bumper stickers promoting fluoridation, which were displayed on

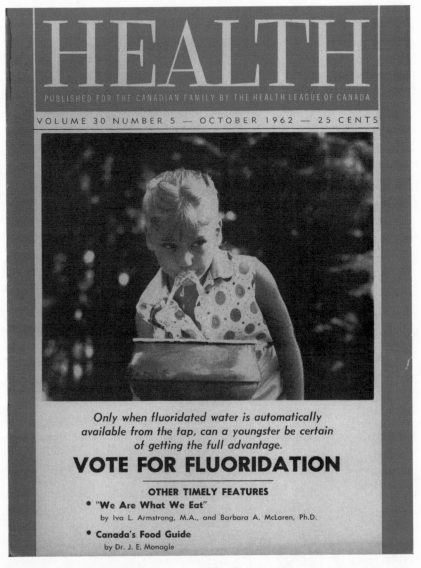

Figure 19 This cover of *Health*, encouraging readers to "vote for fluoridation," was distributed in press kits distributed to newspapers and radio stations. | *Health*, October 1962. LAC, MG 28, I332, vol. 182, file 3.

the backs of taxicabs and the cars of members of the Academy of Dentistry and were distributed to every pharmacy in Metropolitan Toronto.

The Metro Committee also sent a letter to every candidate for office in Metro Toronto. The letter touted the cost savings associated with fluoridation, pointing out that Torontonians spent $17 million each year on dental care, while the cost of fluoridating the water supply would be only ten cents per person per year, and emphasized the danger of tooth loss and of focal infection.[64] Under the name of E.C. Roelofson, its chair, the Metro Committee also sent letters to all members of Home and School Associations. These letters stressed that dental decay affected most children and that it could "seriously affect their health, not only as children, but throughout their life." Roelofson reassured parents that fluoridation was completely safe and urged them, if any doubt remained in their minds, to contact the Metro Committee for Fluoridation.[65]

As part of the campaign, the Metro Committee circulated several pamphlets produced by the Health League, including *The Fluoridation Picture, Facts and Fancies,* and *Summary of Conclusions and Recommendations from the Report of the Ontario Fluoridation Investigating Committee.* All of the pamphlets were printed on cheap paper with little attention to graphic design. *The Fluoridation Picture,* which featured two toddlers grinning on the cover, emphasized that "dental decay is Canada's most widespread chronic ailment" and that dental care cost the average family $20 each year. It promised that fluoridating community water supplies would cost from five to fifteen cents per person and could reduce dental decay by as much as 69 percent. The benefits accrued not only to children: it claimed that adult tooth loss was also much higher in communities without fluoride. The booklet explained that fluorides occurred naturally in underground deposits all over the world, as well as in many fruits and vegetables. Artificial fluoridation merely raised the level of fluoride to the optimum level determined by dental researchers. It concluded that fluoridation had been endorsed by, among other bodies, the World Health Organization, the Department of National Health and Welfare, the Canadian Dental Association, and the Canadian Public Health Association. Finally, the Health League suggested that people interested in "the health of the children of this country should procure authentic literature originating in health departments or from recognized medical and or dental authorities."[66] This, of course, was an obvious stab at the anti-fluoridationists, whose views the Health League believed should not be taken seriously.

The second pamphlet, *Fluorine: Facts and Fancies,* focused on refuting commonly circulated anti-fluoridation arguments. It took an authoritative tone, pronouncing that "the constituted health authorities in North America" and "a great body of scientific opinion" regarded water fluoridation as "a sound and effective means of reducing tooth decay." The pamphlet listed

"Objections" and then countered them. The first was that fluoride would not reduce tooth decay. The Health League asserted "there is most reliable evidence that in every area where there is over one part per million of fluoride in communal water supplies, the tooth decay rate has been greatly reduced." Another objection was that cancer and heart disease had increased in areas where water was fluoridated. The booklet countered that "cancer and heart disease have increased everywhere in fluoridated and unfluoridated areas alike. Anti-fluoridationists have produced false statistics by picking out special areas where heart disease and rates have been higher in fluoridated areas disregarding the fact that in subsequent years, the reverse is true."[67] The pamphlet provided little actual detail in refuting the claims of anti-fluoridationists. Instead, it simply asserted that anti-fluoridationist research was poorly done, and that "constituted health authorities" ought to be trusted. For people who were educating themselves on the issue, the pamphlet may have seemed patronizing, especially when the anti-fluoridation material was often much more detailed about research findings. Moreover, this pamphlet may have been more than a little frightening to people who knew little about fluoridation, as it served to raise concerns that most people had probably never heard of.

The final piece of literature produced by the Health League was a summary of the royal commission's Report of the Ontario Fluoridation Investigating Committee, often referred to as the Morden Commission. The pamphlet emphasized the severity of the problem of dental decay in Ontario. It recognized that better nutrition and better oral hygiene were part of the solution but argued that water fluoridation could play a dramatic role in reducing the incidence of decay. It insisted that water fluoridation "was not harmful to bodily health" and that fluoride could be delivered safely and effectively. It concluded, "THESE ARE THE FACTS: Water fluoridation is effective, safe, costs little, gives lifelong protection, has no health hazards, strikingly reduces tooth decay, saves money on dental bills, is approved by dental, medical and public health organizations."[68]

Somewhat surprisingly, the Health League regarded *Facts and Fancies* as a better pamphlet than *The Fluoridation Picture*. This may be because Bates found it hard to refrain from a good fight and was infuriated by what he saw as the factually incorrect and illogical arguments of the antis. As a result, he may have overemphasized countering the anti-arguments in preference to putting forward the more positive reasons in favour of fluoridation. During the Toronto referendum campaign, the Toronto and District Trades and Labour Council distributed *Facts and Fancies* to its members.

Twelve of the thirteen medical officers of health in Toronto distributed *Facts and Fancies* or the Morden summary through public nurses during their daily rounds. Even after the Toronto campaign, *Facts and Fancies* would remain a standby of the league's pro-fluoridation program, although in 1963 the literature subcommittee of the National Fluoridation Committee (the new name for the league's long-standing Fluoridation Committee) criticized *Facts and Fancies* for being too negative. It recommended that it should be given out only to professional groups.[69] Even so, the league continued to circulate it.[70]

Thanks in large part to the massive publicity campaign led by the Health League, Toronto voted narrowly in favour of water fluoridation. The league trumpeted that the campaign had succeeded because the Metro Committee "sold the value and benefits of fluoride to two groups of citizens – those with young families and those with high intelligence and better than average financial means. Both these groups, the majority of whom live outside Toronto proper, voted overwhelmingly in favour of fluoridation."[71] Such boasts, of course, reflected the Health League's pursuit of what it believed to be the most intelligent, most forward thinking, and therefore most health-minded portion of the Canadian citizenry.

Ultimately, the Health League paid heavily for its advocacy of fluoridation. While there were other factors at work, as will be described in Chapter 8, the United Community Fund greatly reduced its grant to the league. In 1962, the league received $78,463 from the Fund; by 1964, that had fallen to $39,250; and in 1965, it received no United Fund grant at all. Although this grant represented a substantial portion of its budget, the Health League maintained a strong commitment to its pro-fluoridation activities.[72] It continued to employ Lloyd Bowen until 1967, when it could no longer afford his salary. Bowen then joined the staff of the Canadian Dental Association, but he remained the honorary secretary of the National Fluoridation Committee and kept the two organizations in close contact. Moreover, despite falling revenues, the league continued to spend substantial sums on fluoridation education.[73] It provided pamphlets for fluoridation campaigns in other parts of the country as well as a guide for interested community members with recommendations on how to organize a campaign for community water fluoridation. But, in its annual report for 1965, the National Fluoridation Committee complained that, even though it was recognized as the leading body promoting fluoridation in Canada, its effectiveness was limited. The report warned that the committee "dare not advertise generally the availability of its facilities as it could not begin to cope with the latent demand." Instead, it merely responded to requests as they arrived.[74]

After the Toronto campaign, the Health League tended to be more reactive than proactive with respect to the fluoridation movement. In particular, it continued its fight against the arguments of the antis, which were becomingly increasing sophisticated. In 1963, three scientists from the National Research Council (NRC), J.R. Marier, Dyson Rose, and Marcel Boulet, published an article in the *Archives of Environmental Health* suggesting that fluoride could accumulate in bones.[75] This article received widespread publicity when John Lear, the science editor for the highbrow *Saturday Review*, used it as the centrepiece of an anti-fluoridation article. Gordon Sinclair crowed, "The most impartial scientific body in my country, the National Research Council in Canada, has found that fluorides injected into the water supply are injurious."[76] Bates wrote to the head of the NRC to complain that the article was a "blazing indiscretion."[77] He asked a leading American nutritionist and long-time ally of the Health League, Frederick Stare, to address the safety of fluoridation in his comments to the Voluntary Committee on Health of the Senate and House of Commons. While Stare did not specifically address the work by scientists at the NRC, he made it clear that only certain voices should be listened to on the issue of fluoridation.[78] In another letter of complaint about the NRC paper, Bates questioned whether research in rats was relevant to humans and claimed that he had read some of the details of the research and that "it was very badly done."[79] In fact, the NRC article was a review that dealt with fluoride accumulation in both rats and humans and involved no original research. Bates' reading of the paper was either careless or deliberately dishonest. More positively, after the Royal Commission on Health Services recommended that every community water supply in Canada be fluoridated in 1964, the Health League issued a press release and wrote a letter to the Minister of National Health and Welfare, Judy LaMarsh, to tell her that the Health League heartily endorsed this recommendation.[80]

After Lloyd Bowen moved to the Canadian Dental Association, he continued to work closely with the Health League in his position as honorary secretary to the National Fluoridation Committee. So, in 1969, when Dr. K.A. Baird published an article against water fluoridation in *Canadian Doctor*, a magazine that was provided free to every doctor in the country, Bowen arranged for Carol Buck, the chair of the Department of Community Medicine at the University of Western Ontario, to pen a reply.[81] Bowen wrote letters of protest when it appeared that Fort Erie,

Ontario, might lose its water fluoridation as a result of amalgamation with communities that did not fluoridate their water.[82] In the mid-1970s, both he and Mabel Ferris wrote to the National Council of Women to express their stern opposition to an anti-fluoridation motion being put forward by the Provincial Council of Women of British Columbia, which would potentially overturn the National Council's long-term endorsement of fluoridation.[83] When the Canadian Dental Association tried to push Bowen into retirement, the Health League urged the Department of National Health and Welfare to continue his work promoting fluoridation.[84] In 1973, the Health League wrote to every minister of health in the country, urging them to pass legislation requiring communities to fluoridate their water. (This was after the Liberals in Quebec had introduced legislation to this effect but had withdrawn it in the face of opposition.)[85] A few years later, when the Liberals in Quebec did pass legislation requiring compulsory fluoridation, Bowen issued a press release celebrating their decision and indicating that there "could be no more suitable tribute to the memory of Gordon Bates."[86]

***

Fluoridation activism became a major aspect of Health League activities in the mid-1950s. The league's decision to take on fluoridation reflected broader developments in the field of public health. By this time, there had been huge improvements in child and maternal health, most parents believed in the value of vaccination, and milk pasteurization had become the norm. By the 1950s, fluoridation had become the most promising new public health intervention, as well as the most controversial. It is not surprising that the Health League, and its head, Gordon Bates, who throve on controversy, took up the cudgel in favour of fluoridation. As in previous campaigns, the league urged Canadians to listen to the advice of experts and support water fluoridation as part of their duties as health citizens. It had often exaggerated the benefits of the measures it promoted, and it rarely shied from controversy, but it took a particularly confrontational and somewhat idiosyncratic approach to fluoridation. Its emphasis on the dangers of focal infection and its optimistic view of sugar consumption separated it from mainstream medical and dental bodies. At the same time Bates, and, by extension, the Health League, brought remarkable energy and persistence to the cause, especially during the 1962 fluoridation referendum in Toronto. Bates had a talent for building networks, rallying troops, and skewering opponents. At the same time, his extreme style likely alienated many erstwhile allies. Without doubt, the Health League paid the price for its fluoride activism, and it would never recover from cuts to, and then the loss of, its United Fund grant. By the late 1960s, the league was becoming a shadow of its former self.

8

Circling the Drain
The League's Slow Decline

In 1975, Gordon Bates was in hospital, recovering from a serious stroke, but his passion and zeal for public health, particularly its moral aspects, was undampened. From his bed, Bates expressed outrage at TV Ontario's plan to produce a thirteen-part series on sexual problems, designed for high school or college sex education classes and hosted by journalist June Callwood and Dr. Stuart Smith. The episodes were to deal with subjects such as masturbation, sex and childhood, premature ejaculation, female orgasm, and sex without commitment.[1] Bates complained to Premier Bill Davis, "The contents of these films are so outrageous, and in my opinion, so indecent, that I go on record protesting their showing." He instructed Mabel Ferris to circulate this letter to politicians, service clubs, and the media.[2] By this point, the Health League of Canada was bruised and battered: its budget and staff were a fraction of what they had been in the 1950s and early 1960s, and its networks were frayed. Moreover, on issues related to sexuality and morality, the views of younger Canadians significantly diverged from those of Bates. The organization would peter out, going dormant in the 1980s, but the organization's decline was in evidence well before then.

In 1964, as a result of ongoing conflicts, including its active support for water fluoridation, the Health League was expelled from Toronto's United Community Fund. It never recovered financially. At the same time, its stance on social, moral, and political issues, including publicly funded physician care, made the organization seem out of date. The league opposed universal state-funded health insurance in the 1950s and 1960s. While it was far from alone in its opposition, its stand alienated the league from potential supporters, as Canadians quickly embraced publicly funded physician care. This alienation was exacerbated by Bates' inflated rhetoric on the need for improved moral standards. The league's troubles were further compounded by internal difficulties that compromised its programming, finances, and organizational structure. Finally, a lack of organizational flexibility and failing social networks meant that the league's support system and capacity to govern itself was crumbling.

The Financing of the Health League

The league (and it precursor Canadian Social Hygiene Council) initially received the majority of its funding through government grants – the main sources were the federal government, the Ontario government, and the city of Toronto.[3] It generated additional revenues from film showings and the sale of its educational materials. Beginning in 1939, the league organized yearly "tag days," in which volunteers took to the streets asking for funds to support the organization.[4] During the Second World War, funding significantly increased when the league decided to join Toronto's United Welfare Chest (later known as the Community Chest and the United Community Fund, and today known as the United Way).[5] During the 1920s and 1930s, members of charitable organizations and business people formed Community Chests to centralize fundraising appeals, thereby avoiding the duplication and unnecessary expense of each charity having to fundraise separately.[6] Another advantage of such federated funds is that they had the resources to evaluate the quality of the organizations they supported. Because federated fundraising was organized on a municipal scale, it was never an easy fit for national organizations (even purportedly national organizations like the Health League). Moreover, one of the requirements of joining the federated fundraising movement was that member organizations could not run separate fundraising campaigns in the city in which they were receiving funds.[7] While the league happily took money from federated funds, its relationship with federated fundraising organizations was always rocky, in large part because Bates believed that the united appeals paid too much attention to charity and relief and not enough to prevention.[8] He believed that federated fundraising perverted the meaning of charity and voluntarism, was cowardly in the face of controversy, and placed too much power in the hands of social workers. Also, he was continuously unhappy with the amount of money offered by federated funds – perhaps not surprising, as the Toronto federated fund regularly fell short of its fundraising goals and was unable to finance its member organizations to the extent that it would have liked.[9] After the league was excluded from the Toronto Community Fund, Bates' hostility grew; his subsequent actions ensured that the league would never be invited to return to the fund.[10] As a result, the league's revenues plummeted and never recovered.[11]

Bates' criticisms of the federated fund were certainly coloured by his organization's difficulties, but he was not alone in his animosity towards this new form of charitable fundraising. Some of Bates' contemporaries, as well as scholars of federated fundraising, have argued that organizations such as Community Chests and United Funds made giving less meaningful because donors lacked a sense of connection to an individual charity or cause. Moreover, because federated fundraising often involved raising funds through payroll deductions, some have argued that it was coercive: some workers felt that they must give but, at the same time, they had no choice over what charities received their largess.[12] As Shirley Tillotson has argued in the Canadian context, "in its ease and efficiency, payroll deduction deprived employees of the privacy in which they could make free choices about charity."[13] Bates and his contemporaries had a similar critique. In 1957, Rev. William P. Jenkins wrote an article in *Maclean's* entitled "Why I Am against the United Fund," in which he argued that such simplified and "painless" methods made charitable giving so coercive that it was not a matter of personal morality at all, but rather a private tax strategy that kept donors distant from the social issues their donations allegedly tackled.[14] In a 1969 *Saturday Night* article, journalist Peter Desbarats described the federated fundraising movement as "an archaic, inefficient and self-centred system which coolly defrauds the public of millions every year and perpetrates the social evils it pretends to attack." He complained that, through the use of payroll deductions, annual appeals took money from the working poor and gave it back to them in the form of "charity."[15]

Bates' biggest quarrel with federated fundraising was that it prioritized "relief" over prevention. Throughout his career, Bates quoted the Fabian socialists Sidney and Beatrice Webb as saying that "sickness has been the greatest single cause of poverty."[16] Bates was certainly not a Fabian, but he strongly believed that sickness led to poverty (rather than vice versa). (Of course, Bates' view is strongly contradicted by today's scholars of the social determinants of health: being poor greatly increases your risk of illness.)[17] He critiqued the federated fundraising movement for failing to recognize that, if illness could be prevented, there would be little need for old people's homes, settlement houses, and many other organizations that federated funds supported.[18] He complained that it "is far easier to build a hospital than it is to persuade people that preventive measures such as compulsory pasteurization of milk or medical examinations before marriage will keep hospitals empty."[19] He also believed that, by removing the need for organizations to run their own fundraising campaigns, federated fundraising weakened the relationship between the organization receiving funds and its supporters. Volunteers no longer had to go door to door or stand in the streets to raise funds, but neither did they have to convince their fellow citizens that their cause was worthwhile.[20] Bates also protested that voluntary health organizations functioned primarily on a national scale, while federated fundraising organizations tended to prioritize the local. As a result, voluntary health agencies were not receiving the support they deserved.

Bates believed that professional social workers controlled the federated fundraising movement and used it to further their own ends, to the detriment of worthy organizations like his own. He worried that federated fundraising organizations run by social workers could not possibly understand health agencies. On at least one occasion, Bates expressed outraged at the notion that social workers would rate his organization's success, writing to a league board member in 1963 that a "Miss Florence Philpott – a Social Worker" was to rank priorities among the voluntary health agencies. He added, "What in the world she knows about it, I don't know, but I certainly know that the Health Agencies are not going to be very happy."[21] Bates resented that social work expertise would garner greater respect and authority than his own medical expertise. In fact, most scholars have argued that federated fundraising represented the views of business people above all. As Gale Wills argues in her history of federated fundraising in Toronto, federated funds were heavily inflected with business values at the expense of social workers' ideals.[22] Wills maintains that the United Community Fund took over from the Community Chest in 1957 in part to shake off social work influences and woo prominent business people, big donors, and large national agencies.[23] Bates had little objection to recognizing business expertise – he filled his own board with prominent members of the business community – but he did not understand why the federated funds paid so little attention (from his perspective) to health and to the expertise of physicians.

Bates created additional conflict when, in 1952, the Toronto Welfare Council (TWC), a planning committee of the Community Chest, established a special committee in the hope of clarifying whether the league's work should be considered national or local and how it related to the TWC's own Health Committee.[24] Bates refused to meet with the Welfare Council: he thought that he should be able to put the league's case directly before the Community Chest's board of directors. His grandstanding delayed the special committee's work and created significant irritation among its members. Nonetheless, the committee eventually concluded that the league's work was not redundant and congratulated it on its publicity work, especially *Health* magazine, which it regarded as an excellent resource, although it questioned whether "aspects of its program are particularly applicable to the Greater Toronto area."[25] Despite this general stamp of approval, Bates' refusal to cooperate with the special committee had won him few allies within the Community Chest. Adding fuel to the fire, he was carrying out a behind-the-scenes lobbying campaign against the Community Chest/United Community Fund. In 1956, he met with Pierre Berton, then the managing editor of *Maclean's*, and another critic of the federated fundraising movement. Berton invited him to submit an article criticizing federated fundraising. The article was never published, but Bates shared it with numerous friends and allies, sometimes unsolicited and sometimes upon request.[26]

A few years later, Bates continued his obstreperous behaviour by refusing to participate in a review that was to be undertaken by the National Agency Review Board (NARC). NARC was designed to review and advise on national agencies' budgets, providing its findings to Canadian Community Chests/United Funds as well as corporate donors and giving advice to the agencies themselves.[27] Every other national organization in Toronto's United Community Fund had agreed to participate in this review.[28] It is unclear why the league refused: perhaps it feared that the results of the review would be negative, or perhaps its intransigence was due to Bates' ongoing hostility towards the Community Fund.[29] Eventually, the league agreed to participate, and the Community Fund generously agreed to push back a decision that was to be made about the league's ongoing funding. Although NARC reported positively on its activities, it recommended that the league join other federated funds outside of Toronto and that it work on its leadership-succession plan. The point about succession was fair: Bates was in his late seventies at this point, with no successor in sight.[30]

A final bone of contention with the federated agency was the league's support for water fluoridation, which we discussed in Chapter 7. Bates believed that a public health education organization like the league had to advocate for water fluoridation, which medical and dental authorities agreed would substantially improve children's oral health. Yet the federated fund had become increasingly adverse to controversy, as it attempted to reach as many donors as possible.[31] During the late 1950s, the United Community Fund began to receive protest letters about the league's pro-fluoridation activities.[32] For example, a disgruntled dentist, J.H. Johnson, wrote to the fund's executive director, John Yerger, in 1959, asking why the league was getting an allocation from the fund. He complained that the league primarily propagandized in favour of fluoridation, "a project with which more than fifty percent of the community are not in sympathy. If you persist in providing funds from the charity purse for these free lance kibitzers ... you must surely expect to alienate the good will and contribution of a large segment of the community."[33] In this instance, a fund representative met with Johnson and defended the league, explaining that water fluoridation was widely endorsed by medical and dental authorities.[34] In 1961, W.K. Long of the Ontario Citizens' Rights Association (an anti-fluoridation group) wrote to the fund to complain about its support of the league.[35] Yerger responded that he would place Long's letter in a file for the review committee's consideration. He copied this correspondence to Bates, who responded furiously. Yerger shot back that the league's fluoridation program could harm fundraising and that the fund could not take sides on such controversial issues.[36] The fluoridation controversy highlighted significant and growing ideological differences between Bates and the federated fund leaders. Bates felt strongly that it was the role of a voluntary organization like the Health League to push for measures that would improve public health, even if they were unpopular, while the Community Fund leadership preferred member agencies to be inoffensive and uncontroversial. This episode illustrates Bates' growing obstinacy: in the 1920s, he had steered his organization away from controversial positions in the hopes of attracting allies and building consensus; now, he no longer seemed willing to compromise.

The Health League and the federated fundraising movement were an ill fit. Clearly, Bates' views on charity's purpose and voluntary associations' responsibilities did not match the federated fundraising movement's model. These conflicts, coupled with Bates' stubbornness, practically ensured that the Health League would be expelled from the United Fund. This independence meant that Bates and his organization could remain true to their vision, but it crushed the league financially. In 1963, the last year of full support from the United Fund, the league had revenues of $132,320, more than half of which ($77,700) came from the fund. By 1965, the league was struggling, with just under $60,000 a year in revenue.[37]

The League and other Organizations in the Voluntary Sector

The league's problems with the United Fund need to be understood in the context of the changing landscape for voluntary health organizations in this period. As concern about chronic disease began to overshadow that about infectious disease, a host of new organizations were established in Canada, including the Canadian Arthritis and Rheumatism Society (1947), the Canadian Cancer Society (1938), and the Canadian Heart Foundation (1956).[38] The league was also interested in chronic disease, but its general approach to health could not compete with the work of these new organizations. These associations generally funded research as well as education, and many provided services to the sufferers of these conditions. Such work made them far more attractive to potential donors. They were also far more successful at on-the-ground organization. For example, the Canadian Mental Health Association (CMHA) began to organize provincial branches in 1950 aided by a grant from the federal government. By the mid-1950s, the Saskatchewan branch of the CMHA had 20,000 members and nine branch offices.[39] Christian Smith, the director of health education for Saskatchewan and a former Health League employee, scolded Bates for spending too much time on national media campaigns and not enough on local organizing. He warned that the Health League was being surpassed.[40]

A comparison between the Heath League and the Ontario Diabetic Association indicates how each organization's fortunes changed as the public became more interested in chronic diseases and the associations that targeted them. The league began with the advantage. In 1951, when the league was well established in its office at 111 Avenue Road, Toronto, it received a request from the Canadian Diabetic Association. The association wanted desk space and access to a telephone so it could start an Ontario branch.[41] The league graciously honoured the request, and the branch resided in the Health League's office rent-free until 1956. At that point, the Ontario branch was consolidated into the Canadian Diabetic Association, which by then had a significant staff. By 1972, the Canadian Diabetic Association needed a space twice as large as the league's headquarters.[42] In the meantime, the league had had to sell its building on Avenue Road and move into a rented space down the street.[43] Within a relatively short space of time, a group it had help set on its feet had overtaken the league.

Beginning in the 1950s, the league, aware that its star was falling in comparison to more specialized organizations, attempted to establish a federation of all national health organizations under its leadership. Bates hoped thereby to centralize resources and fundraising.[44] He also hoped that this plan would solve the problem that national health organizations had in meeting the criteria of the federated fundraising movement. But leaders of other health organizations were not convinced that the Health League was the right organization to reorganize Canadian health charities. The general director of the Canadian Mental Health Association agreed with Bates that many Community Chests were not very interested in, and, indeed, were sometimes even "hostile" towards, health charities – or those "'horrible disease boys." But he felt that the Health League was too small to lead such a group and that it might be perceived as having "selfish interests."[45] Even so, Bates continued to work on his plan. He met with representatives of other non-profit organizations in November 1958 and suggested that the organizations buy a new building together to use as group headquarters.[46] Only two national non-profit organizations – the Canadian Council for Crippled Children and Adults and the United Nations Association – expressed interest.[47] Although the league did not buy a building, its executive remained interested in collaborative effort. In 1961, the Health League's national executive considered drawing other health organizations in by including them in National Health Week and offering them access to a new building and *Health* magazine.[48] Over the next several years, the league looked at buying the properties adjacent to its own and expanding its existing facility to accommodate other voluntary health agencies. It does not appear that any other agencies offered to put up money or even confirmed that they would rent space.[49] The Health League president, A.C. Ashforth, questioned why the league was planning to spend so much money on an uncertain project, but Bates craved progress and argued that the league "must have a vision, and we could set an example to the rest of the world ... We either believe in health or we don't."[50] The league's attempts to collaborate with other organizations illustrated its ongoing ambition but also its growing inability to connect with other organizations and influential players in the public health field.

The League and the Medicare Debate

Today, most Canadians see the introduction of publicly funded medical care as one of the country's great achievements.[51] But, in the years prior to its enactment, publicly funded physician care was fiercely debated. Although doctors had expressed some support for the measure in the 1930s and 1940s, when their incomes were low, by the 1960s, when the measure was proposed once again, their incomes had risen, and private insurance (including several non-profit plans) provided a possible alternative to state-funded medicine. The Canadian Medical Association (CMA), which had supported state insurance in the 1940s, backed away from the measure as early as 1949. The Health League followed a similar trajectory. Bates expressed some support for publicly funded health care in the 1930s and 1940s. Indeed, many of the people involved in the Canadian Social Hygiene Council, such as Charles Hastings and J.J. Heagerty, were supporters of publicly funded health care.[52] But by the 1960s, Bates came to believe that publicly funded insurance would pay insufficient attention to prevention. He worried that the health habits that he had encouraged Canadians to adopt for the sake of their health and the nation would be abandoned in the face of free health care. He believed that voluntary groups like his own would lose influence and power, and he feared that the decline of groups such as the Health League would have negative consequences for controversial public health measures like pasteurization and water fluoridation, which he thought governments were too cowardly to enact on their own.

In the 1930s, the league's engagement with publicly funded health insurance was restricted to running a series of articles exploring arguments for and against the measure in *Health*.[53] But, by the 1940s, the league was actively promoting the Heagerty proposals for health insurance. The Heagerty Committee was established in 1942 to advise the Ministry of Pensions and National Health on options for health insurance.[54] The committee proposed to insure all Canadians against the costs of medical and hospital care, pharmaceuticals, and children's dental care. It indicated that physicians' services "should be utilized for prevention as well as treatment." Under the proposed plan, the federal government would also grant money to support the prevention and treatment of venereal disease, tuberculosis, and mental illness; public health improvement; physical fitness; public health research; and training for public health workers.[55] Gordon Bates and J.J. Heagerty had a long-standing relationship and similar philosophies on public health.[56] Throughout his career in the federal government, Heagerty contributed articles to *Health* and kept up a correspondence with Bates.[57] Not surprisingly, given their long relationship, Heagerty called on the league to support his plan. The league issued at least one press release in support of public health insurance.[58] The organization also invited Henry Sigerist to speak on its behalf to members of Parliament.[59] Sigerist was a professor of history at Johns Hopkins University and an authority on socialized medicine; he played an important role in Saskatchewan's revolutionary hospital and health insurance systems.[60] In the speech arranged by the Health League, Sigerist expressed his strong support for the Heagerty proposals. Bates also editorialized in favour of the Heagerty proposals in *Health,* commending them for their strong emphasis on prevention.[61] The Heagerty proposals, though, ultimately failed, a victim of growing opposition within the medical profession, concerns about the cost, and jurisdictional wrangling.

In the years that followed, Saskatchewan beat a path to public health insurance by introducing a hospital insurance program. Other provinces followed suit, and in 1957 the federal government introduced legislation that committed it to providing one-half of the cost of any provincial hospital insurance program, providing that services were available to all residents of the province and that a majority of provincial governments representing a majority of the people in Canada would introduce provincial plans. The other provinces acted quickly, and by 1961, all Canadians had access to public hospital insurance. The league did not take an active role in this debate, although it telegraphed its resistance to the measure in 1956, when it invited the economist W. Wallace Goforth to give a speech at its annual meeting in which he advised Canadians to embrace private insurance plans, which, he pointed out, already operated successfully.[62] The speech was reprinted in *Health* and included as part of the league's submission to the Royal Commission on Health Services in 1962.[63] In an editorial in the issue that reprinted Goforth's address, Bates underlined that the "only true Health Insurance is the prevention of sickness and the promotion of health." He recommended that, instead of funding hospital insurance, the federal government should increase its grants to the Health League for popular education that would keep people well and make them into "valuable producing assets in the body politic."[64]

After public hospital insurance became a fact, the next major step in creating the health care system that Canadians know today was universal coverage of physicians' visits. Again, Saskatchewan paved the way. In 1961, it passed legislation that would cover all medical visits. Panicked, the CMA, which was by this time fully opposed to publicly funded physician care, asked the federal government to appoint a royal commission to study and report on the "health needs and resources of Canada."[65] The Hall Commission was established in 1961 and reported in 1964. The league's brief to the royal commission encouraged the government to put money into preventive medicine and voluntary organizations. It held that only voluntary groups could educate the public about controversial issues like fluoridation and milk pasteurization. The Hall Commission apparently paid little mind to the Health League's brief, which, after all, was only one among hundreds. Moreover, by this time, the league wielded little influence, compared to many of the other organizations that submitted briefs, including the CMA, the Canadian Dental Association, the Canadian Tuberculosis Association, and the Canadian Red Cross. The Hall Commission ultimately recommended that universal coverage for medical services, prescription drugs, prostheses, and home care be instituted through federal-provincial cooperation, and that dental and optical services be available to children and indigent people.[66] The commission paid relatively little attention to prevention.[67] It did see an important role for voluntary organizations but made no specific mention of the Health League.[68]

Bates strongly opposed the Hall Commission's recommendations. In October 1964, he published an editorial that condemned health insurance's projected costs. "Erroneously called 'health insurance,'" he raged, such a measure "does not insure the health of anybody." "Such a procedure," he concluded, "should be called by its true name, sickness insurance. The only real health insurance rests in the application of the principles of preventive medicine."[69] Two years later, *Health* ran an article by two doctors complaining that the Hall report had paid insufficient attention to the views of doctors and that publicly funded health insurance would threaten the medical profession and the "rights of the patient" and would lead to mediocre medical care.[70] Another physician-authored article claimed that publicly funded health insurance would create so much work for general practitioners that they were at risk of an early death.[71] In 1968, National Health Week's theme was a jab at medicare: "Your Health Is YOUR Responsibility." In an editorial marking that event, Bates wrote: "There has been a great deal of confusion ... We talk about Health Insurance when we mean Sickness Insurance and plan to spend vast sums on trying to restore sick people to health when we should exert ourselves to keep people from getting sick at all."[72] In this, and in other writings, Bates appeared to regard publicly funded physician care as a direct affront to the league. In a 1970 letter to John Diefenbaker, who was then a member of Parliament, lobbying for an increase in the league's grant from the federal government Bates complained that the money he was asking for was "a modest sum" when "one considers that it is estimated that the cost of Medicare ... during the first year will be $2 billion."[73] Two years later, Bates complained to Senator William M. Benedickson that "the sum that we are receiving from the Government is completely out of line" compared to the "enormous expenditures on welfare and relief."[74]

Bates' obdurate opposition to medicare would win him support from the Canadian Medical Association. In May 1965, the CMA promoted Bates to senior membership, a distinction bestowed on "the Association's good and faithful servants."[75] In December of that year, the CMA officially endorsed the Health League.[76] But both the CMA and the league were on the losing side of this debate. Despite the high cost, publicly funded health insurance quickly gained the support of Canadians. The league's opposition to the measure helped ensure the organization's growing irrelevance.

The League Confronts the New Morality

While the league was embroiled with Toronto's federated fund and opposing health insurance, it was also making enemies in the press and within the public health community over sexually transmitted infections. Throughout the "swinging sixties," Bates argued that venereal disease needed to be treated as a moral problem, not a medical one. He blamed penicillin and the birth control pill (which became available in Canada in 1961) for "making promiscuity and prostitution comparatively safe."[77] He critiqued governments and public health workers for placing too much effort on contact tracing and treatment and not enough on inculcating moral values. In the early 1970s, when there was growing public alarm about the venereal disease problem, Bates tried to position the Health League to take charge of a renewed educational campaign. Although the league did receive funds to carry out a survey of venereal disease rates in Ontario, it was otherwise unsuccessful at leading the charge against venereal disease. By this point, the Health League had little standing in public health circles, and health departments preferred to launch their own educational campaigns.

The rift between the Health League, public health organizations, and the public on moral issues dated back to at least 1960, when Bates campaigned against the publication of a new paperback edition of *Lady Chatterley's Lover* by D.H. Lawrence. The novel – featuring a passionate love affair between an upper-class woman and the groundskeeper of her estate – had first been published in hardcover in 1928, but the release of the paperback edition in 1960 led to obscenity court cases in Britain and the United States as well as Canada.[78] In a news release and in *Health*, Bates described the book as "notorious and obnoxious," and he claimed that it appealed to those with a "penchant for the prurient and pornographic." He accused Canadian literary icons Morley Callaghan and Hugh MacLennan of contributing to "adultery, prostitution and venereal disease" because they had testified in favour of the work's literary merit.[79] In response, several newspapers, including the *Kingston Whig-Standard*, the *Oshawa Times*, and the *Peterborough Examiner* questioned why the Health League received public funds: "The literature and propaganda spread by this League and uttered by its director is so antiquated and reactionary that its validity could frequently be called into question." They described Bates as "a one-man league of decency."[80] The *Toronto Telegram* editorialized that "a health magazine seems to be taking in quite a bit of territory when it decides what the people should or shouldn't read."[81]

Not surprisingly, public opposition only strengthened Bates' resolve to educate Canadians about morality. In 1962, *Health* published a long piece by Jenkin Lloyd Jones, the editor of the *Tulsa Tribune*. In it, Jones praised Russia for its high moral standards, while condemning the communist economic system. He complained about the progressive education system in the United States, which, in his view, was not asking American students to do their best, and savaged modern art for being talentless and meaningless. Most serious of all, for Jones, was "our collapse of moral standards and the blunting of our capacity for righteous indignation." He condemned the lack of morality in American movies, asserting that Hollywood was increasing the sexual content of films to draw people away from their televisions. He was outraged by the easy availability of books like *Lady Chatterley's Lover* and Henry Miller's *Tropic of Cancer*.[82] The publication of this piece proved to be a significant success for *Health*: the league received more mail on this article than on any other it had published, and it had so many requests for reprints that it began offering them at the price of $2.50 for one hundred copies.[83] This response shows that Bates was in alignment with many of his readers, and that he was not a lone voice in expressing concern about the decline in moral standards. Indeed, as Mary Louise Adams has shown for a slightly earlier time period, many Canadians were worried about licentious magazines and pornographic literature.[84] But, it was clear that norms were changing, and Bates was the voice of a generation that was increasingly seen as irrelevant and backward.

By the late 1960s, Bates, who had made his career championing instruction in the "facts of life" as a VD-prevention measure, feared that sex education was being overemphasized. He fretted that sex education without moral direction would promote promiscuity, and in a 1969 *Health* editorial he claimed that "most sex delinquents know too much about sex already and not enough about the virtues of honesty and respect for one's parents."[85] In another editorial in *Health*, he urged doctors to take responsibility for teaching morality, claiming that the only way of reducing venereal disease was to reduce the contact rate: "Careful training of young people in the principles of morality is the real cure ... High moral standards are the ultimate answer."[86] To make his point that VD was a moral, not a medical, issue, Bates frequently claimed that "I've seen thousands of cases and I've never seen a clergyman with VD."[87]

Bates kept up a stream of criticism against developments that he believed would be harmful to morality. In this, he tended to view morally neutral or non-judgmental material on sexuality as actively immoral. When the Scarborough Board of Health recommended the distribution of contraceptives to young people in the spring of 1971, Bates wrote a furious letter to the *Toronto Telegram,* saying the board "had violated the principles of both education and health." He argued, "We should all be engaged in maintaining the moral and spiritual standards which have to be characteristic of our civilization."[88] In 1971, when the *Toronto Star* hosted a forum on venereal disease, Bates stood out from the other panellists by demanding a "moral crusade" against venereal disease, while others focused on the need for better education about sex in schools.[89]

To convince people of the importance of the issue, he often exaggerated the threat posed by these diseases in the antibiotic era. So, in a 1972 *Health* editorial, he claimed that gonorrhea and syphilis "are dangerous and fatal. Here are some of the results: blindness, deafness, insanity and infection of the bones. The ultimate result is too frequently disability or death."[90] Bates was not alone in such claims: a 1966 pamphlet produced by the federal government also underlined that untreated syphilis could lead to mental illness, paralysis, and heart disease.[91] In fact, while cases of latent syphilis continued to occur, there were few deaths as a result of the disease, and even serious complications were fairly unusual.[92] During the charmed time period between the development of antibiotics and the appearance of HIV/ AIDS, public health authorities expressed concern about infertility and other complications of venereal disease, but, overall, they took the view that it would be better to reduce the stigma associated with sexually transmitted diseases and emphasized the value of treatment.[93] Bates, meanwhile, was unwilling or unable to adjust his rhetoric to account for the vastly diminished danger of these diseases.

He was also unable to adjust his message to make it more appealing to a younger generation. Alan Petigny has argued that the sexual revolution was more about talk than action and that sexual behaviour actually changed relatively little from the 1950s to the 1970s.[94] Even so, the conversation about sex changed dramatically. The Kinsey Reports, published in 1948 and 1953, had made it clear that sexual behaviour did not match sexual norms, and by the 1960s the media was abuzz with discussions of premarital sex.[95] Yet Bates continued to utilize material that was entirely unsuited to baby boomers. He wanted to show the silent film *The End of the Road* (1919) to teenagers who had grown up on technicolour.[96] He also reprinted an editorial originally published in the *Toronto Globe* at the end of the First World War. Entitled "She Might Have Been Your Daughter," it told of the tragic marriage of a pure and noble young woman who was infected with venereal disease by her husband. "Never again was she to know happiness, or purity, or health. Children came to the home – one, two, three each with its own entail of sorrow and bearing, seen or unseen, the brand more inescapable, more inevitable, more mysteriously persistent than any brand of Cain."[97] Not only was the piece vastly out of date in terms of the likely consequences of venereal disease, but the rhetoric of female purity and the idea that women's happiness came from their maternal duties made the piece seem desperately out of touch in an era of second-wave feminism. Similarly, as part of National Health Week in 1974, the league put out a press release claiming that:

> gonorrhoea and syphilis are the most dangerous and long-lived of all diseases. Syphilis was named by Sir William Osler as "Captain of the Men of Death" and may be fatal if it is not treated. Death may come from such a variety of causes that the disease has also been called "The Great Imitator" because it hits every section of the human body ... Sometimes there are no symptoms for years, the first indication being a mental abnormality which ends in general paralysis of the insane which only a few years ago killed every victim.[98]

Again, such rhetoric bore little resemblance to medical reality in the antibiotic era. And the reference to the famous Canadian physician Sir William Osler, who had been dead for more than half a century, likely meant little to the younger generation. Such approaches accomplished little in the Health League's quest to put itself in the forefront of the fight against venereal disease.

In the interwar years, the Canadian Social Hygiene Council and then the Health League had conducted several influential surveys on venereal diseases. Bates believed that a new survey would be helpful, as he thought that the actual incidence of venereal disease was vastly underreported (the federal Department of Health and Welfare agreed).[99] It took years for the league to acquire the necessary funding to undertake the survey, but it was finally able to complete it in 1974.[100] In the end, only 40 percent of the physicians who were sent the survey responded (this compared to a 98 percent response rate when the CSHC had conducted a survey of Toronto physicians in 1929).[101] The sparse response may speak to growing survey fatigue, may reflect the Health League's declining influence, or may be the result of the growing desire of physicians to keep the confidentiality of their patients who were seeking treatment for venereal disease. It may also be that doctors did not see the point of the survey. At a 1968 meeting, when Bates raised the idea of a survey with the directors of VD clinics, they saw little advantage of such a plan, even though they acknowledged that the number of cases in their clinics was rising.[102]

If the league's outdated attitudes and approaches were not enough to compromise its role in new anti-VD campaigns, by this point, governments were increasingly carrying out their own initiatives. In the 1920s, government departments had been happy to have the CSHC undertake this educational work because the government had fewer available staff and was uneasy about undertaking education on venereal disease, but, by the 1970s, they felt that it was more effective to do this work in-house. They had far more staff and resources than they had had fifty years earlier, there was less stigma attached to sexually transmitted infections, and doing the work themselves meant that they could exert more control over the message. Over the course of the 1960s and 1970s, pamphlets became increasingly explicit and often included diagrams of genital organs. A succession of pamphlets issued by the federal government highlights the evolution in such materials and how they modified the strict moral stance that had characterized earlier pamphlets produced by the Health League. In 1960, a pamphlet produced by the federal government blamed prostitutes and "good time girls" for spreading disease, and warned that venereal disease "threatens marital happiness, endangers the health and future of innocent children, wives and husbands." A revised version produced in 1966 still warned that easy pick-ups spread disease, and cautioned that untreated syphilis could lead "to disaster," but the rhetoric was significantly toned down from the version published just six years earlier.[103] In 1971, a pamphlet acknowledged that societal mores were changing and that, in the past, attitudes towards premarital sex were "simple and rigid." Even so, the pamphlet argued, promiscuity had its dangers.[104] A pamphlet produced by National Health and Welfare a few years later dropped any discussion of promiscuity and emphasized the value of early treatment.[105] The league did not produce any pamphlets during this time period, because it never received any funding to do so. Yet, given Bates' oft-expressed views on the need for moral teaching, one can imagine any new pamphlet would have closely resembled those that the league had circulated in the interwar years.

By the late 1960s, it was clear that the provincial and federal governments saw little role for the Health League in VD education. In 1969, when Bates was writing to senior politicians trying to garner funds for a survey of the venereal disease problem, the minister of health and welfare for New Brunswick wrote back to say that the "Federal Department of National Health and Welfare is much better equipped to carry out statistical and epidemiological surveys in conjunction with the provinces," while the Ontario Minister of Health responded that "I believe that our Department is adequately equipped to carry out such studies."[106] Several provinces responded that adequate statistics were already gathered by the Dominion Bureau of Statistics and published by the Department of National Health and Welfare.[107] By the 1970s, Bates was an isolated voice, and public health authorities saw little role for the league in addressing rising rates of venereal disease. Moreover, the Health League's disgust at the more open discussion of sexuality and venereal disease had little resonance with young people, although it undoubtedly appealed to some cranky elders who were baffled by the younger generation and its new norms.

The Decline of the League's Supporters and Network

The league's decline was also hastened by its unwieldy structure. The organization's constitution and bylaws, and Bates' desire for a large network, meant that it technically had a huge collection of directors, honorary advisory directors, and committee members, but those individuals' lack of time and commitment meant that a small handful of individuals actually conducted the league's business.[108] The Honorary Advisory Board of Directors emblemizes this issue. The board was established in 1925 and existed throughout the league's lifetime, but it did not hold regular meetings, and its value was largely nominal.[109] Writing to Lady Eaton in 1949, Bates noted that "the only responsibility of these directors is that they may occasionally be asked for advice."[110] But, like many leaders of voluntary organizations, especially those in need of funds to carry out their work, Bates was eager to recruit elites who were willing to associate their name with the organization. He used the list of Honorary Advisory Board members to recruit other members, framing the organization as an exclusive club.[111]

Initially, Bates was able to entice members of Canada's elite to lend their names to his cause. Many members of the Honorary Advisory Board were part of Peter C. Newman's "Canadian establishment" and lived at the top of John Porter's "vertical mosaic."[112] Business leaders were particularly prominent, followed by elite doctors. An analysis of board members shows that they were primarily Protestant and tended to be members of elite sporting groups like golf, hunt, and yacht clubs, of the Freemasons, and of prestigious men's clubs, such as the York, Toronto, and National Clubs.[113] Membership in these men's clubs indicates wealth, as they required costly dues, but they also signify social cachet and recognition from other members of the elite.[114] Out of 195 known members of the Honorary Advisory Board, nearly half belonged to at least one of these three clubs.[115] Bates put a strong emphasis on recruiting businessmen for the advisory board, partly because he respected their success and knowledge, but also because he likely hoped that they could enhance the league's prominence – and perhaps its fortunes. Of the 161 Honorary Advisory Board members whose occupations are known, 55 percent (89 individuals) worked in business while 11 percent (17 individuals) worked in medicine. Among the businessmen were 57 company presidents, 30 chairmen of boards, and 7 vice-presidents. The rest were identified as founders, partners, board managers, chief executive officers, vice-chairs, managing directors, general managers, or senior consultants. Some of these men led major corporations. When A.C. Ashforth joined the Honorary Advisory Board, he was president of the Toronto-Dominion Bank, while H.D. Burns joined during his tenure as chairman of the board at the Bank of Nova Scotia.[116] S.G. Dobson, president of the Royal Bank, served on the board, albeit briefly, as did Gordon Ball, a president and CEO of the Bank of Montreal.[117] The board also included presidents of major insurance firms – the Confederation Life Association, the Imperial Life Insurance Company of Canada, and Sun Life Assurance.[118] E.P. Taylor, president of the massive Argus Corporation, the man whom Peter C. Newman identified as the avatar of the Canadian establishment, served on the Honorary Advisory Board for three decades, from 1950 onward.[119]

Another rich avenue for analysis is the generational shift in membership, which helps to explain the Health League's decline. As Figure 20 indicates, most Honorary Advisory Board members were born between 1860 and 1889. Bates, born in 1885, built associations with people of his own generation and the one before, who came of age in the late Victorian and Edwardian eras.[120] As the older generation passed away or retired from active involvement in the league, Bates was unable to replace them with younger people.

The period between 1945 and 1954 saw an increase in members on the Honorary Advisory Board. But, starting in the late 1950s, more board

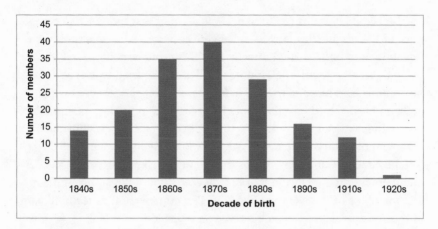

Figure 20 Years of birth of Health League of Canada Honorary Advisory Board members
Sources: See note 113.

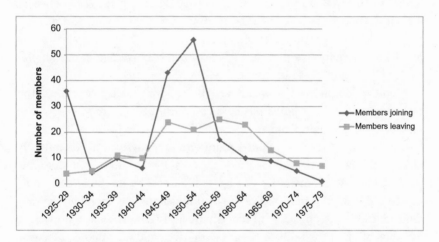

Figure 21 Members joining and leaving the Health League's Honorary Advisory Board, 1925–79
Sources: 1929 CSHC Annual Report, LAC, MG28, I332, vol. 9, file 14; minutes of the CSHC Annual Meetings for 11 December 1925, 7 May 1926, 13 June 1927, and , 14 June 1928 (LAC, MG28, I332, vol. 10, files 23–26); "Report of the Nominating Committee," 1930, LAC, MG28, I332, vol. 10, file 31; a list of Honourary Advisory Board members from one issue of each year of *Health* magazine (1933–81).

members were dying or resigning than joining. Though Bates remained active into his ninetieth year, his generation trickled out of public life over his last two decades, and his Honorary Advisory Board did not recuperate fully from those losses.[121]

The National Board of Directors was a larger and more active component of the league's leadership. At any given time, the league was to have twenty-five to one hundred directors.[122] This group was supposed to meet once a year.[123] As with the Honorary Advisory Board, involvement could be nominal, and many of the 292 listed members are largely invisible in the archival files. Yet others contributed a great deal to the league's functioning.[124] The National Board of Directors was composed of a slightly different demographic than the Honorary Advisory Board. For one, it included fewer "establishment" Canadians. While 156 out of 195 Honorary Advisory Board members merited inclusion in *The Canadian Who's Who*, only 122 out of 292 members of the National Board of Directors were thus featured; and, of those national board members who were listed in *Who's Who*, far fewer belonged to elite clubs.[125] Moreover, the percentage of business people was lower: only 17 percent of national board members were in business. These findings confirm that the Honorary Advisory Board was largely a networking body, while the national board was meant to run the league. Not surprisingly, then, the largest known occupational group on the national board was physicians. Twenty-five percent of board members were doctors, supplemented by a handful of nurses and dentists.[126]

Membership on the National Board of Directors could be nominal. The real support for the league's business came from two committees, whose members were drawn from the national board – the National Executive Committee and the Sub-Executive Committee. Analysis of the (admittedly incomplete) files on these bodies indicates that the Sub-Executive Committee had 142 distinct members during its lifetime, and the Executive Committee had 238.[127] From these, we can distinguish the core membership who ran the league. It is possible to identify thirty-five individuals who were a member of either or both of these committees and attended eighteen or more documented meetings. Interestingly, this list did not line up with the organization's executive, indicating that some executive appointments were more nominal than active. All presidents but one made the list, as did some vice-presidents, while few treasurers did. These individuals' service ranged from seven to fifty-four years, with an average length of seventeen and a half years.[128]

This core group was an interesting cross-section of the national board. Some were leaders in large businesses: such members included A.C. Ashforth, a president of the TD Bank, H.H. Bishop, vice-president of the Commercial Life Assurance Company, and R.C. Berkinshaw, president of Goodyear Tire and Rubber Company of Canada.[129] Others were prominent physicians: Dr. J.W.S. McCullough was the chief officer of health for Ontario from 1910 to 1935, while Drs. F.O. Wishart and John R. Brown were both professors at University of Toronto.[130] The Health League's long-time president, Justice William Renwick Riddell, a judge on Ontario's Supreme Court, was included as well.[131] Yet, several other of these core members did not enjoy such fame. Only sixteen of the thirty-five people on this list merited inclusion in *Canadian Who's Who*.[132]

The most notable thing about this group is the number of women. Only 10 percent of the members of the National Board of Directors, from which this group was drawn, were women. By contrast, 31 percent of this core, committed group were women. Many of these women were distinguished professionals. Helen Cleveland, for example, was an Investment Advisor at Wood Gundy – she opened the first-ever "Women's Department" at Wood Gundy and after the Second World War ran a series of lectures educating women about investing.[133] Appropriately, she served on the Health League's Business Committee, which existed partially to advise on investments.[134] Mary McNab came from a wealthy family but worked as an organizer with the Trades and Labour Congress in Hamilton and Toronto.[135] She was a member of the Program Division of the Executive Committee and joined the league's 1963 deputation to the National Agency Review Committee.[136] Reginae Tait, at various points in her career, served as national president of the Imperial Order Daughters of the Empire, an executive member of the National Action Committee on the Status of Women, and governor of Frontier College.[137] She also served as a vice-president of the league, and, briefly, as president of the organization in 1981.[138]

Clearly, the league was able to recruit talented and successful people, including many women, to serve on its various boards and committees. The elite status of so many of these individuals probably helps to account for the fact that the league represented its ideal health citizen as white and middle class, and that its efforts to reach out to the working classes were often patronizing. The generational homogeneity of this group was also striking. As Bates himself aged, these people, drawn largely from his own generation, were increasingly difficult to replace. By the 1960s, the league would be seriously weakened by the decline in the number of people involved. From the late 1950s onward, the league's leadership was aware that the organization had structural problems: attendance at meetings was poor, the number of board members was declining, and it was finding it increasingly difficult to recruit enough volunteers to staff committees.[139] Initially, the league attempted to deal with these problems by weeding out inactive members and ensuring that there was enough parking at meetings, but these strategies met with limited success.[140]

During the 1960s, the league reorganized its committee structure to try to improve the level of participation. Bates seemed to want to deal with the situation by appointing even more committees, but, when the league reached out for professional advice, it was told to shrink the board of directors and reduce the number of committees.[141] The executive, perhaps missing the point, appointed a new committee to study these recommendations.[142] In the meantime, the league's staff was also shrinking. By the mid-1960s, the only full-time time people working for the league in management or professional positions were Bates and Mabel Ferris. The only other professional staff person left was Murdoch McIver, the organizer of Health Week, and he was being paid less than a third of what he had received in the 1950s and early 1960s, indicating that he was probably working only on a very limited part-time basis.[143] Bates was so central to the league's operation that the board seriously considered shutting the organization down when he was incapacitated by illness in 1966 and not expected to recover.[144] Bates did return to work, but the league continued to struggle to recruit and retain staff and volunteers.

After Bates' death in 1975, the Executive Committee considered shutting down the league and using its monies to establish a Gordon Bates Foundation for Preventive Medicine at the University of Toronto. Arguably, that option would have been ideal: it would have secured Bates' legacy and afforded Ferris a well-deserved retirement. In the end, though, the executive opted to continue the league, which crumbled over the next five years.[145] A few months after the executive decided to continue, it become apparent that the financial situation was dire. A meeting resolved that "the annual audited statement be approved, with the suggestion that the item 'Bad Debts' be transferred to 'Miscellaneous Expense' in order to avoid criticism from our supporters."[146] Ferris took over the league after Bates' death, but in 1980 she retired due to health problems. Donald F. Damude, a past president of the Ontario Public Health Association, replaced her. Damude's background was in veterinary public health, and he does not appear to have had any previous connection with the Health League. As a result of the interest and enthusiasm of a new board president, David M. Garner, the league turned its attention to eating disorders. This new work resulted in a slight increase in grants, and in 1986 the league established the National Eating Disorder Information Centre in collaboration with the Toronto General Hospital's Eating Disorder Day Centre.[147] It also continued to educate people about sexually transmitted infections. But in 1987, after conducting a review process that described the group as "an anacronysm [sic] – out of touch," the federal government withdrew the small grants that the league had continued to receive.[148] The organization went dormant, although, over the past several years, it has been trying to reinvent itself to focus on the health threats posed by international air travel. It remains to be seen if this will be successful.[149]

***

Beginning as far back as the late 1950s, there were clear signs that the Health League was in decline. Although its boards required little involvement, it was increasingly difficult to recruit people to serve on them: the boards greyed alongside Bates and Ferris. The league took no steps to renew its leadership: Bates and Ferris continued to be the lifeblood of the organization and failed to find and nurture possible successors. Bates' intransigence and inability to change further contributed to the problem. All of the elite names the league had mustered could not prevent its expulsion from the United Community Fund – Bates' combativeness had driven a wedge between the fund and the league. The league's support for the teaching of morality made it a laughing stock among young people (insofar as they were aware of its existence), while public health officials increasingly distanced themselves from it. Its opposition to publicly funded health insurance also alienated the organization from possible new supporters. The loss of support from the federated fund meant that the league struggled on with few financial resources. By the late 1960s, it had far fewer prominent allies in the worlds of business and public health. It muddled on through the late 1960s and early 1970s, but it no longer had the same prominence or influence. By the late 1960s, *Health* was publishing only sporadically, and it stopped altogether from 1969 to 1972. The league stopped holding its annual meeting and publishing an annual report. National Immunization Week ended in 1971. While National Health Week continued, it did not receive nearly as much publicity and advertising as it had in its heyday in the 1940s, 1950s, and early 1960s.[150] While the league briefly transformed itself in the 1980s to provide education about eating disorders, its major endeavours had ceased by the early 1970s.

Conclusion
The Successes and Failures of Preventive Health

In the early years of the twentieth century, the "new public health" shifted attention away from the environmental causes of disease towards the individual. This shift involved the embrace of the "entrepreneurial self" – an individual who was expected to take responsibility for his or her own health – and the notion of the health citizen. It assumed that those who had not assumed the duties of health citizenship were in some way responsible if they fell ill. The Health League of Canada, first established as an anti-venereal disease organization, was in a perfect position to take advantage of this transition: it believed that adopting the health behaviours advised by doctors and other health experts, including dentists and nutritionists, was crucial to ensuring ongoing good health. As a result, it urged parents, especially mothers, to vaccinate their children and feed them well; workers to avoid colds; and executives to care for their heart health. These new health behaviours could be time consuming: they involved careful meal planning, exercise, and regular trips to physicians and dentists. The Health League was not alone in urging these activities, but it was an important voice in trying to convince Canadians to change their behaviours and assume individual responsibility for their health. While the league itself did not survive, the ideology that it played a role in fostering has continued: Canadians are still urged to carefully monitor their health habits and behaviours in order to live longer (and happier) lives and to continue to contribute to the country through productive work.

Throughout its history, including its early years as the Canadian National Council for Combatting Venereal Disease and the Canadian Social Hygiene Council (CSHC), the league believed that good health included living what it considered to be a moral life. It campaigned against the sexual double standard, urging men to suppress their urges for the good of the race and of the country. It encouraged parents to be open with their children about sex, believing that lack of knowledge was an important factor behind why young people went astray. Heavily influenced by the eugenics movement, particularly its more positive variants, it urged healthy recreational and physical activities to help guarantee the health of future generations. Finally, it tried to persuade those who were already infected with venereal disease to get treated. The expansion of venereal disease clinics at this time significantly reduced the number of Canadians infected with secondary and tertiary syphilis. Fewer people suffered from mental illness, locomotor ataxia, and other complications of later-stage syphilis. Reducing the suffering associated with this serious disease represented an important victory for public health, although it came at a cost in terms of promoting a very narrow vision of what sexuality should look like.

The lessening of the venereal disease problem, and the success it had had in educating Canadians about the issue, encouraged the CSHC to branch into new areas of health education. Indeed, the ideology of social hygiene, which aimed to improve the race by combining medicine and morality, made it easy for the CSHC, and then the Health League, to extend its advocacy into other arenas. In the late 1920s, the council partnered with the Toronto Public Health Department to encourage parents to have their children toxoided against diphtheria, a disease that was then a major cause of child death. While its methods of persuasion drew primarily on guilt and fear, the CSHC/Health League did persuade many parents to have their children vaccinated, and, as a result, in 1940, Toronto became one of the first major world centres to not have a child die from diphtheria over the course of a year. The CSHC/Health League became an important voice in the campaign for mandatory milk pasteurization and was an important player in Ontario's decision to mandate pasteurization throughout the province in 1938. It began a more general health education program through its magazine *Health* (which it established in 1933), substantial radio programming, and regular press releases. While its message was often highly moralistic and judgmental, much of its advice was sound and may have encouraged Canadians to learn more about health and to take measures that would protect their health and that of their children.

At the same time, it encouraged a mindset that assumed that health was an individual or family responsibility rather than viewing ill health as a consequence of economic and social inequality.

With the outbreak of the Second World War, the league was able to consolidate the gains it had made during the difficult years of the Great Depression. Its government grants increased, and its decision to join Toronto's federated fund brought about a period of relative financial security for the organization. During the war, it renewed its anti–venereal disease campaign, although, unlike its earlier campaign, which had been influenced by figures in the feminist movement, the league placed more blame on women for spreading the disease. Encouraged by the new treatments developed during the war, especially penicillin, it launched a major campaign encouraging Canadians to be tested and treated. After the war, it urged provinces to pass legislation requiring premarital syphilis testing. Even though it had started as an anti–venereal disease group, there were already some small signs that other public health authorities regarded the league as too moralistic on this issue and were growing hesitant about cooperating with it.

But, by this point, the Health League had several other important and much less controversial projects on the go. Like the Red Cross, Women's Institutes, and some other groups, the league launched a major nutrition education program during the war. This program followed the lead of the Canadian Council on Nutrition and later the Nutritional Services Division of the Department of National Health and Welfare. The league also established an Industrial Health Division, which was geared towards reducing absenteeism in the workforce. In this program, it assumed that employers did their best by their employees and that workers who were ill largely had themselves to blame. The league also launched National Immunization Week and National Health Week – major publicity campaigns that encouraged Canadians to vaccinate their children and to take personal responsibility for their health. In all of these programs, the league continued to take a moralistic stance towards health: it encouraged Canadians to adopt menus and health habits that would increase their value as citizens by making them more productive workers. At the same time, it urged Canadians to get involved in their communities: it hoped to create a collective commitment to health by getting people to attend nutrition classes, by encouraging their involvement in Health League branches, and by persuading organizations such as women's groups and male-dominated service clubs to sponsor health-related speakers and programming.

From the 1940s to the early 1960s, the league had several notable successes. National Immunization Week and National Health Week were important events on the public health calendar. *Health* magazine increased in size, published more regularly, and provided considerable material for press releases, which the league sent to media outlets across the country. The organization used its magazine and annual events to argue that Canadians needed to visit their doctors and dentists regularly, to eat better, to exercise regularly, and to take time for rest and relaxation.

The campaign for water fluoridation represented a mixed success for the league. Bates had long been interested in dental health, and the league was quick to support fluoridation. While the league played an important role in Toronto's successful fluoridation referendum in 1962, its support for the controversial measure drove a wedge between it and Toronto's United Community Fund. This rift, combined with Bates' belief that voluntary health groups like his own were being disadvantaged by the federated fund movement, and his unwillingness to cooperate with the fund's regular processes, eventually resulted in the league's expulsion from the fund, with devastating consequences for the league's financial health.

By the 1960s, it was clear that the league was increasingly out of touch. As rates of venereal disease began to increase in the late 1960s and early 1970s, the league resurrected materials it had used in the 1920s, with little recognition that the cultural and sexual landscape had changed considerably over the intervening half century. The league also showed itself out of touch in its opposition to medicare – which Bates viewed as "sickness insurance" rather than health insurance – although that opposition was at least consistent with the league's emphasis on the importance of individual responsibility for health. Yet, the league's opposition to a measure that rapidly obtained favour among Canadians alienated potential supporters. Moreover, the league itself was shrinking as the generations that had supported it were dying off or retiring from public life. In the 1960s and 1970s, it found it difficult to recruit new members, and its vast committee structure shrank while its staff diminished due to lack of funds.

Clearly, the league had a mixed record. Even so, its story has much to tell us about the history of voluntary groups in Canada and of public health. When the Canadian Social Hygiene Council began its work, the federal Department of Health had just been created and many provincial departments were still small. As a result, there was a real role for the council, and later the league, to play in health education. But, as time went on, and governments significantly expanded their public health apparatus, there was less space or use for an organization like the Health League. Although Bates persisted in his belief that voluntary groups could best carry out this work, the function was increasingly taken over by the state. At the same time, the federated fundraising movement that evolved in the middle decades of the twentieth century was an awkward fit for health organizations, especially those with a national mandate (or, in the case of the Health League, national ambitions). The league was also disadvantaged by the establishment of disease-focused charities – the Canadian Cancer Society, the Canadian Heart Foundation, and others – which were able to play on people's emotions more effectively than could an organization like the Health League, with its broad attention to preventive health. The history of the Health League also teaches us how important it is for voluntary groups to renew their leadership over time: the league's long reliance on Gordon Bates and Mabel Ferris and its growing inability to recruit new board members meant that little by way of new ideas or energy was being injected into the organization.

Preventive health has much to commend it. Clearly, it is much better to avoid getting sick than to cure an illness once it has struck. The Health League's efforts to encourage people with venereal disease to get tested and treated and its campaigns in favour of childhood immunization likely reduced the burden of disease and suffering. But its promotion of healthy diets, regular exercise, and leisure and relaxation were, at times, shockingly ignorant of the realities of poverty. Such advice fed into a tendency to blame the sick for having failed in their health responsibilities, ignoring the fact that much ill health was the result of poverty, trauma, and other forms of social marginalization. The league's moralistic hectoring of Canadians to assume the responsibilities of health citizenship demanded that people place health above pleasure and valued responsibility over freedom. Its labelling of people who did not assume these responsibilities as ignorant or apathetic was condescending and paternalistic. Also, the value that the league attached to medical expertise undermined other understandings of what health could be: most Canadians likely had their own views of what it meant to have a healthy body and a healthy mind, and might prefer to follow the advice of their families, respect the traditions of their culture, or simply be true to their own sense of self. The Health League generally did not recognize that these alternative understandings existed, but even if it had, they would have been no match for its unshakable faith in medical expertise. Indeed, the history of the Health League exemplifies the rise in medical power and prestige, the growing emphasis on "health citizenship," and the increased complexity of the interaction between the state and voluntary organizations in the middle decades of the twentieth century.

Notes

Introduction

1 Steven Bratman, *Health Food Junkies: Orthorexia Nervosa – Overcoming the Obsession with Healthful Eating* (New York: Broadway, 2001); Moyra Sidell, Linda Jones, Jeanne Katz, Alyson Peberdy, and Jenny Douglas, eds., *Debates and Dilemmas in Promoting Health* (Houndsmills, UK: Palgrave Macmillan, 2003). Michael Fitzpatric also provides compelling accounts of undue anxiety in his *Tyranny of Health* (New York and London: Routledge, 2001).

2 Ruth A. Lanius, Eric Vermetten, and Claire Pain, eds., *The Impact of Early Live Trauma on Health and Disease: The Hidden Epidemic* (Cambridge: Cambridge University Press, 2010); Michael Marmot and Jessica Allen, "The Social Determinants of Health Equity," *American Journal of Public Health* 104, Supplement 4 (2014): S514–16.

3 For scholarship on the new public health, see Alison Bashford, *Imperial Hygiene: A Critical History of Colonialism, Nationalism and Public Health* (Basingstoke, UK: Palgrave Macmillan, 2014), 11; Christopher Sellers, "The Dearth of the Clinic: Lead, Air, and Agency in Twentieth-Century America," *Journal of the History of Medicine and Allied Sciences* 58, 3 (2003): 255–91; Hibert Hill, *The New Public Health* (New York: Macmillan, 1916).

4 Sarah Glassford, "Marching as to War: The Canadian Red Cross Society" (PhD diss., York University, 2007); Canada, Royal Commission on Health Services, *Voluntary Health Organizations in Canada 1965* (Ottawa: Queen's Printer, 1966); Geoffrey Reaume, *Lyndhurst: Canada's First Rehabilitation Centre for People with Spinal Cord Injuries, 1945–1998* (Montreal and Kingston: McGill-Queen's University Press, 2007); Shirley Tillotson, *Contributing Citizens: Modern Charitable Fundraising and the Making of the Welfare State* (Vancouver: UBC Press, 2008).

5 Minutes of the Canadian Social Hygiene Council, Library and Archives Canada (hereafter LAC), MG28, I322, vol. 1, file 10.

6 Christina Simmons, "African-Americans and Sexual Victorianism in the Social Hygiene Movement, 1910–1940," *Journal of the History of Sexuality* 4, 1 (1993): 51–75.

7 Kristin Luker, "Sex, Social Hygiene and the State: The Double-edged Sword of Social Reform," *Theory* 27 (1998): 612.

8 David Evans, "Tackling the 'Hideous Scourge': The Creation of the Venereal Disease Treatment Centres in Twentieth-Century Britain," *Social History of Medicine* 5, 3 (1992): 414–15.

9 Greta Jones, *Social Hygiene in Twentieth Century Britain* (London: Croom Helm, 1986).

10 Gordon Bates, "The Value of Social Hygiene to a Community," *Public Health Journal* (Canada) 17, 1 (1926): 17–26.

11 "Canada's Unique Crusade for Better Health," 1957, LAC, MG28, I332, vol. 1, file 1.

12 Laura Lovett's and Erica Boudreau's work on "fitter family" contests underlines the importance of these aspects of positive eugenics. Laura Lovett, *Conceiving the Future: Pronatalism, Reproduction and the Family in the United States, 1890–1938* (Chapel Hill: University of North Carolina Press, 2007), 131–62; Erica Bicchieri Boudreau, "'Yes, I Have a Goodly Heritage': Health versus Hereditary in the Fitter Family Contests, 1920–1928," *Journal of Family History* 30, 4 (2005): 366–87. The diversity of the eugenics movement is well described in Alison Bashford and Philippa Levine's edited collection *The Oxford Handbook on the History of Eugenics* (New York: Oxford University Press, 2010).

13 Frank Dikötter, "Race Culture: Recent Perspectives on the History of Eugenics," *American Historical Review* 103, 2 (1998): 467.

14 Philippa Levine and Alison Bashford, "Introduction: Eugenics and the Modern World," in Bashford and Levine, *Oxford Handbook of the History of Eugenics*, 3–24.

15 Alan Peterson and Deborah Lupton, *The New Public Health: Health and Self in the Age of Risk* (London: Sage, 1997), xiii.

16 James Colgrove, *State of Immunity: The Politics of Vaccination in Twentieth-Century America* (Berkeley: University of California Press, 2006), 94.

17 John Burnham, "American Medicine's Golden Age: What Happened to It?" *Science* 215 (March 1982): 1474–79; Paul Starr, *The Social Transformation of American Medicine* (New York: Basic Books, 1982).

18 John Ward and Christian Warren, *Silent Victories: The History and Practice of Public Health in Twentieth-Century America* (Oxford: Oxford University Press, 2007); Roy Porter, *The Greatest Benefit to Mankind* (New York: W.W. Norton, 1997); Ivan Illich, *Medical Nemesis* (New York: Pantheon, 1976); Thomas McKeown, *The Role of Medicine: Dream, Mirage or Nemesis* (London: Nuffield Provincial Hospitals Trust, 1976).

19 Statistics Canada, Life Expectancy at Birth, by Sex, by Province (table), http://www.statcan.gc.ca/tables-tableaux/sum-som/l01/cst01/health26-eng.htm.

20 David Gagan and Rosemary Gagan, *For Patients of Moderate Means: A Social History of the Voluntary Public General Hospital in Canada, 1890–1950* (Montreal and Kingston: McGill-Queen's University Press, 2002).

21 The growth of pre-payment plans began in the 1930s and expanded rapidly after the Second World War. C. David Naylor, *Private Practice, Public Payment: Canadian*

Medicine and the Politics of Health Insurance, 1911–1966 (Montreal and Kingston: McGill-Queen's University Press, 1986), 100–1, 160–62.

22 Dorothy Porter, *Health Citizenship: Essays in Social Medicine and Biomedical Politics* (Berkeley: University of California Press, 2011).

23 Dominique Clement has traced the origins of the rights revolution in *Canada's Rights Revolution: Social Movements and Social Change* (Vancouver: UBC Press, 2008). Earlier conceptions of citizenship as a "contribution" can be seen in Shirley Tillotson, *Contributing Citizens*. Of course, several scholars have also pointed out the extent to which Canada's welfare state was also built on the principle of claiming rights on behalf of citizenship. See, for example, Lara Campbell, *Respectable Citizens: Gender, Family and Unemployment in Ontario's Great Depression* (Toronto: University of Toronto Press, 2009) and James G. Snell, *The Citizen's Wage: The State and the Elderly in Canada, 1900–1951* (Toronto: University of Toronto Press, 1996). Catherine Gidney argues that the shift towards the rights of citizenship can be traced back to the interwar years and sees this coming to greater fruition by the 1960s. Catherine Gidney, *Tending the Student Body: Youth, Health and the Modern University* (Toronto: University of Toronto Press, 2015).

24 Robert Putnam, *Bowling Alone: The Collapse and Revival of American Community* (New York: Simon and Shuster, 2000), 93–95.

25 Tillotson, *Contributing Citizens;* Len Kuffert, *A Great Duty: Canadian Responses to Modern Life and Mass Culture 1939–1967* (Montreal and Kingston: McGill-Queen's University Press, 2003); Patricia Roy, *The Triumph of Citizenship: The Japanese and Chinese in Canada, 1941–1967* (Vancouver: UBC Press, 2008); Veronica Strong-Boag, Sherrill Grace, Joan M. Anderson, and Avigail Eisenberg, eds., *Painting the Maple: Essays on Race, Gender, and the Construction of Canada* (Vancouver: UBC Press, 1999); José Igartua, *The Other Quiet Revolution: National Identities in English Canada, 1945–1971* (Vancouver: UBC Press, 2007); Matthew Hayday, *Bilingual Today, United Tomorrow: Canadian Federalism and Official Languages in Education* (Montreal and Kingston: McGill-Queen's University Press, 2005).

26 Gordon Bates, "Canada's Destiny," *Health,* Winter 1941–42, 3.

27 Gordon Bates, "Health Is Your Business," *Health,* November/December 1952, 33.

28 See, for example, extensive correspondence with Christian Smith in LAC, MG28, I332, vol. 45, file 21.

29 Bashford, *Imperial Hygiene* 5.

30 A large literature has drawn attention to how the Chinese, Indigenous people, and other racial minority groups were seen as sources of contagion. Maureen Lux, *Separate Beds: A History of Indian Hospitals in Canada* (Toronto: University of Toronto Press, 2016); Adele Perry, *On the Edge of Empire: Gender, Race and the Making of British Columbia, 1849–1871* (Toronto: University of Toronto Press, 2001), 110–23; Mona Gleason, "Race, Class and Health: School Medical Inspection and 'Healthy' Children in British Columbia, 1890–1930," *Canadian Bulletin of Medical History* 19 (2002): 95–112; Mary-Ellen Kelm, "Diagnosing the Discursive Indian: Medicine, Gender and the 'Dying Race,'" *Ethnohistory* 52, 2 (2005): 371–406; Megan Davis, "Night Soil, Cesspools, and Smelly Hogs on the Streets: Sanitation, Race and Governance in Early British Columbia," *Histoire sociale/Social History* 38, 75 (2005):

1–35; James B. Waldram, D. Ann Herring, and T. Kue Young, *Aboriginal Health in Canada* (Toronto: University of Toronto Press, 2006).

31 See, for example, a letter from Kingsley Kay, acting chief of the Division of Industrial Hygiene in the Department of National Health and Welfare, to Gordon Bates, 17 April 1941, saying that "the committee's value would be diminished if representatives from outside of Toronto were to feel that the nucleus committee was mainly responsible for the Committee's policy and work ... I believe that one or two active meetings per year, at which a scheme of work would be laid out and some of which would be handled by each representative in his own territory would have advantages over advising representatives far afield of plans that had been decided without their direct participation." LAC, RG29, vol. 617, file 343-10-11.

32 Bethany Philpott, "The Greater Vancouver Health League" (unpublished paper, 2014).

33 Bethany Philpott, "Quebec Division" (unpublished paper, 2014).

34 "Biographical Sketch of Gordon Bates," n.d. [c. 1975], LAC, MG28, I332, vol. 79, file 19.

35 Letter from Christian Smith to Gordon Bates, 24 October 1945, LAC, MG28, I332, vol. 45, file 19.

36 For example, Maurice Seymour, the commissioner of public health in Saskatchewan, wrote that he did not see a need for a branch of the CNCCVD in that province, although he appreciated receiving educational materials. He wrote, "the complicated programme which you have outlined in the letter to me, may be very suitable to Toronto with its large industrial works and extensive aggregations of workers, but it would not be suitable at all to an agricultural, sparsely settled Province, such as is Saskatchewan." Letter from Maurice Seymour to Gordon Bates, 3 February 1921, LAC, MG28, I332, vol. 45, file 9. Later attempts to organize in Saskatchewan faltered on similar grounds, with local people feeling that the Health League was insufficiently attentive to the unique conditions in their province. See LAC, RG29, vol 45, file 16 and 17. In Winnipeg as well, local leaders complained that the league was insufficiently attentive to local conditions. Letter from Lillian Halfpenny to Gordon Bates, 2 February 1926, LAC, RG29, vol. 46, file 14. When Charles Fenwick made a trip to Nova Scotia and New Brunswick to re-invigorate league organizing there, he discovered that "they are most courteous and willing to accept suggestions as long as the suggestion is not one of trying to show them how things are done in other parts of Canada and as to how we think they should do their own work." "Visit to New Brunswick by Dr. Fenwick," n.d. [early 1930s], LAC, MG28, I332, vol. 70, file 6. A trip to the Maritimes by another League worker a decade latter also confirmed that people had little interest in being dictated to by Toronto. "Report of Field Trip, March 9–22, 1947," LAC, MG28, I332, vol. 70, file 10.

37 Lynda Jessup, "The Group of Seven and the Tourist Landscape in Western Canada, or The More Things Change," *Journal of Canadian Studies* 37, 1 (2002): 144–79; Sylvia Bashevkin, *True Patriot Love: The Politics of Canadian Nationalism* (Toronto: Oxford University Press, 1991).

38 The lack of female volunteers is particularly noticeable in contrast to the Hospital for Sick Children, which mobilized dozens of volunteers in the same time period. David Wright, *SickKids: The History of the Hospital for Sick Children* (Toronto: University of Toronto Press, 2017), 212–14.

39 For more detailed information about the Health League's administrative structure, see Sara Wilmshurst, "'The Dust-up which Dr. Bates Appears Intent on Creating': Changes in the Health League of Canada's Support, Funding, and Status, 1944–1975" (MA thesis, University of Guelph, 2015).

40 Sidney Katz, "The Doctor Who Won't Take 'NO' for an Answer," *Maclean's*, 26 November 1955, 12.

41 Michael Bliss, "Pure Books on Avoided Subjects: Pre-Freudian Sexual Ideas in Canada," *Historical Papers/Communications historiques* 5, 1 (1970): 89–108; Christabelle Sethna, "The Facts of Life: The Sex Instruction of Ontario Public School Children, 1900–1950" (PhD diss., University of Toronto, 1995).

42 CSHC 10th Annual Report, July 1929, LAC, MG28, I332, vol. 9, file 4; Voluntary Committee of the Senate and the House of Commons, 1973–76, and letter from Mabel Ferris to Stanley Haidasz, 30 June 1976, LAC, MG28, I332, vol. 150, file 19.

43 HLC Report for the Year 1958, LAC, MG28, I332, vol. 10, file 8.

44 Health League of Canada, Thirty-Fourth Annual Meeting, 30 November–2 December 1953, LAC, MG28, I332, vol. 10, file 4.

45 G.D.W. Cameron, "The Department of National Health and Welfare," in *The Federal and Provincial Health Services in Canada*, ed. R.D. Defries (Toronto: Canadian Public Health Association, 1962), 7, 16.

46 W.G. Brown, "The Ontario Department of Health," in ibid., 75–87. Also see the annual reports of the Department of Health of Ontario. In 1956, for example, the department distributed more than a million pieces of literature in addition to showing films at the Canadian National Exhibition, Ottawa's Central Canada Exposition, and the International Plowing Match in Brooklin. *The 32nd Annual Report of the Department of Health, Ontario for the Year 1956* (Toronto: Ontario Department of Health, 1957), 7–8.

47 "The Health League of Canada, A Brief to Justify the Adequate Financing of Their Organization ...," n.d. [c. 1957], LAC, MG28, I322, vol. 128, file 10; Health League of Canada, *National Voluntary Health Associations in Canada* (Toronto: Health League of Canada, 1956).

48 Angus McLaren and Arlene Tigar McLaren, *The Bedroom and the State: The Changing Practices and Politics of Contraception and Abortion in Canada, 1880–1997* (Toronto: Oxford University Press, 1997); Gary Kinsman and Patrizia Gentile, *The Canadian War on Queers: National Security as Sexual Regulation* (Vancouver: UBC Press, 2010); Tom Warner, *Never Going Back: A History of Queer Activism in Canada* (Toronto: University of Toronto Press, 2002).

49 "Ontario's First Chief Provincial Health Officer," http://resources.cpha.ca/CPHA/ThisIsPublicHealth/profiles/item.php?l=e&i=1392; Gordon Bates, "A Tribute to the late J.W.S. McCullough," *Health*, December 1940–January 1941, 102; Heather MacDougall, "Creating Medicare," http://www.historymuseum.ca/cmc/exhibitions/hist/medicare/medic-5h18e.shtml; Heather MacDougall, *Activists and Advocates: Toronto's Health Department, 1883–1983* (Toronto: Dundurn Press, 1990), 26–31.

50 Catherine Carstairs and Rachel Elder, "Expertise, Health and Popular Opinion: Debating Water Fluoridation, 1945–1980," *Canadian Historical Review* 89, 3 (2008): 348.

51 Defries, *The Federal and Provincial Health Services in Canada*, 6; Eugene Vayda and Raisa B. Deber, "The Canadian Health-Care System: A Developmental Overview," in

Canadian Health Care and the State: A Century of Evolution, ed. C. David Naylor (Montreal and Kingston: McGill-Queen's University Press, 1992), 128.

52 Kirsta McCraken, "Crumbling Communities: Declining Service Club Membership," *Active History,* 12 November 2012, http://activehistory.ca/2012/11/crumbling -communities-declining-service-club-membership/; Elections Canada, "Estimation of Voter Turnout by Age Group and Gender at the 2011 Federal General Election," http://www.elections.ca/content.aspx?section=res&dir=rec/part/estim/41ge& document=report41&lang=e; Reginald Bibby and Merlin Brinkerhoff, "Circulation of the Saints, 1966–1990: New Data, New Reflections," *Journal for the Scientific Study of Religion* 33, 3 (1994): 273–80.

53 "Dr. Gordon A. Bates: Founder of Health League Made Preventive Medicine His Career," *Globe and Mail,* 8 November 1975, 5; "Health League of Canada: Dr. Gordon Bates," http://www.healthleagueofcanada.com/founder/.

54 Allan Brandt, "'Just Say No': Risk, Behavior, and Disease in Twentieth-Century America," in *Scientific Authority and Twentieth-Century America,* ed. Roland Walters (Baltimore: Johns Hopkins University Press, 1997), 95.

55 Benoît Gaumer, *Le système de santé et des services sociaux au Québec: une histoire recente et tourmentée, 1921–2000* (Quebec: Presses de l'Université Laval, 2008); Peter Keating and Othmar Keel, *Santé et société au Québec* (Montreal: Boréal, 1995); François Guérard, *Histoire de la santé au Québec* (Montreal: Boréal, 1996); Georges Desrosiers, Benoît Gaumier, and Othmar Keel, *Vers un système de santé publique au Québec* (Montreal: Université de Montréal, 1991); Benoît Gaumer, Georges Desrosiers, and Othmar Keel, *Histoire du Service de santé de la ville de Montréal, 1865–1975* (Sainte-Foy: Les Presses de L'Université Laval, 2002).

56 Christopher Rutty and Sue Sullivan, *This Is Public Health: A Canadian History* (Ottawa: Canadian Public Health Association, 2010), https://cpha.ca/sites/default/ files/assets/history/book/history-book-print_all_e.pdf.

57 MacDougall, *Activists and Advocates,* 12.

58 Katherine Arnup, *Education for Motherhood: Advice for Mothers in Twentieth-Century Canada* (Toronto: University of Toronto Press, 1994); Cynthia Comacchio, *Nations Are Built of Babies: Saving Ontario's Mothers and Children, 1900–1940* (Montreal and Kingston: McGill-Queen's University Press, 1993); Denise Baillargeon, *Babies for the Nation: The Medicalization of Motherhood in Quebec, 1910– 1970,* trans. W. Donald Wilson (Waterloo, ON: Wilfrid Laurier University Press, 2009); Mona Gleason, *Small Matters: Canadian Children in Sickness and Health, 1900–1940* (Montreal and Kingston: McGill-Queen's University Press, 2013).

59 Jay Cassel, *The Secret Plague: Venereal Disease in Canada 1838–1939* (Toronto: University of Toronto Press, 1987); Dorothy Chunn, "A Little Sex Can Be a Dangerous Thing: Regulating Sexuality, Venereal Disease and Reproduction in British Columbia, 1919–1935," in *Challenging the Public/Private Divide: Feminism, Law and Public Policy,* ed. Susan Boyd (Toronto: University of Toronto Press, 2016), 62–86; Renisa Mawani, "Regulating the 'Respectable' Classes: Venereal Disease, Gender, and Public Health Initiatives in Canada, 1914–35," in *Regulating Lives: Historical Essays on the State, Society, the Individual, and the Law,* ed. John McLaren, Robert Menzies, and Dorothy E. Chunn (Vancouver: UBC Press, 2002), 170–95; Janice Dickin McGinnis, "Law and the Leprosies of Lust: Regulating Syphilis and AIDS," *Ottawa*

Law Review 22, 1 (1990): 49–75; Suzann Buckley and Janice Dickin McGinnis, "Venereal Disease and Public Health Reform in Canada," *Canadian Historical Review* 63, 3 (1982): 337–54.

60 Mark Humphries, *The Last Plague: Spanish Influenza and the Politics of Public Health in Canada* (Toronto: University of Toronto Press, 2013); Madga Fahrni and Esyllt Jones, *Epidemic Encounters: Influenza, Society, and Culture in Canada, 1918–20* (Vancouver: UBC Press, 2012); Esyllt Jones, *Influenza 1918: Disease, Death and Struggle in Winnipeg* (Toronto: University of Toronto Press, 2007); Ian Mosby, *Food Will Win the War: The Politics, Culture, and Science of Food on Canada's Home Front* (Vancouver: UBC Press, 2014); Caroline Durand, *Nourrir la machine humaine: nutrition et alimentation au Québec, 1860–1945* (Montreal and Kingston: McGill-Queen's University Press, 2015).

61 Jane E. Jenkins, "Politics, Pasteurization and the Naturalizing Myth of Pure Milk in 1920s Saint John, New Brunswick," *Acadiensis* 37, 2 (2008): 86–105; Andrew Ebejer, "'Milking' the Consumer? Consumer Dissatisfaction and Regulatory Intervention in the Ontario Milk Industry during the Great Depression," *Ontario History* 52, 1 (2010): 20–39; Marion McKay, "'The Tubercular Cow Must Go': Business, Politics and Winnipeg's Milk Supply, 1894–1922," *Canadian Bulletin of Medical History* 23, 2 (2006): 355–80; Lisa Cox, "'Reasonable Tact and Diplomacy': Disease Management and Bovine Tuberculosis in North America, 1890–1950" (PhD diss., University of Guelph, 2013).

62 Tillotson, *Contributing Citizens*; Gale Wills, *A Marriage of Convenience: Business and Social Work in Toronto* (Toronto: University of Toronto Press, 1995).

Chapter 1: "Tell Your Children the Truth"

1 In her description of the film, Paula Bartley stresses the similarity between "Vera" and "venereal." Paula Bartley, *Emmeline Pankhurst* (London: Routledge, 2002), 215. *End of the Road* (1919), University of Michigan Historical Health Films Collection. Thanks to Marty Pernick for making the film available to us.

2 See, for example, Donica Belisle, "A Labour Force for the Consumer Century: Commodification in Canada's Largest Department Stores, 1890–1940," *Labour/Le Travail* 58 (Fall 2006): 107–44.

3 John Parascandola, *Sex, Sin and Science: A History of Syphilis in America* (Westport, CT: Praeger, 2008), 65; Bartley, *Emmeline Pankhurst*, 215.

4 The British Social Hygiene Council started as the Council for Combatting Venereal Disease. It changed its name in 1925. Greta Jones, *Social Hygiene in Twentieth Century Britain* (London: Croom Helm, 1986), 27. The American Social Hygiene Association was founded in 1913. Allan Brandt, *No Magic Bullet: A Social History of Venereal Disease in the United States since 1880* (New York: Oxford University Press, 1985), 38. There is considerable material from these two organizations in the papers of the Canadian Social Hygiene Council/Health League. The CSHC was represented at the Imperial Social Hygiene Council in Wembley in 1924. "International Congress on Social Hygiene," *Social Health* 1, 3 (1924): 3.

5 The recent literature on eugenics includes Laura Lovett, *Conceiving the Future: Pronatalism, Reproduction and the Family in the United States, 1890–1938* (Chapel Hill: University of North Carolina Press, 2007); Alexandra Minna Stern, *Eugenic Nation:*

Faults and Frontiers of Better Breeding in Modern America (Berkeley: University of California Press, 2005); Erika Dyck, *Facing Eugenics: Reproduction, Sterilization and the Politics of Choice* (Toronto: University of Toronto Press, 2013). A recent addition to the history of eugenics in Ontario suggests that, despite the fact that much-studied proponents of sterilization such as Helen MacMurchy and C.K. Clarke played a prominent role in the public debate over eugenics, there were also more moderate voices and that attempts to achieve sterilization legislation in Ontario failed four times. C. Elizabeth Koester, "An Evil Hitherto Unchecked: Eugenics and the 1917 Ontario Royal Commission on the Care and Control of the Mentally Defective and Feeble-Minded," *Canadian Bulletin of Medical History* 33, 1 (2016): 59–81.

6 Jay Cassel, *The Secret Plague: Venereal Disease in Canada, 1838–1939* (Toronto: University of Toronto Press, 1987).

7 Carolyn Strange and Tina Loo, *Making Good: Law and Moral Regulation in Canada, 1867–1939* (Toronto: University of Toronto Press, 1997); Carolyn Strange, *Toronto's Girl Problem: The Perils and Pleasures of the City, 1880–1930* (Toronto: University of Toronto Press, 1995); Joan Sangster, *Regulating Girls and Women: Sexuality, Family and the Law in Ontario, 1920–1960* (Toronto: Oxford University Press, 2001); Mariana Valverde, *The Age of Light, Soap and Water: Moral Reform in English Canada, 1885–1925* (Toronto: McClelland and Stewart, 1991); Dorothy Chunn, "A Little Sex Can Be a Dangerous Thing: Regulating Sexuality, Venereal Disease and Reproduction in British Columbia, 1919–1935," in *Challenging the Public/Private Divide: Feminism, Law and Public Policy*, ed. Susan Boyd (Toronto: University of Toronto Press), 62–86; Renisa Mawani, "Regulating the 'Respectable' Classes: Venereal Disease, Gender, and Public Health Initiatives in Canada, 1914–35," in *Regulating Lives: Historical Essays on the State, Society, the Individual, and the Law*, ed. John McLaren, Robert Menzies, and Dorothy E. Chunn (Vancouver: UBC Press, 2002), 170–95; Janice Dickin McGinnis, "Law and the Leprosies of Lust: Regulating Syphilis and AIDS," *Ottawa Law Review* 22, 1 (1990): 49–75; Suzann Buckley and Janice Dickin McGinnis, "Venereal Disease and Public Health Reform in Canada," *Canadian Historical Review* 63, 3 (1982): 337–54; Cassel, *Secret Plague*; Christabelle Sethna, "The Facts of Life: The Sex Instruction of Ontario Public School Children, 1900–1950" (PhD diss., University of Toronto, 1995).

8 Jay Cassel, "Making Canada Safe for Sex: Government and the Problem of Sexually Transmitted Disease in the Twentieth Century," in *Canadian Health Care and the State: A Century of Evolution*, ed. C. David Naylor (Montreal and Kingston: McGill-Queen's University Press, 1992), 147. This estimate may be a little high. During the war, J.G. Fitzgerald estimated that 6–10 percent of the population treated at general hospitals were infected with syphilis. J.G. Fitzgerald, "The Advisory Committee on Venereal Diseases for Military District No. 2," *Public Health Journal* 9, 2 (1918): 50. These statistics may also have been on the high side. A large number of ailments can result in a false positive Wassermann reaction, including viral and bacterial infections. Rafal Bialynicki-Birula, "The 100th Anniversary of the Wassermann-Neisser-Bruck Reaction," *Clinics in Dermatology* 26 (2008): 79–88; "International Conference on the Standardisation of Sera and Serological Tests," *Lancet* 200, 5180 (1922): 1238–40.

9 Gordon Bates, "Some Broader Aspects of the Venereal Disease Problem," *Public Health Journal* 9, 11 (1918): 497–98.

10 Untitled memo, n.d. [c. 1937–39], Library and Archives Canada (hereafter LAC), MG28, I332, vol. 134, file 3.

11 Buckley and McGinnis, "Venereal Disease," 337–54. Sethna shows that the Woman's Christian Temperance Union was addressing venereal disease long before the war. Sethna, "Facts of Life," 80–86; Gordon Bates, "Venereal Disease Control in Canada: A General Survey of the Movement in Canada," October 1933, LAC, MG28, I332, vol. 140, file 18.

12 Cassel, *Secret Plague*, 122–23. Rates remained high throughout the war. By the end of the war, the Canadian Expeditionary Force had treated 66,346 cases of venereal disease, compared to 45,460 cases of influenza. Desmond Morton, *When Your Number's Up: The Canadian Soldier in the First World War* (Toronto: Random House, 1993), 200.

13 Cassel, *Secret Plague*, 124–25.

14 Brandt, *No Magic Bullet*, 40.

15 Ibid., 40.

16 Cassel, *Secret Plague*, 56; Edna Moore, "Venereal Disease Control in Ontario," *Public Health Journal* 14, 2 (1923): 74–75. By the 1940s, neosarsphenamine seems to have been the most common drug used. *Venereal Diseases, Diagnosis, Treatment and Laboratory Methods* (Ottawa: Department of Pensions and National Health, n.d [c. 1943]).

17 David Evans, "Tackling the 'Hideous Scourge': The Creation of Venereal Disease Treatment Centres in Early Twentieth-Century Britain," *Social History of Medicine* 5, 3 (1992): 413–33.

18 See, for example, Tim Cook, "Wet Canteens and Worrying Mothers: Alcohol, Soldiers and Temperance Groups in the Great War," *Histoire sociale/Social History* 35, 70 (2002): 310–30; see also "Dr. Chown and His Critics," *Globe*, 27 September 1917; "Back to a Clean Canada," *Globe*, 15 November 1918; and "Must Not Be Blind to Sex Problem," n.d, n.p., LAC, MG28, I332, vol. 238, part I.

19 "'Cleansing the Portals of Life': The Venereal Disease Campaign in the Early Twentieth Century," in *Crisis in the British State, 1880–1930*, ed. Mary Langan and Bill Schwarz (London: Hutchinson, 1985), 192–208.

20 For a discussion of this, see John W.S. McCullough, "The Scourge of the World," *Maclean's*, 15 October 1937; Gordon Bates, "The Venereal Disease Problem from the Military Standpoint," *Public Health Journal* 8, 2 (1917): 43–46.

21 Cassel, *Secret Plague*, 124. Also see Tim Cook, *Shock Troops: Canadians Fighting the Great War, 1917–1918* (Toronto: Viking, 2008): 173–77. Angela Woollacott argues that many adolescent girls were caught up in the excitement of flirtation and sex during the early days of the war: "'Khaki Fever' and Its Control: Gender, Class, Age and Sexual Morality on the British Homefront in the First World War," *Journal of Contemporary History* 29, 2 (1994): 325–47. Edward H. Beardsley agrees about the widespread availability of sex for soldiers: "Allied against Sin: American and British Responses to Venereal Disease in World War I," *Medical History* 20, 2 (1976): 192–93.

22 Cassel, *Secret Plague*, 123–26.
23 Ibid., 130; Andrea Tone, *Devices and Desires: A History of Contraceptives in America* (New York: Hill and Wang, 2001).
24 Cassel, *Secret Plague*, 142.
25 Ibid., 141–43; Carol Lee Bacchi, *Liberation Deferred? The Ideas of the English-Canadian Suffragists* (Toronto: University of Toronto Press, 1993).
26 Cassel, *Secret Plague*, 141–43.
27 Sidney Katz, "The Doctor Who Won't Take 'NO' for an Answer," *Maclean's*, 26 November 1955, 13. Frank Dewitt Bates is listed as an oculist and auralist in the 1885 City of Hamilton Directory, http://archive.org/stream/cityofhamiltondi1885hamiuoft/cityofhamiltondi1885hamiuoft_djvu.txt.
28 Oral interviews conducted with Bates' granddaughter Pippa Wysong on 21 January 2014, and Bates' son, John Bates, and his family, on 27 January 2014. Bethany Philpott, "Bates: Personal Life and Education" (unpublished paper, 2015).
29 Gordon Anderson Bates biography, *Torontonensis* 9 (1907): 151, https://archive.org/details/torontonensis1907univ.
30 Ibid. In his fourth year, he ranked ninth out of twelve in "Group I – medicine, clinical medicine, pathology and therapeutics," ninth out of nineteen in "Group III – obstetrics, gynecology and pathology," and fourth out of forty-one in "Group IV – medical jurisprudence, toxicology, hygiene and medical psychology." Class and Prize Lists, 1900–1907. University of Toronto Archives, P78.0158.(01)-(03).
31 Sethna, "Facts of Life," 141.
32 Angus McLaren, *Our Own Master Race: Eugenics in Canada* (Toronto: McClelland and Stewart, 1990), 108; Sethna, "Facts of Life," 145.
33 "Social and Personal: Academy of Medicine," *Toronto Star*, 27 October 1911, 10; "Feeble-Minded a Ghastly Menace: Many Potential Murderers at Large," *Globe*, 1 December 1916, 6; "Academy of Medicine Officers," *Toronto Star*, 11 May 1917, 11.
34 C.S. McVicar, Gordon Bates, and George Strathy, "Laboratory Tests in the Diagnosis of General Paresis," *Canadian Medical Association Journal* 2, 7 (1912): 563–67.
35 Gordon Bates, George S. Strathy, and C.S. McVicar, "The Treatment of Tabes Dorsalis and General Paresis with Salvarsan," *Canadian Medical Association Journal* 4, 3 (1914): 197–200.
36 Letter from Gordon Bates to Major Foulds, 5 April 1918, LAC, MG28, I332, vol. 133, file 10; Gordon Bates, "The Venereal Disease Problem," *Public Health Journal* 9, 8 (1918): 356.
37 Letter from Gordon Bates to Vincent Massey, 6 August 1918, LAC, MG28, I332, vol. 133, file 10.
38 Brandt, *No Magic Bullet*, 52–95.
39 Memo from Officer for Venereal Disease, Military District No 2 to ADMS for Military District, 17 June 1918, LAC, MG28, I332, vol. 132, file 21.
40 For a recent account of the creation of the Department of Health, see Mark Humphries, *The Last Plague: Spanish Influenza and the Politics of Public Health in Canada* (Toronto: University of Toronto Press, 2013). Free VD treatment began to be provided in Britain just a few years earlier. Evans, "Tackling the 'Hideous Scourge.'"
41 Cassel, *Secret Plague*, 176.

42 The initial grant was $5,000 per year. In 1921–22, this was increased to $10,000. It ranged between $5,000 and $20,000 from 1922 to 1927, when it was increased to $20,000 year. Memorandum concerning the Canadian Social Hygiene Council, n.d., LAC, MG28, I332, vol. 34, file 4. This was a substantial grant. The entire budget of the Social Service Council of Canada was $10,000 in 1918. Richard Allan, *The Social Passion: Religion and Social Reform in Canada, 1914–1928* (Toronto: University of Toronto Press, 1971), 64.

43 For example, in 1928, Minister of Health James King told the House that

> We cannot do anything more than to subsidize an organization like this, which through propaganda and education is doing a very good work in Canada, work that the federal government might not be able to do. The people are sensitive in regard to suggestions in the matter of health and their home affairs, and especially sensitive of government interference but men like Dr. Bates can through their organization and through the county and municipal councils carry on an effective campaign which is undoubtedly improving the condition in Canada and interesting the people in health affairs.

Canada, House of Commons, *Debates*, 5 June 1928.

44 "Social Hygiene and Venereal Disease Control in Canada," n.d. [c. mid-1920s], LAC, MG28, I332, vol. 133, file 8; Bates, "The Venereal Disease Problem," 357–58; J.J. Heagerty, "Venereal Disease Situation in Canada," *Public Health Journal* (Canada) 13, 11 (1922), 485–96. Heagerty noted that people in Quebec seemed more likely to seek treatment, indicating that compulsory notification backfired.

45 "Social Hygiene and Venereal Disease Control in Canada," LAC, MG28, I332, vol. 133, file 8.

46 Heagerty, "Venereal Disease Situation in Canada," 494.

47 Velma Demerson, *Incorrigible* (Waterloo, ON: Wilfrid Laurier University Press, 2004).

48 Carolyn Strange, "'Velvet Glove: Maternalistic Reform at the Andrew Mercer Ontario Reformatory for Females, 1874–1931" (MA thesis, University of Ottawa, 1983), cited in Constance Backhouse, *Carnal Crimes: Sexual Assault Law in Canada, 1900–1975* (Toronto: Osgoode Society for Legal History, 2008), 348*n*16.

49 Kathy Southee, "The Story of Florence Gooderham Hamilton Huestis" (unpublished paper, 17 April 2009), http://www.gooderham-worts.ca/showmedia.php?mediaID=198&tngpage=7. Huestis was treasurer in the early years of the CNCCVD. See "Executive: The National Council for Combatting Venereal Disease," n.d. [c. 1921], LAC, MG28, I332, vol. 1 file 9; History Committee, *Nothing New Under the Sun: A History of the Toronto Council of Women* (Toronto: Local Council of Women of Toronto, 1978), 37–38; "Barnett Robert Brickner," *The Encyclopedia of Cleveland History*, https://case.edu/ech/articles/b/brickner-barnett-robert/; Rabbi Barnett Brickner, "Immigration and Colonization," *Empire Club of Canada Addresses*, 16 March 1922, http://speeches.empireclub.org/60887/data?n=2; William K. Klempa, "The College and the North: Andrew S. Grant," in *Still Voices – Still Heard: Sermons, Addresses, Letters and Reports. The Presbyterian College, Montreal, 1865–2015*, ed.

J.S. Armour, Judith Kashul, William Klempa, Lucille Marr, and Dan Shute (Eugene, OR: WIPF and Stock, 2015), 81–94.

50 John Farley, *To Cast Out Disease: A History of the International Health Division of the Rockefeller Foundation, 1913–1951* (Oxford: Oxford University Press, 2004), 235.

51 Jérôme Boivin, "De la protection de la santé publique dans le Québec de l'entre-deux-guerres," in *Autour de la médicalisation*, ed. Joceline Chabot, Daniel Hickey, and Martin Pâquet (Quebec: Presses de l'Université Laval, 2012), 149–65.

52 Minutes of the Executive Committee, CNCCVD, 17 May 1921, LAC, MG28, I332, vol. 1, file 9; Jane E. Jenkins, "Baptism of Fire: New Brunswick's Public Health Movement and the 1918 Influenza Epidemic," *Canadian Bulletin of Medical History* 24, 2 (2007): 317–342; "John W.S. McCullough: Ontario's First Chief Provincial Health Officer," http://resources.cpha.ca/CPHA/ThisIsPublicHealth/profiles/item.php?l= E&i=1392.

53 Russell Johnston, "Defining an Era," *Marketing Magazine*, 11 February 2008, http:// marketingmag.ca/media/defining-an-era-13213; Euclid Herie, *Journey to Independence: Blindness, the Canadian Story* (Toronto: Dundurn Press, 2005), 42–43.

54 Martin Pernick, "More Than Illustrations: Early Twentieth-Century Health Films as Contributors to the Histories of Medicine and of Motion Pictures," in *Medicine's Moving Pictures: Medicine, Health, and Bodies in American Film and Television*, ed. Leslie J. Reagan, Nancy Tomes, and Paula Treichler (Rochester, NY: Rochester University Press, 2007), 19.

55 "Social Hygiene and Venereal Disease Control in Canada," n.d. [c. 1924–25], LAC, MG28, I332, vol. 133, file 8.

56 Pernick, "More Than Illustrations," 26.

57 Jeffrey Moran, *Teaching Sex: The Shaping of Adolescence in the 20th Century* (Cambridge: Harvard University Press, 2000), 43–44.

58 Action Committee Meeting, 23 November 1971, LAC, MG28, I332, vol. 135, file 2.

59 Christable Pankhurst, *The Great Scourge and How to End It* (London: E. Pankhurst, 1913).

60 Bartley, *Emmeline Pankhurst*, 212.

61 Ibid., 214.

62 "First Duty of British to Stamp Out Disease," *Toronto Star*, 23 April 1921, 10.

63 Lucy Bland, *Banishing the Beast: Sexuality and the Early Feminists* (New York: New Press, 1995), 236–37, 243–46.

64 "Social Hygiene: A Tabooed Subject, Explained by Mrs. Pankhurst, Dr. Heagerty and Others," Woodstock [name of paper illegible], 20 January 1923, LAC, MG28, I332, vol. 238, part II. "Mrs. Pankhurst Now Becomes a Canadian," *Toronto Star*, 9 January 1922, 12. Additional clippings from talks across the country are available in LAC, MG28, I332, vol. 239.

65 Cassel, *Secret Plague*, 215.

66 "Social Hygiene and Venereal Disease Control in Canada," n.d. [c. 1924–25], LAC, MG28, I332, vol. 133, file 8.

67 Cassel, *Secret Plague*, 215.

68 Bartley, *Emmeline Pankhurst*, 215.

69 "Health Crusaders Off on 1,500 Mile Tour," *Toronto Telegram,* 14 July 1923; "Mrs E. Pankhurst and Party Upset; Train Misses Car," *Bellville Intelligencer,* 14 December 1923.

70 Bartley, *Emmeline Pankhurst,* 219. Also see reports by Hewson in LAC, MG28, I332, vol. 48, files 1–8.

71 Gordon Bates, "The Results of Venereal Disease Control in Canada," *American Journal of Public Health,* February 1939, 146.

72 For example, see Gordon Bates, "Women in Politics," *Health,* Spring 1941, 2.

73 "Membership Campaign Results in Increase of Several Hundreds" *Social Health* 5, 1 (1928): 2, 4. The Ottawa Social Hygiene Council, praised as one of the most active councils, engaged in a similar array of talks, films, and exhibits. "Ottawa Council a Model" *Social Health,* October 1924, 1–2.

74 "Report of the Winnipeg Health League to the Executives and Members of the Canadian Social Hygiene Council," 12 June 1928, in LAC, MG28, I332, vol. 10, file 26.

75 "Report on the Social Hygiene Activities in Montreal for 1925," LAC, MG28, I332, vol. 10, file 24.

76 "Report of the Western Branches, 1929," LAC, MG28, I332, vol. 10, file 28.

77 "Report of the Work Carried Out in the Province of Alberta and British Columbia for the year ended 30th April 1930," LAC, MG28, I332, vol. 10, file 30.

78 Letter from Estelle Hewson to William C. Smith, 11 January 1926, LAC, MG28, I332, vol. 48, file 16. Fenwick was the son-in-law of J.W.S. McCullough. He would serve the Canadian Social Hygiene Council for many years before enlisting in the Second World War. "Maj-Gen. Fenwick to Quit Army; Takes C.P.R Post," *Globe and Mail,* 25 January 1946, 9; "Fenwick-McCullough," *Globe,* 9 June 1921, 10. In contrast to others involved in the CSHC, Fenwick believed in promoting prophylaxis. "Co-Education Is Discussed," newspaper clipping, 25 June 1929, LAC, MG28 I332, vol. 10, file 29. Fenwick later became the director general of the Canadian Army Medical Services, "Army Medical Chief Named," *Globe and Mail,* 8 December 1944, 10.

79 The league stayed in this location for five years. Materials produced by the league later indicated that "it was during these 5 years that the League had its greatest impact on opinion in the City of Toronto." See a brief suggesting that the Health League of Canada embark immediately on a Program to adequately finance its activities, n.d. [c. 1959], LAC, MG28, I332, vol. 102, file 3.

80 Letter from Estelle Hewson to Frances Mayer, 9 January 1926, LAC, MG28, I332, vol. 48, file 16. For fuller details of the CSHC's financial picture, see the financial statements in LAC, MG28, I332, vol. 23, files 6–8. Interestingly, J.J. Heagerty wrote to A.C. Joust, the provincial officer for health for Ontario, to say that he wished that the Metropolitan Life Insurance grant had actually been given to the province for the "development of work of the social service nurse in the clinics and especially in its relation to the delinquent girl." He also expressed his despair about the short-lived nature of many of the social hygiene councils that had been established after his tour with the social hygiene council in 1923. See letter from J.J. Heagerty to A.C. Joust, 7 April 1925, LAC, RG29, vol. 216, file 1.

81 William G. Rothstein, *Public Health and the Risk Factor: A History of an Uneven Medical Revolution* (Rochester, NY: Rochester University Press, 2003), 146–75.

82 See correspondence in LAC, MG28, I332, vol. 17, file 22.

83 Peter Sandiford was particularly active. In 1926 he gave six lectures on social hygiene education at the Ontario College of Education. This was the fourth such course he had offered. See letter from Alex D. Hardie to J.J. Heagerty, 2 September 1926, LAC, RG29, vol. 216, file 311-V3–22, part 4. For more on Sandiford, see Jennifer Stephen, *Pick One Intelligent Girl: Employability, Domesticity and the Gendering of Canada's Welfare State* (Toronto: University of Toronto Press, 2007), 68. Edna Guest's brutal treatment of women has been documented by several feminist historians. See, for example, Backhouse, *Carnal Crimes,* 105–30 and Demerson, *Incorrigible.*

84 LAC, MG28, I332, vol. 48, file 1.

85 For more on the early years of the Wayside House, see Shirley Frances Payment, "The Big Project: James M. Shaver at All Peoples' Mission, Winnipeg, 1921–1941" (MA thesis, University of Manitoba, 1999), 50–51.

86 Health League of Canada, LAC, MG28, I332, vols. 49–56.

87 Kristin Luker, "Sex, Social Hygiene and the State: The Double-edged Sword of Social Reform," *Theory* 27 (1998): 601–34.

88 Carolyn Strange, *Toronto's Girl Problem: The Perils and Pleasures of the City, 1880–1930* (Toronto: University of Toronto Press, 1995); Joan Sangster, *Regulating Girls and Women: Sexuality, Family and the Law in Ontario, 1920–1960* (Toronto: Oxford University Press, 2001); Karen Dubinsky, *Improper Advances: Rape and Heterosexual Conflict in Ontario, 1880–1929* (Chicago: University of Chicago Press, 1993); Andrée Lévesque, *Making and Breaking the Rules: Women in Quebec, 1919–1939* (Montreal: McClelland and Stewart, 1994); Tamara Myers, *Caught: Montreal's Modern Girls and the Law, 1869–1945* (Toronto: University of Toronto Press, 2006).

89 David Pivar, *Purity and Hygiene: Women, Prostitution and the "American Plan," 1900–1930* (Westport, CT: Greewood Press, 2002), 147–55.

90 Cyril Greenland, "C.K. Clarke: A Founder of Canadian Psychiatry," *Canadian Medical Association Journal* 95 (22 July 1966), 155; Ian Dowbiggin, "'Keeping This Young Country Sane': C.K. Clarke, Immigration Restriction and Canadian Psychiatry, 1890–1925," *Canadian Historical Review* 76, 4 (1995): 598–627.

91 Murphy carried out a significant correspondence with Bates, but she was not involved in on-the-ground organizing, other than helping with Pankhurst's visit to Alberta in 1921. LAC, MG28, I332, vol. 45, files 1–3. The Alberta Division of the CSHC was not very active.

92 "Hastings, Charles," *Eugenics Archive,* http://eugenicsarchive.ca/discover/connectio ns/5232a8235c2ec5000000001f.

93 McLaren, *Our Own Master Race,* 107–26. McLaren includes a list of members of the Eugenics Society at 202n34.

94 "The Fit and the Unfit to Carry on the Race," *Social Health,* March 1924, 1.

95 "Child Immigration Investigated," *Social Health,* October 1924, 2; Dowbiggin, "Keeping This Young Country Sane," 605–6.

96 Clarence Hincks, "The Relation between Mental and Social Hygiene," *Social Health,* November/December 1925, 2.

97 "Medical Examination of Immigrants," 12 June 1928, LAC, MG28, I332, vol 10, file 26.

98 American Social Hygiene Association, *Healthy Happy Womanhood*, n.d. [c. 1942], LAC, MG28, I332, vol. 139, file 8. A pamphlet of the same title was also published by the US Public Health Service.

99 For more on the influence of positive eugenics in the interwar period in North America, see, Wendy Kline, *Building a Better Race: Gender, Sexuality and Eugenics from the Turn of the Century to the Baby Boom* (Berkeley: University of California Press, 2001) and Stern, *Eugenic Nation*.

100 "National Board Supports Pre-Marriage Regulation for Control of Disease," *Social Health*, April/May 1928, 2. A number of activists in the organization, including Murray Thompson (the western organizer) and Toronto's Rabbi Isserman, spoke out in favour of them.

101 Brandt, *No Magic Bullet*, 19–20.

102 See Strange, *Toronto's Girl Problem*, for an extensive discussion of how social reformers in Toronto encouraged girls to pursue healthful recreation.

103 Annual Report of the Toronto Social Hygiene Club, January 1928, in LAC, MG28, I332 vol. 57, file 15.

104 Bates, "Some Broader Aspects of the Venereal Disease Problem"; Bates, "The Venereal Disease Problem," *Public Health Journal* (Canada) 13, 5 (1922): 272.

105 "Jail for Each Party to Vice Advocated," *Social Health*, January/February 1925, 4; "Dr. A.K. Haywood of Montreal General Hospital Favours Wiping Out of Red Light District," *Social Health*, January/February 1925, 3–4.

106 See, for example, "Notes Prepared for Nurses and Social Workers throughout the Province," n.d. [c. 1923], LAC, MG28, I332, vol. 132, file 13; similar arguments are made in Gordon Bates, "The Venereal Disease Problem," 265–79.

107 The first mention of this case may be in Gordon Bates, "Social Investigation and Follow-up in Venereal Disease Cases," *Public Health Journal* 13, 8 (1922): 362–68. Another mention can be found in "Social Hygiene and Venereal Disease Control in Canada," n.d. [c. 1924], LAC, MG28, I332, vol. 133, file 8. It also appears in "Think of It!" *Social Health*, April 1924, 1.

108 David Micklos and Elof Carlson "Engineering American Society: The Lesson of Eugenics," *Nature Reviews Genetics* 1 (November 2000): 153–58.

109 Conference of Representatives of Social Agencies Called by the Dominion Government to Discuss Constructive Social Measure to Combat the Existence of Venereal Disease in the Dominion of Canada, 29–30 May 1919, LAC, MG28, I332 vol. 132, file 14.

110 Garett O'Connor, letter to the editor, "Female Offenders Scarce," *Toronto Star*, 5 May 1919, 12.

111 Edith Houghton Hooker, "The Scapegoat," *Survey* 35, 10 (1915), 254–55. Although this piece is regularly listed as a publication available from the Canadian Social Hygiene Council, we could find no copies in the records of the Health League.

112 *The Gift of Life*, University of Michigan Historical Health Films Collection. Thanks to Marty Pernick for making this film available. A description of *How Life Begins* can be found at http://www.afi.com/members/catalog/DetailView.aspx?s=1&Movie=15960 and in Palle Petterson, *Cameras into the Wild: A History of Early Wildlife and Expedition Filmmaking* (Jefferson, NC: McFarland and Company, 2011), 131–32.

113 *Tell Your Children the Truth,* n.d. [c. 1942], LAC, MG28, I332, vol. 139, file 8.
114 Edith Howes, *The Cradle Ship* (London: Cassell, 1916); D.B. and E.B. Armstrong, "Sex in Life," *Journal of Social Hygiene* 2, 3 (1916): 331–46.
115 Douglas White, "An Open Letter to Young Men," n.d. [c. 1942], distributed for the showing of *No Greater Sin,* LAC, MG28, I332, vol. 139, file 8.
116 Letter from Gordon Bates to T.W. McGarru, 14 November 1918, LAC, MG28, I332, vol. 133, file 9.
117 This description of *Fit to Fight* actually comes from *Fit to Win* – a new version of the film re-titled when the war was over (University of Michigan Historical Health Films Collection). Thanks to Marty Pernick for making the film available. The film is also described in Alexandra Lord, *Condom Nation: The US Government's Sex Education Campaign from World War I to the Internet* (Baltimore, MD: Johns Hopkins University Press, 2010), 29, and in Martin Pernick, "More Than Illustrations," 19–34.
118 Letter from Gordon Bates to Henry E. Spencer, 7 March 1932, LAC, MG28, I332, vol. 33, file 6.
119 As Alison Bashford has noted, and as the CSHC/Health League realized, epidemiology was a powerful tool in the quest to regulate populations through public health programs. Alison Bashford, *Imperial Hygiene: A Critical History of Colonialism, Nationalism and Public Health* (Basingstoke, UK: Palgrave Macmillan, 2014), 9.
120 C.P. Fenwick, "Venereal Disease Survey in Toronto," *Canadian Public Health Journal* 21, 3 (1930): 132–38.
121 Winnipeg Health League and Department of Health and Public Welfare, Manitoba, "A Venereal Disease Survey in Manitoba," *Canadian Public Health Journal* 22, 4 (1931): 189–93.
122 Gordon Bates, "A Survey of the Incidence of Venereal Diseases in Toronto in 1937," *Canadian Public Health Journal* 28, 12 (1937). This survey was carried out with the cooperation of the Toronto Academy of Medicine. Over 97 percent of doctors responded.
123 J.T. Clarke, "A Survey of the Incidence of Venereal Diseases in Ottawa," *Canadian Public Health Journal* 29, 5 (1938): 213–15.
124 Gordon Bates, "The Present Problem in Venereal Disease," paper read before the Section of Preventive Medicine and Hygiene, 25 November 1937, LAC, MG28, I332, vol. 133, file 11. The growing acknowledgment that venereal disease rates were decreasing can also be found in F.S. Parney, "The Venereal Disease Situation in Canada," *Canadian Journal of Public Health* 24, 7 (1933): 553–61.
125 Gordon Bates, "Venereal Disease Control in Canada," *Canadian Public Health Journal* 25, 2 (1934): 63.
126 Cassel, *Secret Plague,* 2.
127 Ibid., 194–96.
128 Bates, "Present Problem in Venereal Disease." In 1925, the grant was reduced to $150,000, in 1926 it was reduced to $125,000, and in 1927 it was reduced to $100,000, where it remained for the next four years before being cut entirely. "Venereal Disease Control," n.d. [c. late 1930s], LAC, MG28 I332, vol. 133, file 8. The CSHC launched a major campaign in 1931 to have the grant continued, and prominent doctors and citizens from across the country wrote to the minister of health to ask that it be

continued. Letters were received from A.K. Haywood, general superintendent, Vancouver General Hospital; H.E. Young, the provincial health officer in British Columbia; William Warwick, district officer of health, Saint John, NB; Emily Murphy, police magistrate, Alberta; Sir Arthur Currie, principal and vice-chancellor, McGill University, among others. Editorials supporting the continuation of the grant were published in the *Toronto Star* and the *Ottawa Morning Journal.* Prime Minister R.B. Bennett felt that the grant to the Social Hygiene Council should be cut because this work was now being done by the federal and provincial Departments of Health. Letter from R.B. Bennett to H.H. Williams, 21 July 1931, LAC, MG28, I332, vol. 35, file 6.

129 Canadian Social Hygiene Council, Sixteenth Annual Meeting, 5 June 1935, LAC, MG28, I332, vol. 9, file 16.

130 Letter from Mabel Ferris to Arthur Kent, 27 June 1933, LAC, MG28, I332, vol. 17, file 24.

131 "Biographical Sketch of Dr. Gordon Bates," n.d. [c. 1950s], LAC, MG28, I332, vol. 148, file 1.

132 *Damaged Lives,* directed by Edgar G. Ulmer, Columbia Pictures, 1933. The quotations in the following discussion are taken from the film.

133 Christabelle Sethna, "Guilty Parties: The Ignorant Husband, the Selfish Wife and the New Woman in 'Damaged Lives'" (paper presented at the Canadian Historical Association Annual Meeting, 3 June 2015).

134 Women's Lecture, n.d. [c. 1933], LAC, MG28, I332, vol. 137, file 6.

135 Men's Lecture, n.d. [c. 1933], LAC, MG28, I332, vol. 137, file 6.

136 Letter from Waldon Picture Corporation to Gordon Bates, 13 October 1933, LAC, MG28, I332, vol. 137, file 4; Eric Schaefer, *"Bold! Daring! Shocking! True! A History of Exploitation Films* (Durham, NC: Duke University Press, 1999), 127.

137 "Comments on Preview of Damaged Lives," n.d. [c. 1933], LAC, MG28, I332, vol. 136, file 11.

138 Lists of audience numbers can be found in LAC, MG28, I332, vol. 137, file 3.

139 "Hygiene Council Sponsors Health Picture," *Charlottetown Guardian,* 28 October 1933, LAC, MG28, I332, vol. 136, file 10. This wording was obviously part of a press release sent out by the Health League, as it is repeated in numerous other articles as well. See, for example, "'Damaged Lives' at the Empress Theatre Next Week," *North Battleford Optimist,* 21 September 1933.

140 Untitled clipping, *Toronto Star Weekly,* 3 June 1933, LAC, MG28, I332, vol. 136, file 10; "A Valuable Lesson," *Saskatoon Star-Phoenix,* 20 September 1933.

141 Letter from Eileen O'Brien to Gordon Bates, 5 September 1933, LAC, MG28, I332, vol. 136, file 12.

142 "A News Dispatch Is Quoted in *Health,*" n.d. [c. 1933], LAC, MG28, I332, vol. 136, file 11; letter from Gordon Bates to Mr. D.L. Merrell, 22 May 1935, LAC, MG28, I332, vol. 136, file 11; report from the British Social Hygiene Council to the Canadian Social Hygiene Council on Circulation of *Damaged Lives,* 1933–34, LAC, MG28, I332, vol. 136, file 7; "Ten Million People View Canadian Film," *Health,* December 1934, 84.

143 Letter from Gordon Bates to K.W. Wise, 23 March 1935, LAC, MG28, I332, vol. 135, file 11.

144 Special Announcement, "A New Social Hygiene Motion Picture," *Journal of Social Hygiene* 29, 7 (1933).
145 Untitled clipping from *Journal of Social Hygiene*, November 1934, 401, LAC, MG28, I332, vol. 136, file 11. See also Jean B. Pinney, "New Brooms and Old Cobwebs," *Journal of Social Hygiene* 22, 4 (1936): 145–64.
146 Schaefer, *Bold! Daring!* 165–216.
147 Letter from Gordon Bates to the Honourable R.B. Bennett, 14 March 1938, LAC, MG28, I332, vol. 133, file 13.
148 Letter from Gordon Bates to C.G. Power, 11 June 1938, LAC, MG28, I332, vol. 133, file 15.
149 Letter from Alan Brown to Charles A. Dunning, 5 June 1939, LAC, MG28, I332, vol. 133, file 18.
150 Letter from Mrs. Edgar Harvey to the Honourable C.G. Power, 16 September 1938; Letter from Gordon Bates to R.A.E. Greenshields, 16 December 1938; Letter from Unknown (initials WG) to Chief Justice Greenshields, 13 December 1938, in LAC, MG28, I332, vol. 133, file 18.
151 Subcommittee report, n.d.; minutes of the Medical and Clergymen's Committee, 24 November 1926, LAC, MG28, I332, vol. 58, file 19. See also "Report of Committee on Medical Examination before Marriage," *Social Health*, May 1930, 8; letter from J.A. Walker to unknown recipient, 2 November 1936, LAC, MG28, I332, vol. 149, file 3.

Chapter 2: Expanding the Mission

1 "Radio Drama No. 1," Library and Archives Canada (hereafter LAC), MG28, I332, vol. 128, file 17.
2 An exchange of letters between Heagerty and Bates in 1928 shows that they both believed that interest in social hygiene was on the decline. Bates mentioned that the CSHC was sending out material on everything except venereal disease and he hoped that Heagerty would have some suggestions for drumming up interest in venereal disease. Letter from Bates to Heagerty, 19 January 1928, LAC, RG29, vol. 216, file 311-V3-22, part 5.
3 Minutes of the National Sub-Executive, 22 December 1930, LAC, MG28, I332, vol. 4, file 15.
4 See, for example, Minutes of the National Sub-Executive Committee, 11 March 1935, LAC, MG28, I332, vol. 4, file 15.
5 Jack Morantz, "Toronto Personalities: Gordon Bates," *Globe and Mail*, 5 December 1932, 9.
6 Dorothy Porter, *Health Citizenship: Essays in Social Medicine and Biomedical Politics* (Berkeley: University of California Press, 2011), 154–81.
7 Minutes of the Sub-Executive of the Canadian Social Hygiene Council, 13 May 1927, LAC, MG28, I332, vol. 4, file 12. A 1937 letter indicates that, while circulation had declined to 350 dailies and weeklies, approximately half of all Canadian newspapers published the columns. Confidential letter to the editor, 13 January 1937, LAC, MG28, I332, vol. 18, file 2.
8 Minutes of the National Sub-Executive of the Canadian Social Hygiene Council, 16 March 1927, LAC, MG28, I332, vol. 4, file 12.

9   This phrasing was used as early as 1937. J.W.S. McCullough, "Health League of Canada Presents Topics of Vital Interest," *Prince Rupert Empire*, 27 November 1937.

10   "Broadcast Stations from Coast to Coast in New Health Chain," *Social Health* 4, 5 (1927): 1.

11   "Department of Publicity," n.d. [1927–28], LAC, MG28, I332, vol. 4, file 14. "Broadcast Chain Increased to Ten Stations," *Social Health* 5, 1 (1928): 1, 3.

12   "Interim Publicity Report," n.d. [c. 1928], LAC, MG28, I332, vol. 4, file 13.

13   "Sunday Night Meetings on Air," *Social Health* 6, 2 (1929): 1, 6. For information on radio at this time, see Mary Vipond, *Listening In: The First Decade of Canadian Radio Broadcasting* (Montreal and Kingston: McGill-Queen's University Press, 1992), 203–4.

14   Minutes of the National Sub-Executive of the Canadian Social Hygiene Council, 30 October 1931, LAC, MG28, I332, vol. 4, file 15.

15   "Newspapers Now Publishing Reports of Our Radio Talks," *Social Health* 7, 5 (1930): 6.

16   "French Radio," *Social Health* 7, 6 (1931): 3.

17   Minutes of the National Sub-Executive Meeting, 17 May 1937, LAC, MG28, I332, vol. 4, file 16.

18   "Health League of Canada: A Series of 13 Dramatic Radio Plays," September 1941, LAC, MG28, I332, vol. 129, file 2.

19   "Let's Talk about Health," May 1945, and "List of Stations Who Will Carry 'Let's Talk about Health Series,'" n.d. [c. 1945], LAC, MG28, I332, vol. 129, file 3.

20   "Infantile Paralysis," n.d. [c. 1934–35], LAC, MG28, I332, vol. 128, file 17.

21   "Germs," n.d. [c. 1934–35], LAC, MG28, I332, vol. 128, file 17.

22   Lara Campbell, *Respectable Citizens: Gender, Family and Unemployment in Ontario's Great Depression* (Toronto: University of Toronto Press, 2009), 42–46.

23   "Goitre," n.d. [c. 1934–35], LAC, MG28, I332, vol. 128, file 17.

24   Ian Dowbiggin, "'Keeping This Young Country Sane': C.K. Clarke, Immigration Restriction and Canadian Psychiatry, 1890–1925," *Canadian Historical Review* 76, 4 (1995): 598–627; Peter Ward, *White Canada Forever: Public Attitudes and Public Policy towards Orientals in British Columbia* (Montreal and Kingston: McGill-Queen's University Press, 1978); Mariana Valverde, *The Age of Light, Soap and Water: Moral Reform in English Canada, 1885–1925* (Toronto: University of Toronto Press, 2008); Esyllt Jones, *Influenza, 1918: Disease, Death and Struggle in Winnipeg* (Toronto: University of Toronto Press, 2007); Isabel Wallace, "*Komagata Maru* Revisited: 'Hindus,' Hookworm and the Guise of Public Heath Protection," *BC Studies* 178 (Summer 2013): 33–50

25   "Typhoid: The Preventable Disease," n.d. [c. 1934–35], LAC, MG28, I332, vol. 128, file 17.

26   "Diptheria," n.d. [c. 1934–35], LAC, MG28, I332, vol. 128, file 17.

27   "Health Drama No 1" and "Tonsils," n.d. [c. 1934–35], LAC, MG28, I332, vol. 128, file 17.

28   "Teeth," n.d. [c. 1939–40], LAC, MG28, I332, vol. 129, file 1.

29   Gilles Dussault and Aubrey Sheiham, "Medical Theories and Professional Development: The Theory of Focal Sepsis and Dentistry in Early Twentieth Century Britain," *Social Science Medicine* 16, 15 (1982): 1405–12.

30 "Arthritis," n.d., LAC, MG28, I332, vol. 129, file 7.
31 "Mental Hygiene," Radio Talk No. 29, n.d. [c. 1934–35], LAC, MG28, I332, vol. 129, file 17.
32 For background on *Hygiea,* see "Newsstand 1925: Hygeia," n.d., http://uwf.edu/dearle/enewsstand/enewsstand_files/Page4115.htm. The AMA changed the name of its magazine to *Today's Health* in 1950.
33 Paul Rutherford, *The Making of the Canadian Media* (Toronto: McGraw-Hill, 1978), 46.
34 *Health,* October 1933, 1, 3.
35 Annual Report of the Canadian Social Hygiene Council for the Year Ending 30 April 1934, LAC, MG28, I332, vol. 9, file 15.
36 Canadian Social Hygiene Council Sixteenth Annual General Meeting, 5 June 1935, LAC, MG28, I332, vol. 9, file 16.
37 Health League of Canada Annual Meeting, 3 June 1942, LAC, MG28, I332, vol. 9, file 17.
38 Twenty-Eight Annual Meeting of the Health League of Canada, 17–19 June 1947, LAC, MG28, I332, vol. 9, file 23.
39 For the 1950 figure, see Thirty-First Annual Report of the Health League of Canada, 6–7 February 1951, p. 56, LAC, MG28, I332, vol. 10, file 1. The circulation of the other magazines is given in Rutherford, *The Making of the Canadian Media,* 82. The later circulation figures are from Annual Reports of the Health League of Canada for the years 1956 and 1957, LAC, MG28, I332, vol. 10, file 7; Annual Report of the Health League of Canada for 1962, LAC, MG28, I332, vol. 10, file 11.
40 A distribution survey in October 1958 showed that 23,369 copies reached Ontarians, while 1,529 copies went to Quebec. Prince Edward Island only received 12 copies. Sara Wilmshurst, "'Tobacco Truths': *Health* Magazine, Clinical Epidemiology, and the Cigarette Connection," *Canadian Bulletin of Medical History* 32, 1 (2015): 165.
41 Letter from Emile Vaillancourt to Gordon Bates, 2 March 1943, LAC, MG28, I332, vol. 110, file 8.
42 Wilmshurst, "Tobacco Truths," 172–73.
43 In 1968 for example, 10,000 copies of *Health* were mailed free of charge to physicians, while there were 16,335 paid subscribers. Letter from Mabel Ferris to the postmaster, 25 March 1969, LAC, MG28, I332, vol. 176, file 6.
44 Wilmshurst, "Tobacco Truths," 165.
45 Frederick Tisdall, "Health in Parliament: An Address," *Health,* September 1946, 20–21, 24–25; "Milk – One of Our Most Valuable Foods," *Health,* September 1936, 68, 79; "Nutrition," *Health,* March 1938, 8, 23–25; "The Nutritional Value of Food," *Health,* December 1935, 76, 84–85.
46 These included Elizabeth Chant Robertson, "Toronto Food Survey," *Health,* March 1959, 14–15, 26–27; "Foods for Fitness," *Health,* June 1963, 14–15, 32; "Advice to Parents," *Health,* September 1955, 6. Books written by Chant Robertson include: Alan Brown and Elizabeth Chant Robertson, *The Normal Child* (Toronto: McClelland and Stewart, 1948), and Elizabeth Chant Robertson, *Nutrition for Today* (Toronto: McClelland and Stewart, 1968). For more on Robertson, see Valerie Korinek, *Roughing It in the Suburbs: Reading Chatelaine Magazine in the 1950s and 1960s* (Toronto: University of Toronto Press, 2000), 216.

47 See, for example, R.G. Bell, "What You Should Know about Alcohol," *Health*, March 1954, 11–12, and "A New Concept of Alcohol Addiction," *Health*, July 1950, 15, 29.

48 See, for example, J.D.M. Griffin, "It's Up to You," *Health*, May/June 1953, 19; "Psychiatry Just Helps," *Health*, March/April 1952, 9, 29; "Youngsters Thrive on It," *Health*, March/April 1953, 19–20. John D. Griffin, *In Search of Sanity: A Chronicle of the Canadian Mental Health Association* (London: Third Eye, 1989).

49 Brooke Claxton, "Frontiers of Health," *Health*, Fall 1945, 9; Paul Martin, "The Dominion Health Proposals," *Health*, July/August 1947, 9.

50 Thomas Parran, "The Next Great Plague to Go," *Health*, December 1936, 96–97, 111; "Starvation! Hitler's Secret Weapon," *Health*, Winter 1941–42, 8, 17, 23.

51 Paul Popenoe, "First Aid for Unhappy Marriages," *Health*, September 1946, 5–6, 29.

52 Henry Sigerist, "Medical Care for All the People," *Health*, March 1944, 5–7, 23–25. On Sigerist's role in the Saskatchewan health commission, see C. Stuart Houston, "Sigerist Commission," *The Encyclopedia of Saskatchewan*, http://esask.uregina.ca/entry/sigerist_commission.html

53 Louis Dublin, "Health and the Challenge to Voluntary Agencies," *Health*, March/April 1948, 9, 26, 34; "Louis I. Dublin: November 1, 1882–March 7, 1969," *American Journal of Public Health* 59, 7 (1969): 1083–85.

54 Katherine Arnup, *Education for Motherhood: Advice for Mothers in Twentieth-century Canada* (Toronto: University of Toronto Press, 1994), 16.

55 "Diphtheria Protection," Radio Talk No. 26, April 1940, LAC, MG28, I332, vol. 91, file 7.

56 Alistair J. Lax, *Toxin: The Cunning of Bacterial Poisons* (New York: Oxford University Press, 2005), 64–65; "Canada Can Help Win the War by Keeping Its People Healthy," n.d. [c. 1940], LAC, MG28, I332, vol. 89, file 14.

57 Christopher Rutty and Sue C. Sullivan, *This Is Public Health: A Canadian History* (Ottawa: Canadian Public Health Association, 2010), 1, 13, https://cpha.ca/sites/default/files/assets/history/book/history-book-print_all_e.pdf.

58 Heather MacDougall, *Activists and Advocates: Toronto's Health Department, 1883–1983* (Toronto: Dundurn Press, 1990), 140; Maurice Macdonald Seymour, "Health Work in Saskatchewan" *Public Health Journal* (Canada) 16, 4 (1925): 158; Catherine Braithwaite, Peter Keating, and Sandi Viger, "The Problem of Diphtheria in the Province of Quebec, 1894–1909," *Histoire sociale/Social History* 29, 57 (1996): 94.

59 Maxine Evelynn Hammonds, *Childhood's Deadly Scourge: The Campaign to Control Diphtheria in New York City, 1880–1930* (Baltimore, MD: Johns Hopkins University Press, 1999), 8; Braithwaite, Keating, and Viger "Problem of Diphtheria," 71–95.

60 William H. Park and May C. Schroder, "Diphtheria Toxin-Antitoxin and Toxoid: A Comparison," *American Journal of Public Health* 22, 1 (1932): 7–16; Gaston Ramon, "How Science Fights Diphtheria," *Health*, September–October 1957, 14–15, 29; Gaston Ramon, "How Science Fights Diphtheria," *Health*, November/December 1957, 17, 30.

61 "The Work of the Toronto Diphtheria Committee, November 1931 to February 1937," n.d., LAC, MG28, I332, vol. 89, file 14.

62 "Mr. Mayor and the Members of the Board of Control," n.d. [c. 1932–34], LAC, MG28, I332, vol. 89, file 10; "The Work of the Toronto Diphtheria Committee."

63 "Publicity in Connection with Diphtheria," n.d. [c. 1944], LAC, MG28, I332, vol. 89, file 11; minutes of the Toronto Diphtheria Committee, 30 March 1944, LAC, MG28, I332, vol. 89, file 9.

64 "Publicity in Connection with Diphtheria."
65 Jane Lewis, "The Prevention of Diphtheria in Canada and Britain, 1914–1945," *Journal of Social History* 20, 1 (1986): 163–76.
66 Sidney M. Katz, "A City without Diphtheria," *Health,* March 1941, 17.
67 "Toronto Diphtheria Committee Report on Toxoid Week 1940," n.d., LAC, MG28, I332, vol. 89, file 11.
68 "A Brief Report on the Activities of This Committee," n.d., LAC, MG28, I332, vol. 89, file 13. A sample billboard is available in LAC, MG28, I332, vol. 91, file 12.
69 "Publicity in Connection with Diphtheria."
70 See LAC, MG28, I332, vol. 90, file 3: "Fewer Born but More Live," *Toronto Star,* 20 April 1938; "Parents Should Realize Proved Benefits of Toxoid," *Toronto Evening Telegram,* 26 April 1938.
71 Untitled document, n.d. [c. 1934], LAC, MG28, I332, vol. 89, file 8; "Memo to Dr. Bates by CP Fenwick," 22 March 1934, LAC, MG28, I332 vol. 89, file 11.
72 Ibid.
73 *Diphtheria: The Prevention and Cure* (pamphlet), 1938, LAC, MG28, I332, vol. 91, file 5.
74 Letter from the associate director of the Health League to the Right Rev. T. Albert Moore, D.D., 14 March 1934, LAC, MG28, I332, vol. 89, file 10.
75 Other publicity material also tried to counter the anti-vivisectionist opposition. Excerpt from the Claire Wallace Program of April 10, 1940, LAC, MG28, I332, vol. 90, file 7; Radio talk, n.d. [probably late 1930s], LAC, MG28, I332, vol. 91, file 9.
76 "Toronto Diphtheria Committee," 9 May 1934, LAC, MG28, I332, vol. 89, file 8.
77 Letter from Gordon Bates to the manager, radio station, 3 April 1940, LAC, MG28, I332, vol. 91, file 7.
78 "Diphtheria Protection," Radio Talk No. 26, April 1940, LAC, MG28, I332, vol. 91, file 7.
79 Ibid.
80 Minutes of the Toronto Diphtheria Committee, 22 September 1932, LAC, MG28, I332, vol. 89, file 8.
81 Letter from Albert Moore to Charles P. Fenwick, 10 March 1934, LAC, MG28, I332, vol. 89, file 10.
82 Gordon Bates, "'Diphtheria-Toxoid Week,' in Toronto," *Canadian Public Health Journal* 29, 12 (1938): 581.
83 "Do Not Wait for Next Week – Do It Now" (poster), 1944, LAC, MG28, I332, vol. 92, file 1. Also see "A Meeting of the Diphtheria Committee," 1933, LAC, MG28, I332, vol. 89, file 8.
84 MacDougall, *Activists and Advocates,* 185; Neil Sutherland, *Children in English-Canadian Society: Framing the Twentieth-Century Consensus* (Waterloo, ON: Wilfrid Laurier University Press, 2000), 79–90.
85 "Toronto Diphtheria Committee," 22 September 1932, LAC, MG28, I332, vol. 89, file 8.
86 Bates, "Diphtheria-Toxoid Week," 579. LAC, MG28, I332, vol. 89, file 8.
87 "Toronto Toxoid Week," April 19–25, 1942, LAC, MG28, I332, vol. 90, file 2.
88 James Colgrove, *State of Immunity: The Politics of Vaccination in Twentieth-Century America* (Berkeley: University of California Press, 2006), 97–98; Hammonds, *Childhood's Deadly Scourge,* 191–220.

89 "An Unwise Suggestion," *Globe and Mail,* 17 February 1928, 4; Gordon Bates, "Diphtheria Prevention," *Globe and Mail,* 23 February 1928, 4; W.L. Hutton, "Diphtheria Prevention," *Globe and Mail,* 1 March 1928, 4.

90 "Toronto Toxoid Week," n.d. [c. 1944], LAC, MG28, I332, vol. 92, file 1.

91 Untitled document, likely radio talk, n.d. [c. 1932], LAC, MG28, I332, vol. 90, file 7.

92 Radio talk, n.d. [likely late 1930s], LAC, MG28, I332, vol. 90, file 7.

93 "Too Late: A True Story," *Prairie Messenger,* 23 April 1942, and "Too Late: A True Story," *Moncton Transcript,* 22 April 1942.

94 "Dr. Gillies: Five Minute Address – Toxoid Week 1945," LAC, MG28, I332, vol. 92, file 3.

95 "Five Minute Address by Gordon Bates," 19 April 1943, LAC, MG28, I332, vol. 91, file 15.

96 Naomi Rogers, "Vegetables on Parade: American Medicine and the Child Health Movement in the Jazz Age," in *Children's Health Issues in Historical Perspective,* ed. Cheryl Krasnick Warsh and Veronica Strong-Boag (Waterloo, ON: Wilfrid Laurier University Press, 2005), 27.

97 "Toronto Achieves Fine Record through Toxoid" (poster), April 1940, LAC, MG28, I332, vol. 91, file 7.

98 Letter from Gordon Bates to J.V. McAree, 21 April 1944, LAC, MG28, I332, vol. 92, file 1; "Getting the Facts Straight," *Brantford Expositor,* 21 April 1942.

99 Letter from Gordon Bates to J.V. McAree, 21 April 1944, LAC, MG28, I332, vol. 92, file 1; clippings from *Toronto Star,* n.d., LAC, MG28, I332, vol. 90, file 10.

100 "City Has Lost Clean Record in Diphtheria," *Toronto Evening Telegram,* 22 April 1941; "Combating Diphtheria," *Globe and Mail,* 14 February 1942.

101 "5 New Toxoid Clinics Ordered by Conboy," *Toronto Star,* 3 February 1942.

102 MacDougall, *Activists and Advocates,* 144.

103 In 1933, E.S. Godfrey, for example, predicted that immunization (through three separate doses of toxoid) of 30 percent of children aged 0–4 and 50 percent aged 5–14 was enough to eradicate the disease. Paul E.M. Fine, "Herd Immunity: History, Theory, Practice," *Epidemiologic Reviews* 15, 2 (1993): 289. E.S. Godfrey, "Practical Uses of Diphtheria Immunization Records," *American Journal of Public Health* 23 (1933): 809–12. It is important to note that this is not the first description of "herd immunity," which was formally discussed in the 1920s. Colgrove, *State of Immunity,* 3.

104 Gordon Bates, "Five Minute Address," 1945, LAC, MG28, I332, vol. 92, file 3.

105 "Report of the Diphtheria Committee," Health League of Canada, Annual Meeting, 3 June 1942, LAC, MG28 I331, vol. 9, file 11.

106 For information on Toxoid Week in cities other than Toronto, see "To Prevent Diphtheria," *Montreal Gazette,* 15 May 1942; "Montreal's Diphtheria 'Toxoid' Week, May 5th to 10th, 1941," LAC, MG28, I332, vol. 92, file 18; "The City Declares War on Diphtheria," 18 May 1942, LAC, MG28, I332, vol. 90, file 10; "Toxoid Week in Sherbrooke" and "Toxoid Week in Montreal," n.d., LAC, MG28, I332, vol. 90, file 6. Lord Athlone's address is "Co-operation Can End Diphtheria," 20 April 1942, LAC, MG28, I332, vol. 90, file 10.

107 "Manual of Instructions for Toxoid Week," n.d. [c. 1943], LAC, MG28, I332, vol. 90, file 6.

108 Letter from R.C. Davison to Gordon Bates, 17 July 1942; "Questionnaire Concerning Toxoid Week: New Brunswick," n.d. [c. 1942]; Letter from A. Marguerite Swan to Gordon Bates, 4 June 1942, LAC, MG28, I332, vol. 90, file 6.

109 *Toxoid Prevents Diphtheria* (pamphlet), 15–21 April 1945, LAC, MG28, I332, vol. 92, file 3.

110 Ibid.

111 "Report of the 21st Annual Toronto Toxoid Week, April 22–28, 1951," LAC, MG28, I332, vol. 92, file 15.

112 John C. Scott, "For Release Anytime during Week of April 24, 1949," 30–31, LAC, MG28, I332, vol. 92, file 13.

113 Letter from C.C. Goldring to Dr. Gordon Bates, 15 April 1953, LAC, MG28, I332, vol. 96, file 7.

114 "Toronto Toxoid Week – 19th Annual Campaign – May 1st–7th, 1949," LAC, MG28, I332, vol. 92, file 13.

115 Editorial, "Controlling Diphtheria," *Canadian Public Health Journal* 30, 10 (1939): 500–1.

116 Public Health Agency of Canada, "Diphtheria," 24 July 2014, https://www.canada.ca/en/public-health/services/immunization/vaccine-preventable-diseases/diphtheria/health-professionals.html.

117 "Toronto Diphtheria Committee from L.A. Pequagnat," 8 May 1934, LAC, MG28, I332, vol. 89, file 8. Children needed three immunizations to be fully protected, so these figures reflect the number of immunizations given, not the number of children fully vaccinated.

118 "Toxoid Figures 1942"; "Toxoid Figures 1943," LAC, MG28, I332, vol. 92, file 17.

119 Report on Toronto's 17th Annual Toxoid Week, 20–26 April 1947, LAC, MG28, I332, vol. 92, file 9.

120 Catherine Carstairs, Paige Schell, and Sheilagh Quaile, "Making the 'Perfect Food' Safe: The Milk Pasteurization Debate," in *How Canadians Communicate VI: Food Promotion, Consumption and Controversy,* ed. Charlene Elliot (Edmonton: Athabasca University Press, 2016); Marion McKay, "'The Tubercular Cow Must Go': Business, Politics, and Winnipeg's Milk Supply, 1894–1922," *Canadian Bulletin of Medical History* 23, 2 (2006): 355–80; Susan Jones, "Mapping a Zoonotic Disease: Anglo-American Efforts to Control Bovine Tuberculosis before World War I," *Osiris* 19, 2 (2006): 133–48; Andrew Ejeber, "'Milking' the Consumer? Consumer Dissatisfaction and Regulatory Intervention in the Ontario Milk Industry during the Great Depression," *Ontario History* 52, 1 (2010): 20–39; Jane Jenkins, "Politics, Pasteurization and the Naturalizing Myth of Pure Milk in 1920s Saint John, New Brunswick," *Acadiensis* 37, 2 (2008): 86–105.

121 E.W. McHenry, "The Nutritional Value of Pasteurized Milk," *Canadian Public Health Journal* 25, 1 (1934): 22–25.

122 A.E. Berry, "A Survey of Milk Control in Cities and Towns in Canada," *Canadian Public Health Journal* 29, 6 (1938): 305–9.

123 R.H. Murray, "Milk Sanitation in Canada," *Canadian Public Health Journal* 23, 6 (1932): 259.

124 "Reports from the Annual Meeting; The Third Annual Report of the Committee on Milk Control," *Canadian Public Health Journal* 28, 9 (1937): 462.

125 Veronica McCormick, *A Hundred Years in the Dairy Industry, 1867–1967* (Ottawa: Dairy Farmers of Canada, 1968); Gordon C. Church, *An Unfailing Faith: A History of the Saskatchewan Dairy Industry* (Regina: Canadian Plains Research Center, 1985).

126 Melanie Dupuis, *Nature's Perfect Food: How Milk Became America's Drink* (New York: New York University Press, 2002), 75–94.

127 Harvey Levenstein, "'Best for Babies' or 'Preventable Infanticide': The Controversy over Artificial Feeding of Infants in America, 1880–1920," *Journal of American History* 70, 1 (1983): 75–94.

128 Helen MacMurchy, *Canadians Need Milk* (Ottawa: Dominion of Canada, 1921).

129 E.W. McHenry, "The Nutritional Value of Raw and Pasteurized Milk," *Canadian Journal of Public Health* 29, 6 (1938): 295. For more about McHenry and his role in Canadian nutrition debates, see Ian Mosby, *Food Will Win the War: The Politics, Culture, and Science of Food on Canada's Home Front* (Vancouver: UBC Press, 2014), 29–33, 167–72, 181–87.

130 *What to Eat to Be Healthy* (pamphlet), n.d. [1930s], LAC, MG28, I332, vol. 107, file 8.

131 M.C. Urquhart, *Gross National Product of Canada, 1870–1926* (Montreal and Kingston: McGill-Queen's University Press, 1993), 114.

132 Statistics Canada, *Handbook of Agricultural Statistics* (Ottawa: Queen's Printer, 1955), 14.

133 "Human and Bovine Tuberculosis," *Journal of the Canadian Medical Association* 16, 4 (1926): 438–39.

134 Katharine McCuaig, *The Weariness, the Fever and the Fret: The Campaign against Tuberculosis in Canada, 1900–1950* (Montreal and Kingston: McGill-Queen's University Press, 1999), 177.

135 "The Montreal Typhoid Fever Situation: Report of a Special Board of the US Public Health Service," *American Journal of Public Health* 17, 8 (1927): 783–90; "Milk News," *Canada's Health News* 1, 3 (1938): 1–2.

136 A. McNabb, "Undulant Fever in Ontario," *Canadian Journal of Public Health* 25, 1 (1934): 10–12.

137 W.H. Marriot, "Infectious Abortion of Cattle in Canada," *Canadian Public Health Journal* 29, 6 (1938): 269.

138 Report on Field Trip, 17 October–7 November 1946, LAC, MG28, I332, vol. 70 file 12.

139 "The Value of Pasteurization," *Social Health*, June 1931, LAC, MG28, I332, vol. 107, file 3.

140 See for example, G.Bates, "Health" and "Pasteurization of Milk for Health," *The Signet* (Elmira, ON), 4 July 1935; G. Bates, "Health" and "Health and the Pasteurization of Milk," *The Star* (Goderich, ON), 20 June 1935; "Pasteurizaiton of Milk," *Sentinel Review* (Woodstock, ON), 2 March 1934; "Milk," *The Era* (Newmarket, ON), 2 March 1934. LAC, MG28, I332, vol. 107, files 27–28.

141 W.J. Bell, "Safe Milk," *Canadian Journal of Public Health* 25, 1 (1934): 1–2.

142 "Preliminary Committee to Consider a Ways & Means of Organizing a National Movement for Safe Milk," 4 November 1935, LAC, MG28, I332, vol. 106, file 14.

143 "Dr. McCullough Dies at Desk; in 73rd Year," *Globe and Mail*, 6 January 1941, 4; Fred Adams, "John W.S. McCullough, M.D., C.M, D.P.H," *Canadian Public Health*

Journal 32, 2 (1941): 89–91; Gordon Bates, "A Tribute to the Late J.W.S. McCullough," *Health*, December 1940, 102.

144 Harry Ebbs, "Alan Brown, the Man" *Canadian Medical Association Journal*, 113 (20 September 1975): 92.

145 Letter from Gordon Bates to J. Robbins, 11 April 1936, LAC, MG28, I332, vol. 106, file 14.

146 Susan E. Lederer and John Parascandola, "Screening Syphilis: *Dr. Ehlich's Magic Bullet* Meets the Public Health Service," *Journal of the History of Medicine and Allied Sciences* 53 (1998): 345–70.

147 *Louis Pasteur's Great Speech* (pamphlet), n.d. [c. 1936], LAC, MG28, I332, vol. 17, file 3.

148 "Health Educational Materials," 1942–43, LAC, MG28, I332, vol. 107, file 12.

149 Annual Report for the year ending 30 April 1949, 27, LAC, MG28, I332, vol. 9, file 25; also see much earlier articles in *Health* by A.E. Berry: "Milk as a Summer Vacation Problem," June 1936, 37, 49–50, and "When Safe Milk Takes a Holiday," June 1937, 34–35, 49. A poster on the dangers of consuming raw milk while on summer holidays was produced during the war: "Going on Holiday?," n.d. [c. 1939–45], LAC, MG28, I332, vol. 107, file 14.

150 "Pasteurization in Port Dover," n.d. [c. 1933], LAC, MG28, I332, vol. 36, file 2; letter from Gordon Bates to Sam Morris, 6 July 1935, LAC, MG28, I332, vol. 106, file 14.

151 Emile Vaillaincourt, "Pasteurization of Milk," 18 May 1943, LAC, MG28, I332, vol. 107, file 18.

152 "Le Ministère de la Santé et du Bien-être social a reçu des resolutions au sujet de la pasteurization du lait dans la Province," n.d. [c. 1943]; Letter from Emile Vaillancourt to Gordon Bates, 2 March 1943, LAC, MG28, I332, vol. 110, file 9.

153 Annual Reports of the Twenty-Fourth Annual Meeting, 6 October 1943, LAC, MG28, I332, vol. 9, file 18; letter from Emile Vaillancourt to Gordon Bates, 2 June 1943, LAC, MG28, I332, vol. 110, file 8.

154 Health League of Canada Annual Meeting, 3 June 1942, LAC, MG28, I332, vol. 9, file 17.

155 See the resolutions in LAC, MG28, I332, vol. 109, file 22.

156 Twenty-Eighth Annual Meeting, 17–19 June 1947, LAC, MG28, I332, vol. 9, file 23, 33.

157 "Manual on the Pasteurization of Milk," n.d., LAC, MG28, I332, vol. 107, file 12. This claim also appeared in *Health*. See, for example, "These Are the Tasks That Demand Action," *Health*, September 1936, 74–75, and "Health League's Activities," *Health*, December 1937, 98.

158 "Letter #1," LAC, MG28, I332, vol. 108, file 18.

159 "Pasteurization of Milk," July 1948, LAC, MG28, I332, vol. 107, file 19.

160 Annual Reports Presented at the Twenty-Fourth Annual Meeting, 6 October 1943, LAC, MG28, I332, vol. 9, file 18.

161 Letter from Gordon Bates to F. Junkinson, 2 October 1939, and from Bates to O.O. Hines, 11 November 1939, LAC, MG28, I332, vol. 107, file 9.

162 Letter from A. Brown to Gordon Bates, 8 January 1948, LAC, MG28, I332, vol. 108, file 20.

163 *Pasteurization of Milk* (pamphlet), n.d. [c. 1936–39], LAC, MG28, I332, vol. 107, file 1.

164 Letter from H.C. Rhodes to Gordon Bates, March 1947, LAC, MG28, I332, vol. 108, file 11.

165 "Pasteurization for Quebec," n.d., LAC, MG28, I332, vol. 110, file 8.
166 "Health League in Action," *Health*, Spring 1972, 21.
167 "Canada's 20th Annual National Health Week," n.d., LAC, MG28, I332, vol. 109, file 1.

Chapter 3: "Stamp Out VD!"

1 In 1939, for example, the government of Ontario created a separate Venereal Disease Division, which was reorganized to provide more extensive service in 1943. R.P. Vivian, "The Public Health Aspects of Venereal Disease Control," *Canadian Journal of Public Health* 36, 2 (1945): 53–57; Quebec also established the Division of Venereal Disease during the war. Elphege Lalande and Jules Archambault, "Administration of a Provincial Venereal-Disease Control Program," *Canadian Journal of Public Health* 25, 2 (1944): 55–58. British Columbia reorganized and expanded its Division of Venereal Disease Control in 1936. Donald H. Williams, "Commercialized Prostitution and Venereal Disease Control," *Canadian Journal of Public Health* 31, 10 (1940): 461–72. In 1943, the federal government re-created its Division of Venereal Disease Control, which had been shuttered in 1932.
2 Elizabeth Fee, "Sin vs. Science: Venereal Disease in Baltimore in the Twentieth Century," *Journal of the History of Medicine and Allied Sciences* 43 (1998): 141–64; Allan Brandt, *No Magic Bullet: A Social History of Venereal Disease in the United States since 1880* (New York: Oxford University Press, 1985), 135–37.
3 Prontylin (a sulpha drug) started to be used for gonorhea treatment in 1937. That year, Bates reports that he has been using it for a few months:

> The spectacular results which have followed its use during the last few months justify the observation, I think, that here we have the most spectacular development in the history of Venereal Disease control. The immediate amelioration of symptoms and apparent rapid cure in a vast majority of acute cases in both males and females will shortly, I believe, result in a rapid fall in the incidence of Gonorrhea.

He is extremely concerned that Prontylin be under the control of physicians and not available through druggists. Gordon Bates, "The Present Problem in Venereal Disease," paper read before the Section of Preventive Medicine and Hygiene, 25 November 1937, Library and Archives Canada (hereafter LAC), MG28, I332, vol. 133, file 11. The VD Clinic at Nôtre-Dame Hospital in Montreal began using sulphapyridine in April 1939. It had considerable success and published results in the *Union médicale* in July 1939 and again in April 1940. Letter from Lucien Sylvestre to Gordon Bates, 15 October 1940, LAC, MG28, I332, vol. 132, file 9. In same file, see articles by Sylvestre, including "Méthode actuelles de traitement de la blennorragie chez l'homme," *Union médicale*, April 1940.
4 A.F.W. Peart, "The Venereal Disease Problem in Canada," *Canadian Journal of Public Health* 44, 5 (1953): 160–66.
5 "Penicillin," *Canadian Journal of Public Health* 36, 3 (1945): 119–21.
6 Peart, "The Venereal Disease Problem in Canada."
7 Ruth Roach Pierson, "The Double Bind of the Double Standard: VD Control and the CWAC in World War II," *Canadian Historical Review* 82, 1 (1981): 44–45.

8   In 1937, a survey documented 3,639 cases of syphilis in Toronto. By 1943, this had
    increased to 4,747, but the population of Toronto had also increased, so that the rate
    per 1,000 population had increased only from 5.6 percent to 6.5 percent. The num-
    ber of cases of gonorrhea fell from 2,549 to 1,595. "Table V: Incidence of Syphilis and
    Gonorrhoea, Toronto, 1929, 1931, 1937, and 1943," LAC, MG28, I332, vol. 145, file 4.

9   Bates, "The Present Problem in Venereal Disease." Indeed, Bates had been promot-
    ing premarital testing since before the National Council for Combatting Venereal
    Disease was established. "Reports of Societies: Academy of Medicine, Toronto,"
    Canadian Practitioner 39 (1914): 177. The CSHC passed a resolution in favour of
    premarital examinations at its 1928 meeting. "Medical Examination before Mar-
    riage," LAC, MG28, I332, vol. 10, file 26; Venereal Disease Control Program of the
    Health League of Canada (Social Hygiene Division), LAC, MG28, I332, vol. 134,
    file 17.

10 Christabelle Sethna, "Cold War and the Sexual Chill: Freezing Girls Out of Sex Edu-
    cation," Canadian Woman Studies 17, 4 (1997): 57–61.

11 For a description of the material released by the federal government and the armed
    forces see Pierson, "The Double Bind," 31–58.

12 Letter from Gordon Bates to Harold J. Kirby, 19 March 1941, LAC, MG28, I332, vol. 132,
    file 8.

13 Minutes of the Venereal Diseases Committee, 25 September 1939, LAC, MG28,
    I332, vol. 132, file 10.

14 Gordon Bates, "Is Venereal Disease a Moral Issue?" Health, July 1941, 54.

15 Gordon Bates, "Venereal Disease Control," Canadian Public Health Journal, July
    1941, 347. In 1930, Bates wrote to all provincial officers of health recommending that
    all venereal disease posters state that people having "illicit contact" should immedi-
    ately visit a doctor. Letters, LAC, MG28, I332, vol. 128, file 16.

16 Letter from Gordon Bates to Harold Orr, 5 October 1942, LAC, MG28, I332, vol. 132,
    file 7.

17 Bates, "Venereal Disease Control," 347.

18 See correspondence in LAC, MG28, I332, vol. 135, file 4.

19 "Teen-Age Tragedy," Modern Digest, November 1943.

20 Minutes of a special committee appointed to study conditions connected with bev-
    erage room abuses and law enforcement, 3 November 1944, LAC, MG28, I332, vol. 58,
    file 11.

21 See, for example, Suggested Feature, "The Churches and VD Prevention August 1944"
    and "Forum on VD Control," n.d. [c. 1944–46], LAC, MG28, I332, vol. 144, file 7.

22 Gene Tunney, "The Bright Shield of Continence," Journal of Social Hygiene 28, 8
    (1942): 473–76, originally published in Reader's Digest, August 1942, as detailed in
    Yves Yvon J. Pelletier, "Fighting for the Chaplains: Bishop Charles Leo Nelligan and
    the Creation of the Canadian Chaplain Service (Roman Catholic), 1939–1945,"
    CCHA Historical Studies 72 (2006): 112.

23 See, for example, Letter from R. Fowlow to the Secretary, Health League of Canada,
    29 November 1943; Letter from Frank Wellington to the Health League of
    Canada, 13 November 1943; Letter from Mabel Ferris to Rev. G. McKinnon,
    30 August 1943, LAC, MG28, I332, vol. 140, file 21.

24 Health League of Canada Annual Report presented at the 24th Annual Meeting, 6 October 1943, LAC, RG29, vol. 216, file 311-V3-22, part 9; *What Are the Venereal Diseases,* n.d., LAC, RG29, vol. 216, file 311-V3-22, part 9, 2, 6–7.

25 Joe Lichstein, "Report Re Junior Chamber of Ontario Regional Conference," LAC, MG28, I332, vol. 134, file 18.

26 Letter from D.E.H. Cleveland to Gordon Bates, 18 January 1943, LAC, MG28, I332, vol. 194, file 21.

27 Minutes of the Social Hygiene Division of the Health League of Canada, 6 June 1944, LAC, MG28, I332, vol. 135, file 7.

28 Letter from Gordon Bates to Mrs. Russell Parks, 1 February 1945, and from Mrs. Russell Parks to Gordon Bates, 16 January 1945, LAC, MG28, I332, vol. 134, file 17.

29 *Fight Syphilis* (film), United States Public Health Service, https://archive.org/details/ FightSyphilis1942.

30 Minutes of the Clergymen's Committee, 13 June 1944, LAC, MG28, I332, vol. 58, file 12.

31 This film has been uploaded to YouTube: https://www.youtube.com/watch?v= 4NovK0vWJIw. Although WorldCat has labelled it as a 1934 anti-STD film, it was released in 1939.

32 American Social Hygiene Association/Willard Pictures, *Health Is a Victory,* 1942, in *Atomic Age Classics,* Volume 4, *Venereal Diseases and You* (Narbeth, PA: Alpha Home Entertainment, 2006).

33 Unfortunately, we were unable to view a copy of *Plain Facts.* This description comes from the WorldCat entry, http://www.worldcat.org/title/plain-facts/oclc/31667931.

34 Health League of Canada, report of activities since March 1942, 6 March 1943, LAC, MG28, I332, vol. 42, file 2; letter from Gordon Bates to N.J. Trow, 2 October 1940, LAC, MG28, I332, vol. 137, file 6.

35 Letter from F.C. Middleton to Gordon Bates, 11 May 1944, LAC, MG28, I332, vol. 134, file 18.

36 "The Health League of Canada: A Brief History of Its Origin," n.d. [c. 1944], LAC, MG28, I332, vol. 134, file 17.

37 Letter P.T.O to Maurice Seymour, 21 June 1921, LAC, MG28, I332, vol. 45, file 12.

38 John C. Scott, "Toronto's VD Fight," *Health,* Autumn 1944, 18, 27–28.

39 Ben Lepkin, "I Like the Movies," *Winnipeg Tribune,* 11 July 1942.

40 "Health League of Canada Sponsors *No Greater Sin,"* *Rouyn Noranda Press,* 10 December 1942.

41 Helen Allen, "At the Movies," *Toronto Telegram,* 18 September 1942.

42 Letter from J.A. Leroux to Gordon Bates, 26 June 1942, LAC, MG28, I332, vol. 135, file 9.

43 Report on attendance to March 15, 1943, LAC, MG28, I332, vol. 141, file 1.

44 Untitled press release, n.d. [c. 1942], LAC, MG28, I332, vol. 139, file 3.

45 Scott, "Toronto's VD Fight," 18; Minutes of National Social Hygiene Division of the Venereal Disease Committee, n.d. [probably 13 October 1944], LAC, MG28, I332, vol. 135, file 7.

46 Letter from Christian Smith to Gordon Bates, 8 June 1944, LAC, MG28, I332, vol. 134, file 18; see "Report on Showings of 'No Greater Sin,'" LAC, MG28, I332, vol. 135, file 4.

47 "Observations and Recommendations Re Showing of 'No Greater Sin' in Massey Hall," 17 October 1944, LAC, MG28, I332, vol. 139, file 14; *No Greater Sin* advertisement, *Welland Post/Colborne Evening Telegram*, 13 June 1942, LAC, MG28, I332, vol. 139, file 7.

48 "Lichstein Heads Junior Chamber VD Campaign," 3 December 1943, LAC, MG28, I332, vol. 134, file 16.

49 "The Health League's Activities in the Voluntary Venereal Disease Education Field," LAC, RG29, vol. 216, file 311-V3-22, part 10.

50 "Achievements," n.d. [ca. 1943], LAC, MG28, I332, vol. 133, file 19.

51 Appendix to Social Hygiene Report, 23 May 1944, LAC, MG28, I332, vol. 134, file 18.

52 Interim Report of the Visit to Prairie Provinces, n.d. [c. May 1944], LAC, MG28, I332, vol. 134, file 18.

53 Inventory Venereal Disease, n.d., LAC, MG28, I332, vol. 140, file 9; also see Social Hygiene Kit, Contents, n.d., LAC, MG28, I332, vol. 140, file 13.

54 The prize followed the lead of the American Social Hygiene Association, which offered a prize to the Jaycees for the best anti-syphilis campaign. See LAC, MG28, I332, vol. 140, file 10. There were some complications, however, and it appears that the prize was never actually awarded. See LAC, MG28, I332, vol. 160, file 18.

55 Report of the National Health Committee to the Ninth Annual Conference of the Junior Chamber of Commerce of Canada, Port Arthur, June 10–11, 1944, on the Junior Chamber's 1943–44 Anti-VD Campaign, LAC, MG28, I332, vol. 134, file 17.

56 Letter from Gordon Bates to F.W. Jackson, 30 December 1943, LAC, MG28, I332, vol. 134, file 16.

57 Letter from Gordon Bates to Mrs. G.E. Dragan, 2 December 1943, LAC, MG28, I332, vol. 140, file 4.

58 "The Community and Venereal Disease for Use on 2 February 1944," LAC, MG28, I332, vol. 129, file 8.

59 "Mass Meeting in Massey Hall," 5 February 1945, LAC, MG28, I332, vol. 134, file 19.

60 "The 1945 Anti-VD Offence," LAC, MG28, I332, vol. 134, file 19.

61 Ibid.

62 Some bad feelings seem to have developed between the Jaycees and the Health League, and in 1946 the Jaycees refused to put forward a representative on the league's council. Letter from K.G. Tremblay to Gordon Bates, 18 April 1946, LAC, MG28, I332, vol. 160, file 18. The withdrawal may have been because of the conflict of interest in having Lichstein work out of the Health League's offices, or it may have been the result of what the Jaycees described as the "failure" of their own national campaign in 1945, although several branches of the Jaycees participated in that campaign. See correspondence in LAC, MG28, I332, vol. 160, file 18.

63 Brooke Claxton, "The Need to Attract Attention to the Health Problem of the Canada," *Health,* Spring 1946, 5.

64 Health League of Canada, Twenty-Eighth Annual Meeting, 17–19 June 1947, LAC, MG28, I332, vol. 9, file 23.

65 Health League of Canada, Twenty-Ninth Annual Meeting, 4–6 November 1948, LAC, MG28, I332, vol. 9, file 24.

66 Health League records indicate that approximately 2,500 drug stores out of a total of 3,865 ran these displays: "Social Hygiene Division Annual Report 1945–6," LAC, MG28, I332, vol. 132, file 4.

67 Health League press release, 15 May 1945, LAC, MG28, I332, vol. 134, file 19; list of newspapers in Sponsored Advertising Campaign, 21–26 May 1945, LAC, MG28, I332, vol. 131, file 23.

68 Press release, 15 May 1945, LAC, MG28, I332, vol. 134, file 19.

69 Interim Report of the Visit to Prairie Provinces.

70 "The Venereal Disease Control Scheme for Canada," n.d. [c. 1943], LAC, MG28, I332, vol. 135, file 5.

71 Memo on the Health League and VD [author unknown], n.d., RG29, vol. 216, file 311-V3-22, part 9.

72 Memo to Gordon Bates from Christian Smith, 14 August 1944, LAC, MG28, I332, vol. 134, file 18.

73 Confidential Report, Venereal Disease Division, n.d., LAC, MG28, I332, vol. 134, file 15.

74 Minutes of the Social Hygiene Division of the Health League of Canada, 6 June 1944, LAC, MG28, I332, vol. 135, file 7.

75 Interim Report of the Visit to Prairie Provinces.

76 *A Case for Pre-Marital Blood Testing* (pamphlet), 1946, RG29, vol. 216, file 311-V3-22, part 12. The Canadian Social Hygiene Council had gone on record as supporting premarital testing as early as 1928. See Ninth Annual Report of the Canadian Social Hygiene Council, 12 June 1928, LAC, MG28, I332, vol. 9, file 13.

77 Joseph Lichstein, "Guard Their Health: Insuring Marriage and the Newborn against Syphilis," *Health*, Summer 1946, 14–15, 27. Boivon argues that premarital syphilis testing gained little traction in Quebec because it would serve as a barrier to marriage. Also, eugenics was less popular in Quebec than elsewhere in Canada. Jérôme Boivin, "État protecteur – état promoteur: La campagne antivénérienne dans le Québec de l'entre deux-guerres" (MA thesis, Université Laval, 2008).

78 Lichstein, "Guard Their Health," 14–15, 27.

79 Ontario, *Legislative Assembly Debates*, 28 February 1951, 3rd session, 23rd Legislature (Mr. Dennison, CCF), H-2.

80 Harold Orr, "The Compulsory Premarital Serological Test in Alberta," *Canadian Journal of Public Health* 38, 5 (1947): 232–35.

81 Brandt, *No Magic Bullet*, 152.

82 E.H. Lossing and R.H. Allen, "Venereal Diseases in Canada," *British Journal of Venereal Disease* 32 (1956): 150–53.

83 Dorothy Chunn, "A Little Sex Can Be a Dangerous Thing: Regulating Sexuality, Venereal Disease and Reproduction in British Columbia" in *Challenging the Public/Private Divide: Feminism, the Law and Public Policy*, ed. Susan Boyd (Toronto: University of Toronto Press, 1997), 62–86.

84 Y.M. Felman, "Repeal of Premarital Tests for Syphilis: A Survey of State Health Officers," *American Journal of Public Health* 71, 2 (1981): 155–59.

85 Jeffrey Keshen, *Saints, Sinners, and Soldiers: Canada's Second World War* (Vancouver: UBC Press, 2004), 194–227.

86 First Meeting of the Subcommittee on Sex Education, 25 July 1944, LAC, MG28, I332, vol. 57, file 18. A year previously, 90 percent of Canadians said that they were

in favour of free treatment for venereal disease. "Gallup Poll of Canada: Should VD Treatment Be Made Compulsory and Free," LAC, MG28, I332, vol. 140, file 1.

87 Letter from Christian Smith to Robin Pearse, W.W. Judd, E.F. Trow, and Black, 3 May 1944, LAC, MG28, I332, vol. 132, file 4. See also First Meeting of the Subcommittee on Sex Education, 25 July 1944, LAC, MG28, I332, vol. 57, file 18.

88 "Program for the Next Six Months," 29 August 1944, LAC, MG28, I332, vol. 132, file 4.

89 A good description of Bates' attitudes towards sex education can be found in "The Place of Sex Education in Life," 13 February 1935, LAC, RG29, vol. 216, file 311-V3-22, part 8.

90 Resolution re sex education passed by the National Social Hygiene Committee, 29–31 October 1945, LAC, RG29, vol. 216, file 311-V3-22, part 11.

91 Sethna, "Cold War and the Sexual Chill," 57–61.

92 Press release, "Teenagers Reckless, Undisciplined Think Largest Group of Grownups," 1 February 1947, and "Think Horse and Buggy Days Had more Successful Families," 29 January 1947, LAC, MG28, I332, vol. 140, file 1.

93 Joan Sangster, *Girl Trouble: Female Delinquency in English Canada* (Toronto: Between the Lines, 2002); Mary Louise Adams, *The Trouble with Normal: Postwar Youth and the Making of Heterosexuality* (Toronto: University of Toronto Press, 1997); Mona Gleason, *Normalizing the Ideal: Psychology, Schooling and the Family in Postwar Canada* (Toronto: University of Toronto Press, 1999).

94 "VD Survey, Toronto, 1950," LAC, MG28, I332, vol. 145, file 6.

95 Spending on the league's venereal disease program dropped from just over $12,000 in the year ending 30 April 1945 to just over $6,500 in the year ending 30 April 1946. Expenditures increased slightly in 1946–47 and then dropped to just over $1,000 for the year ending 30 April 1948. LAC, MG28, I332, vol. 23, file 9.

96 "Sex Education Is Not Enough," *Health*, Summer 1946, 10–11.

97 Jeffrey Moran, *Teaching Sex: The Shaping of Adolescence in the 20th Century* (Cambridge: Harvard University Press, 2000), 123–25.

98 "Sex Education Is Not Enough," 10–11. Some of these claims were based on Herbert Dyson Carter, *Sin and Science* (Toronto: Progress Books, 1945).

99 "Venereal Disease and Morals," *Health*, February 1948, 5.

100 "Health and Moving Pictures," *Health*, May/June 1949, 5.

101 Staff Conference, 1 February 1948, LAC, MG28, I332, vol. 102, file 22.

102 "Health League Urges Banning Kinsey Report," *Globe and Mail*, 1 June 1948, 11.

103 Gordon Bates, "The Kinsey Report," *Health*, March 1950, 5.

104 Minutes of the Toronto Clergy Committee, 7 June 1950, LAC, MG28, I332, vol. 58, file 12.

105 Gordon Bates, "To Ban or Not to Ban," *Health*, March/April 1950, 5.

106 Gordon Bates, "Kinsey at It Again," *Health*, September/October 1953, 34.

107 "A Challenge to Parents," *Health*, September/October 1958, 4.

108 Gordon Bates, "Authors, Publishers and Obscenity," *Health*, September/October 1959, 4.

109 Mary Louise Adams, "Youth, Corruptibility, and English-Canadian Postwar Campaigns against Indecency 1948–55," *Journal of the History of Sexuality* 6, 1 (1995): 89–117.

110 See, for example, two articles by J.V. McAree in the *Globe and Mail*: "Kinsey Report Is Only a Beginning," 10 November 1948, 6; "Trying to Suppress the Kinsey Report," 25 June 1948, 6.

Chapter 4: Preventing Sickness and Absenteeism

1 These posters and pamphlets can be found in Library and Archives Canada (hereafter LAC), MG28, I332, vol. 103, file 9.

2 Jeffrey Keshen, *Saints, Sinners, and Soldiers: Canada's Second World War* (Vancouver: UBC Press, 2004); Ian Mosby, *Food Will Win the War: The Politics, Culture, and Science of Food on Canada's Home Front* (Vancouver: UBC Press, 2014); Jennifer Stephen, *Pick One Intelligent Girl: Employability, Domesticity, and the Gendering of Canada's Welfare State* (Toronto: University of Toronto Press, 2007).

3 For example, in November 1939, the *Canadian Journal of Public Health* devoted a special issue to industrial health. Regular articles continued to appear throughout the war.

4 Peter S. McInnis, *Harnessing Labour Confrontation: Shaping the Postwar Settlement in Canada, 1943–1950* (Toronto: University of Toronto Press, 2002), 26.

5 Allan Brandt, *No Magic Bullet: A Social History of Venereal Disease in the United States since 1880* (New York: Oxford University Press, 1985), 79 and 134.

6 Ontario, *Thirty-Ninth Annual Report of the Provincial Board of Health of Ontario, Canada, for the Year 1920: Division of Industrial Hygiene: Annual Report* (Toronto: King's Printer, 1921), 61; Ontario, *Forty-second Annual Report of the Provincial Board of Health of Ontario, Canada, for the Year 1923: Annual Report, 1923, Division of Industrial Hygiene* (Toronto: Clarkson W. James, Printer to the King's Most Excellent Majesty, 1924), 43–44; Canada, *Department of National Health and Welfare Annual Report for the Fiscal Year Ended March 31, 1948: Division of Industrial Hygiene* (Ottawa: King's Printer, 1948), 44–45.

7 This reflected the direction of the field more generally. See J. Allan Walters, "The Clinical Study of Neurotic Disorders in the Plant," *Canadian Journal of Public Health* 38, 3 (1947): 118–23; C.H. Gundry, "Industrial Psychiatry," *Canadian Journal of Public Health* 40, 1 (1949): 7–12.

8 Eric Tucker, *Administering Danger in the Workplace: The Law and Politics of Occupational Health and Safety Regulation in Ontario, 1850–1914* (Toronto: University of Toronto Press, 1990); Doug Smith, *Consulted to Death: How Canada's Workplace Safety System Fails Workers* (Winnipeg: Arbeiter Ring, 2000); Cynthia Comacchio, "Mechanomorphosis: Science, Management and 'Human Machinery' in Industrial Canada, 1900–1945," *Labour/Le Travail* 41 (Spring 1998): 35–67; Nancy Forestell, "'And I Feel Like I Am Dying from Mining for Gold': Disability, Gender and the Mining Community," *Labour: Studies in Working Class History of the Americas* 3, 3 (2006): 77–93; Alain Pontaut, *Santé et sécurité: Un bilan du régime québécois de santé et sécurité du travail, 1885–1985* (Montreal: Boréal, 1985); Joy Parr, "A Working Knowledge of the Insensible? Radiation Protection in Nuclear Generating Stations, 1962–1992," *Society for the Comparative Study of Society and History* 48, 4 (2006): 820–51; Stephen, *Pick One Intelligent Girl*; Jessica van Horssen, *A Town Called Asbestos: Environmental Contamination, Health, and Resilience in a Resource Community* (Vancouver: UBC Press, 2016).

9 Eric Tucker, "Making the Workplace 'Safe' in Capitalism: The Enforcement of Factory Legislation in Nineteenth-Century Ontario," *Labour/Le Travail* 21 (Spring 1988): 45–85.

10 Smith, *Consulted to Death*.

11 "The Industrial Physician's Services to Industry," *Public Health Journal* 18, 6 (1927): 295–96; Vicky Long, *The Rise and Fall of the Healthy Factory: The Politics of Industrial Health in Britain* (London: Palgrave, 2011).

12 J.G. Cunningham, "Industrial Hygiene in Ontario," *Canadian Public Health Journal* 30, 11 (1939): 524–26.

13 Cynthia Comacchio, "Industrial Hygiene," in *Oxford Companion to Canadian History*, ed. Gerald Hallowell (Toronto: Oxford University Press, 2004), http://www.oxfordreference.com/view/10.1093/acref/9780195415599.001.0001/acref-9780195415599-e-785?rskey=HpKPXi&result=1. She claims that the federal government established an industrial health branch program in 1924, but J.J. Heagerty makes no mention of it in his description of the National Health Division of the Department of Pensions and National Health. J.J. Heagerty, "The National Health Division of the Department of Pensions and National Health," *Canadian Public Health Journal* 26, 11 (1935): 528–40. Instead, Heagerty indicates that the Industrial Hygiene Division was created in the late 1930s. J.J. Heagerty, "The Activities of the National Health Section," *Canadian Public Health Journal* 30, 3 (1939): 120–23. F.J. Tourangeau, "Industrial Hygiene in the Province of Quebec," *Canadian Public Health Journal* 30, 11 (1939): 527–29; "The Health Officer and Industrial Hygiene," *Canadian Public Health Journal* 30, 11 (1939): 558–60.

14 "The Health Officer and Industrial Hygiene," *Canadian Public Health Journal* 30, 11 (1939): 448–60. In 1924, a doctor in the employ of the Spanish River Pulp and Paper Company described the company as being one of the first companies in the province to operate an industrial health plan. Frank L. McCarroll, "Industrial Health," *Public Health Journal* (Canada) 15, 8 (1924): 352–59. In the late 1930s, an industrial doctor indicated that two decades earlier, Canada had almost no industrial physicians. He indicated that, by 1936, "nearly all" major industries and many smaller ones had some sort of plan. Grant L. Bird, "The Doctor in Industry," *Canadian Public Health Journal* 27, 7 (1936): 333–36.

15 Health League of Canada, "Industrial Health Plan: A Vital Service for Canadian Industry," LAC, MG28, I332, vol. 102, file 20.

16 J.G. Cunningham, "Industrial Health and National Defense," *Canadian Public Health Journal* 31, 11 (1940): 556–59; F.S. Parney, "The Division of Industrial Hygiene," *Canadian Public Health Journal* 30, 3 (1939): 149–50.

17 Christopher Sellers, *The Hazards of the Job: From Industrial Disease to Environmental Health Science* (Chapel Hill: University of North Carolina Press, 1997); Long, *Rise and Fall of the Healthy Factory*; Claudia Clark, *Radium Girls: Women and Industrial Health Reform* (Chapel Hill: University of North Carolina Press, 1997). Clark argues that industrial hygiene in the United States split into several different occupations and fields in the 1930s. One of these, industrial medicine, focused on providing medical services to factories.

18 Clark, *Radium Girls*, 96.

19 Letter to 4,000 Key Executives, n.d., LAC, MG28, I332, vol. 101, file 9.

20 "Dividends from Health," *Health*, Summer 1942, 5; *Prevention of Sickness among Industrial Workers*, n.d., LAC, MG28, I332, vol. 102, file 20.

21 McInnis, *Harnessing Labour Confrontation*.

22 "James Stanley McLean," *Canadian Encyclopedia,* http://www.thecanadianen cyclopedia.ca/en/article/james-stanley-mclean/.

23 Ian MacLachlan, *Kill and Chill: Restructuring Canada's Beef Commodity Chain* (Toronto: University of Toronto Press, 2001): 219–21; Smith, *Consulted to Death,* 71–77.

24 "The Human Factory," *Health,* Summer 1945, 18. Canadian Glazed Papers had approximately fifty employees.

25 F.D. Cruickshank and J. Nason, *History of Weston* (Weston: Times and Guide, 1937).

26 A list of paid-up subscribers to *Industrial Health* indicates that a small minority of subscribers came from outside of Ontario. LAC, MG28, I332, vol. 102 file 20.

27 Letter from Mabel Ferris to Madame Paul Hamel, 6 February 1948, LAC, MG28, I332, vol. 102, file 22. Minutes from the National Industrial Health Committee, 21 January 1950 refer to them as providing insufficiently "adequate health messages" and suggest that they were available only in French, LAC, RG29, vol. 617, file 343–10–11.

28 See posters in LAC, MG28, I332, vol. 102, file 8.

29 "Catalogue of Educational Material Available," n.d. [c. 1946], LAC, MG28, I332, vol. 101, file 7.

30 Industrial Health Plan promotional letters, 1943–44, LAC, MG28, I332, vol. 102, file 20; a list of paid-up industrial clients contains numerous cards from companies requesting posters, leaflets, and books, LAC, MG28, I332, vol. 103, file 11.

31 For cheesecake images of women in the labour movement, see Craig Heron and Steve Penfold, *The Workers' Festival: A History of Labour Day in Canada* (Toronto: University of Toronto Press, 2005), 207–15, and Donica Belisle, *Retail Nation: Department Stores and the Making of Modern Canada* (Vancouver: UBC Press, 2011).

32 "Watch Out for Summer Gremlins" (poster), LAC, MG28, I332, vol. 232.

33 *Watch Out for Sumer Gremlins* (pamphlet), LAC, MG28, I332, vol. 232.

34 This idea may have reflected the influence of the chief of the Federal Division of Industrial Hygiene, F.S. Parney, who had published on "neuroses" at work. F.S. Parney, "Neuroses in a Large Office Group" (paper presented at a Meeting of the Canadian Public Health Association, June 1939), LAC, RG29, vol. 617, file 454–10–9.

35 *TB Is Dangerous* (pamphlet), LAC, MG28, I332, vol. 232.

36 *Worry Causes Sickness: Have a Talk with the "Doc"* (pamphlet), n.d., LAC, MG28, I332, vol. 102, file 16.

37 "Get 8 Hours Sleep Every Night" (poster and pay envelope insert), LAC, MG28, I332, vol. 232.

38 Ontario, *Sixteenth Annual Report of the Department of Health: Ontario, Canada for the Year 1940: Division of Industrial Hygiene* (Toronto: King's Printer, 1941), 157.

39 "Beware of Constipation" (pay envelope insert), LAC, MG28, I332, vol. 232.

40 "Don't Sag" (pay envelope insert), LAC, MG28, I332, vol. 232.

41 For a selection, see Hammett A. Dixon, "Athlete's Foot," *Health,* March 1934, 6, 16–17; F.R. Griffin, "Footnotes for Health," *Health,* September/October 1944, 8; "Young Feet Deserve Care," *Health,* September 1952, 13; Arthur Byron, "Fit the Shoe," *Health,* September/October 1954, 11, 30; "10 Steps to Foot Health," *Health,*

January 1955, 16; C.G. Cameron, "Chiroprody with Industrial Medicine," *Health,* September/October 1956, 19–21.

42 "Caring for Your Feet" (poster), LAC, MG28, I332, vol. 232, part 2.

43 "Keep On Your Toes by Caring for Your Feet" (pay envelope insert), LAC, MG28, I332, vol. 232, part 2.

44 "Health Depends on Cleanliness" (poster), LAC, MG28, I332, vol. 232, part 2.

45 "Health Depends on Cleanliness" (pay envelope insert), LAC, MG28, I332, vol. 232, part 2.

46 "Avoid Colds" (poster), LAC, MG28, I332, vol. 232.

47 "Avoid Colds" (pay envelope insert), ibid. On "cold vaccines," see Lemuel McGee, J.E. Andes, C.A. Plume, and S.H. Hinton, "'Cold Vaccines' and the Incidence of the Common Cold," *Journal of the American Medical Association* 124, 9 (1944): 555–57; J.G. Cunningham, "Industrial Health Problems Encountered in the War," *Canadian Medical Association Journal* 56 (January 1947): 34–36.

48 "Don't Be Shortsighted" (poster), LAC, MG28, I332, vol. 232.

49 "Don't Be Shortsighted" (pay envelope insert), ibid.

50 "See Your Dentist Twice a Year" (pay envelope insert), ibid.

51 "Eat a Nourishing Breakfast" (poster), ibid.

52 "A Nourishing Snack" (poster), ibid.

53 "A Nourishing Snack Is Better for You" (pay envelope insert), ibid.

54 "Pack Power in Every Meal" (pay envelope insert), ibid.

55 "Start Your Victory Garden Today!" (pay envelope insert), ibid.

56 "Keep Strong with Whole Grain Products" (poster), ibid.

57 *Syphilis Strikes One Out of Forty Canadians* (pamphlet), ibid.

58 This was John Bruce of the United Association of Plumbers and Steamfitters. See Minutes of the Steering Committee of the Industrial Hygiene Committee, various dates, LAC, MG28, I332, vol. 101, files 9 and 10. On his appointment, see Margaret Gould to Gordon Bates, 17 September 1942, and Gordon Bates to Margaret Gould, 18 September 1942, LAC, MG28, I332, vol. 102, file 7.

59 Minutes of the Industrial Hygiene Committee, 17 June 1941, LAC, MG28, I332, vol. 101, file 9.

60 Minutes of the Industrial Hygiene Committee, 24 September 1940, LAC, MG28, I332, vol. 101, file 9.

61 Untitled Health League press release, 23 November 1943, LAC, MG28, I332, vol. 103, file 10.

62 Ian Dowbiggin, "Prescription for Survival: Brock Chisholm, Sterilization and Mental Health in the Cold War Era," in *Mental Health and Canadian Society,* ed. David Wright and James E. Moran (Montreal and Kingston: McGill-Queen's University Press, 2006), 176–92.

63 Third Annual Conference program, 4 December 1945, LAC, MG28, I332, vol. 102, file 1.

64 Letter from S.E. Caldwell to R.C. Batson, 11 May 1944, LAC, MG28, I332, vol. 102, file 14.

65 Health League of Canada, "Industrial Health Plan."

66 "Dividends from Health," *Health,* Summer 1942, 5.

67 Stephen, *Pick One Intelligent Girl,* 16.
68 H.W. Irquhart, "The Value of Medical Services in Industry," *Health,* May/June 1951, 13.
69 Minutes of the Industrial Health Division Meeting, 16 April 1947, LAC, MG28, I332, vol. 102, file 22.
70 C.A. Massey, "The Soldier's Return," *Health,* Fall 1945, 9; "Men at Work: Veterans in Jobs Can Be Easily Assisted," *Health,* Fall 1945, 16.
71 F.W. Dunn, "What Do Employees Think about Health Service in Industry," *Industrial Health* 4, 1 (1946): 1–2; "Can Your Plant Afford a Health Program," *Industrial Health* 4, 2 (1946): 1–3; Christopher Sellers, "The Public Health Service's Office of Industrial Hygiene and the Transformation of Industrial Medicine," *Bulletin of the History of Medicine* 65 (1991): 42–73; Forestell, "And I Feel Like I Am Dying," 88–89. Vivienne Walters' study of industrial physicians in the 1980s underlines that workers had good reason to be suspicious: "Company Doctors' Perceptions of and Responses to Conflicting Pressures from Labour and Management," *Social Problems* 30, 1 (1982): 1–12.
72 Van Horssen, *A Town Called Asbestos,* 53–64.
73 H.M. Harrison, "Morale in the Factory," *Industrial Health* 3, 11 (1945): 2.
74 Mona Gleason, *Normalizing the Ideal: Psychology, Schooling and the Family in Postwar Canada* (Toronto: University of Toronto Press, 2003); Terry Copp and Bill McAndrew, *Battle Exhaustion: Soldiers and Psychiatrists in the Canadian Army, 1939–1945* (Montreal and Kingston: McGill-Queen's University Press, 1990).
75 Harold M. Harrison, "Cured by Changing His Shirt," *Health,* March/April 1953, 7.
76 "Industrial Health Plan: A Vital Service for Canadian Industry," n.d., LAC, MG28, I332, vol. 102, file 20; D.H. Williams, "VD Control in Industry," *Health,* Spring 1944, 23.
77 Williams, "VD Control in Industry," 23.
78 Katherine McCuaig, *The Weariness, the Fever and the Fret: The Campaign against Tuberculosis in Canada, 1900–1950* (Montreal and Kingston: McGill-Queen's University Press, 1999), 187–209.
79 Health League of Canada, "Industrial Health Plan."
80 Mosby, *Food Will Win the War.*
81 Health League of Canada, "Industrial Health Plan."
82 Florence Ignatieff, "Food for Workers," *Health,* Winter 1942–43, 6.
83 This concern was in keeping with broader trends in the industrial health field. See A. John Nelson, "The Physician and Industry," *Canadian Medical Association Journal* 91 (19 December 1941): 1307–09.
84 Peter Neary and J.L. Granatstein, *The Veteran's Charter and Post–World War II Canada* (Montreal and Kingston: McGill-Queen's University Press, 1998); Christopher Dummitt, *The Manly Modern: Masculinity in Postwar Canada* (Vancouver: UBC Press, 2007).
85 Stanley Caldwell, "Men at Work: No Good National Plan for Rehabilitation," *Health,* Autumn 1944, 10; "Men at Work: Veterans in Jobs Can Be Easily Assisted," *Heath,* Autumn 1945, 14; "Men at Work: Laws Alone Can't Help Handicapped Veterans," *Health,* Winter 1945–46, 24–25.

86 Copp and McAndrew, *Battle Exhaustion;* Stephen, *Pick One Intelligent Girl.*

87 C.A. Massey, "The Soldiers Return" *Health,* Fall 1945, 8.

88 Magda Fahrni makes similar arguments in her article "The Romance of Reunion: Montreal War Veterans Return to Family Life, 1944–1949," *Journal of the Canadian Historical Association* 9, 1 (1998): 187–208.

89 Capt. F.E. Coburn, "The Soldier's Return," *Health,* Spring 1945, 8–9, 22–23, 26.

90 S.E. Caldwell, "When Johnny Comes Back to Work," *Health,* July 1944, 9.

91 Ibid., 25.

92 Industrial medicine was recognized as a specialty by the American Medical Association only in 1955. W.P. Shepard, "Industrial Medicine: A New Specialty," *Canadian Medical Association Journal* 77, 3 (1957): 206–8. Doug Smith argues that very few Canadian doctors had any training in occupation health until the 1980s. Smith, *Consulted to Death,* 60.

93 Exceptions are Brigadier J.C. Meakins, "The Returning Serviceman and His Problems," *Canadian Medical Association Journal* 51, 3 (1944): 195–203, and Editorial, "The Return of the War Veteran to Industry," *Canadian Medical Association Journal* 52, 4 (1945): 409–10, but these articles dealt only peripherally with the disabled veteran, and their arguments in favour of employing the injured veteran were not nearly as strong as those in *Health.*

94 Caldwell, "Men at Work: Laws Alone." The Department of Veterans Affairs had a series of pamphlets on employing disabled workers, including *Employment of Canada's Disabled: Veterans and Others, Part 1: Basic Considerations,* n.d. [c. 1945], LAC, MG28, I332, vol. 102, file 21.

95 Health League of Canada, "Industrial Health Plan."

96 Caldwell, "When Johnny Comes Back to Work," 25.

97 Lois Keith, *Take Up Thy Bed and Walk: Death, Disability and Cure in Classic Fiction for Girls* (Toronto: Routledge, 2001); Paul Longmore, *Why I Burned My Book and Other Essays on Disability* (Philadelphia: Temple University Press, 2003), 138–39.

98 "Everyone's Handicapped!" *Health,* May/June 1955, 16.

99 Frances P. Collier, "Industrial Rehabilitation," *Health,* March/April 1958, 20.

100 D.C. Bews, "Role of Industrial Medicine in Rehabilitation," *Health,* May/June 1956, 10.

101 Collier, "Industrial Rehabilitation," 20–21, 26; Enoch Evans, "Senior Citizens Must Work," *Health,* May/June 1959, 20–21, 26.

102 *Final Report of the Special Committee of the Senate on Aging 1st Session, 27th Parliament* (Ottawa: Queen's Printer, 1966); James Snell, *The Citizen's Wage: The State and the Elderly in Canada, 1900–1951* (Toronto: University of Toronto Press, 1996).

103 Sidney Katz, "At 85 the Old Health Warrior Pleads for Morality," *Toronto Star,* 20 March 1971.

104 Letter from Gordon Bates to Dr. L.A. Weissgerber, 8 March 1961, LAC, MG28, I332, vol. 86, file 15.

105 Ibid.; letter from Bates to Mr. E.D. Bate, 22 July 1970, LAC, MG28 I332, vol. 87, file 10.

106 J.B. McGeachy, "Let Live ... and Let Work," *Health,* September 1953, 3; L.F. Koyl, "Health at Work: The Employment of Older Workers," *Health,* July 1958, 20; Anthony Salamone, "Health at Work: Geriatrics and Retirement," *Health,* November 1958, 22.

107 Dwight S. Sargent, "Health at Work: An Employer Views the Older Worker," *Health*, November 1954, 19.
108 "Royal Commission on Health Services: A Submission by the Health League of Canada," October 1964, LAC, MG28, I332, vol. 186, file 8.
109 Robert Collier Page, "Health at Work: *Without* Health – Why Live to Retire?" *Health*, May 1956, 17; Dr. R.B. Robson, "'R' Day Can Hurt You if You Don't Prepare," *Health*, January 1953, 7; R.F. Buchan, "How to Plan for Retirement," *Health*, January 1954, 16 and March 1954, 24; William M. Mercer, "When Should a Man Retire?" *Health*, March 1957, 16; Charles G. Johnson, "Retirement: Will You Know How to Make the Best Use of Leisure Time When You Become a Senior Citizen?" *Health*, October 1968, 20.
110 Wilder Penfield, "Here's Why You Should Look Forward to: A Second Career – Instead of Retirement," *Health*, January 1960, 19; L.F. Koyl, "What Will You Do after You Retire?" *Health*, March 1957, 18; M. Straker, "After Retirement: What Are the Health Problems Then?" *Health*, November 1961, 18.
111 "Industry Protects the Workers," *Health*, January/February 1947, 12.
112 W.H. Cruickshank, "Industry Protects the Workers," *Health*, March/April 1947, 16.
113 "Industry Protects the Worker," *Health*, November/December 1947, 24–5.
114 Copies of *Industrial Health* are in LAC, MG28, I332, vol. 103, file 5. When it first suspended publication, one of the reasons it gave was the overlap with the publication produced by the Department of National Health and Welfare. Minutes of the Industrial Health Committee, 17 February 1951, LAC, RG29, vol. 617, file 343-10-11.
115 Report of the Industrial Health Division for the year ending 31 December 1961, LAC, MG28, I332, vol. 103, file 1.
116 Health Conservation in Industry, n.d. [c. summer 1942], LAC, MG28, I332, vol. 103, file 4.
117 Circulation of *Health* in 1940–41 averaged 11,762 (LAC, MG28, I332, vol. 178, file 15). In 1944, it was approximately 13,000. See Annual Reports at the Twenty-Fifth Annual Meeting, 23–24 November 1944, LAC, MG28, I332, vol. 9, file 19.
118 Industrial Health Membership Plan, n.d., LAC, MG28, I332, vol. 104, file 13.
119 LAC, MG28, I332, vol. 18, file 6. The Trades and Labour Congress (the predecessor of the CLC) had endorsed Health League activities in the past, and the CLC would be a strong promoter of National Health Week. Greta Jones has found that some union groups in the United Kingdom also supported industrial hygiene: see *Social Hygiene in Twentieth Century Britain* (London: Croom Helm, 1986), 67.
120 *What Your Personal Membership Means* (pamphlet), n.d., LAC, MG28, I332, vol. 104, file 13.
121 "Restaurant Health Education Plan" in *Twenty-Eight Annual Meeting of the Health League of Canada, 17–19 June 1947* [annual report], LAC, MG28, I332, vol. 9, file 23.
122 Health League of Canada balance sheet, 30 April 1948, LAC, MG28, I322, vol. 9, file 24.
123 Letter from Gordon Bates to James W. Meredith, 30 March 1959, LAC, MG28, I322, vol. 104, file 20.
124 "Industrial Health Membership Plan and Its Possibilities," LAC, MG28, I332, vol. 104, file 15.

125 "The Industrial Membership Plan," 19 October 1953, LAC, MG28, I332, vol. 104, file 15.
126 "Current Attitudes of Top Management Medical Directors and Personnel Managers," n.d. [c. 1959–60], LAC, MG28, I332, vol. 104, file 16.
127 Minutes of the National Executive Committee, 11 March 1958, LAC, MG28, I332, vol. 2, file 2, Part 1.
128 Memo from Gordon Bates to Ross Mackenzie, 4 March 1959, LAC, MG28, I332, vol. 16, file 20.
129 "Course for Foodhandlers, First Session," Foodhandling Restaurant Plan Details, 1946–47, LAC, MG28, I332, vol. 85, file 6.
130 Nancy Tomes, *Gospel of Germs: Men, Women and the Microbe in American Life* (Cambridge, MA: Harvard University Press, 1998).
131 H.C. Rhodes, "Eating Out," *Health*, November/December 1946, 22; H. Cecil Rhodes, "Regulation + Education = Sanitation," *Health*, March/April 1948, 10–11, 20.
132 *Our Health Is in Your Hands* (pamphlet), n.d. [c. 1946–47], LAC, MG28, I332, vol. 85, file 6.
133 H.C. Rhodes, Journal, 1945–50, LAC, MG28, I332, vol. 190, file 18; "Food Handling at C.N.E. '65," n.d., LAC, MG28, I332, vol. 186, file 1.

Chapter 5: "The Human Factory"

1 George Weisz, *Chronic Disease in the Twentieth Century* (Baltimore: Johns Hopkins University Press, 2014); Helen Zoe Veit, "'Why Do People Die?' Rising Life Expectancy, Aging, and Personal Responsibility," *Journal of Social History* 45, 4 (2012): 1026–48; Laura David Hirschbein, "Masculinity, Work, and the Fountain of Youth: Irving Fisher and the Life Extension Institute, 1914–31," *Canadian Bulletin of Medical History* 16 (1999): 89–124; Helen Zoe Veit, "'So Few Fat Ones Grow Old': Diet, Health and Virtue in the Golden Age of Rising Life Expectancy," *Endeavour* 35, 2–3 (2011): 91–98.
2 For comparisons of human bodies to machines, see S.A. Davidson, "Why All the Fuss about Fitness," *Health*, May/June 1963, 16, and Doris W. Plewes, "Fitness Is Their Heritage," *Health*, March 1950, 12, 16, 26.
3 For more on the league's lack of attention to women and aging, see Bethany Philpott, "'The First Wealth Is Health': The Health League of Canada, 1935–80" (MA thesis, University of Guelph, 2014), 98–104.
4 Barbara Ehrenreich, *The Hearts of Men: American Dreams and the Flight from Commitment* (New York: Anchor, 1983), 68–87.
5 Statistics Canada, "Life Expectancy at Birth, by Sex, by Province," http://www.statcan. gc.ca/tables-tableaux/sum-som/l01/cst01/health26-eng.htm.
6 "Report of Committee on Periodic Health Examination," *Social Health* 7, 3 (1930): 2.
7 Paul Starr, *The Social Transformation of American Medicine* (New York: Basic Books, 1982), 193; Audrey B. Davis, "Life Insurance and the Physical Examination: A Chapter in the Rise of American Medical Technology," *Bulletin of the History of Medicine* 55, 3 (1981): 392–406. The American Medical Association endorsed periodic exams in 1922. Paul K.J. Han, "Historical Changes in the Objectives of the Periodic Health Examination," *Annals of Internal Medicine* 127 (1997): 912.

8 "Your Death May Be Postponed," *Social Health* 7, 4 (1930): 4.

9 Ibid. Charles R. Hayter, David Payne, and Gunes Ege, "Radiation Oncology in Canada, 1895–1995," *International Journal of Radiation Oncology* 6, 2 (1996): 487–96.

10 "And Pamphlets, Too," *Social Health* 7, 5 (1950): 8.

11 "The Social Hygiene Booth Went on Tour," *Social Health* 7, 5 (1930): 5.

12 J.H. MacDermot, "The Value of the Periodic Health Examination," *Health*, September 1936, 69; F.C. Middleton, "A Periodic Health Examination While Apparently Well," *Health* 4, 4 (1936): 91.

13 Periodic Health Examination Committee members listed on Health League letterhead, Library and Archives Canada (hereafter LAC), MG28, I332, vol. 127, file 2; minutes of various Periodic Health Examination Committee meetings, 1937, LAC, MG28, I332, vol. 127, file 3.

14 Minutes of the Medical Committee of the Toronto Health League, 22 February 1934, LAC, MG28, I332, vol. 127, file 5.

15 Canadian Medical Institute Periodic Health Examination form, n.d. [c. 1933–34], LAC, MG28, I332, vol. 127, file 5; H.M. Harrison, "The Practice of Preventive Medicine by a General Practitioner among Employees in a Small Factory," *Canadian Public Health Journal* 30, 11 (1939): 541–44.

16 Periodic Health Examination Form A, Part 1, LAC, MG28, I332, vol. 127, file 2.

17 Periodic Health Examination Form A, Part 2, LAC, MG28, I332, vol. 127, file 2.

18 Periodic Health Examination Form B, Parts 1 and 2, LAC, MG28, I332, vol. 127, file 2.

19 Letter from S.J. Newton Magwood to Gordon Bates, 23 June 1937, and letter from Gilbert Parker to Gordon Bates, 3 July 1934, LAC, MG28, I332, vol. 127, file 4.

20 Letter from secretary of the Periodic Health Examination Committee to Toronto doctors, 3 January 1938, LAC, MG28, I332, vol. 127, file 2; minutes of the Periodic Health Examination Committee, 12 November 1937, LAC, MG28, I332, vol. 127, file 3.

21 Memo to Dr. A.J. Mackenzie, n.d. [c. 1938], LAC, MG28, I332, vol. 127, file 2.

22 Letters from Gordon Bates to Rowena G. Hume, 13 December 1938, from Gordon Bates to Gordon C. Cameron, 13 December 1938, and from H.M. Harrison to R.J.W. Brooke, 9 September 1938, LAC, MG28, I332, vol. 127, file 6.

23 Letter from R.J.W. Brooke to Jessie I.A. Archer, 8 October 1938, LAC, MG28, I332, vol. 127, file 6.

24 Frederick Edwards, "Exit Doctors' Bills," *Maclean's*, 1 June 1939, 14.

25 See, for example, Glenn I. Sawyer, "Every Family Needs a Doctor," *Health*, May/June 1953, 9; R.G. Warminton, "Why Is the Periodic Examination so Important to Health," *Health*, March/April 1954, 19; Milton G. Townsend, "Keeping the Executive Fit," *Health*, July/August 1961, 19; Leslie G. Robertson, "That 5,000 Hour Checkup," *Health*, November/December 1953, 12–13, 26; Stewart MacGregor, "An Ounce of Prevention," *Health*, January/February 1948, 30.

26 Robertson, "That 5,000 Hour Check-Up," 12–13.

27 Valerie Korinek, *Roughing It in the Suburbs: Reading* Chatelaine *Magazine in the Fifties and Sixties* (Toronto: University of Toronto Press, 2000), 178–95.

28 "Editorial: The Need for Action in Nutrition," *Canadian Journal of Public Health* 32, 6 (1941): 317.

29 Rima D. Apple, *Vitamania: Vitamins in American Culture* (New Brunswick, NJ: Rutgers University Press, 1996), 10–11.

30 Amy Bentley, *Eating for Victory: Food Rationing and the Politics of Domesticity* (Urbana: University of Illinois Press, 1998), 2–4; Ian Mosby, *Food Will Win the War: The Politics, Science, and Culture of Food on Canada's Home Front* (Vancouver: UBC Press, 2014).

31 Biography of Margaret E. Smith, n.d., LAC, MG28, I332, vol. 21, file 27.

32 The large literature on the emerging science of nutrition includes Harvey Levenstein, *Revolution at the Table: The Transformation of the American Diet* (Berkeley: University of California Press, 2003); Charlotte Biltekoff, *Eating Right in America: The Cultural Politics of Food and Health* (Durham, NC: Duke University Press, 2013); Laura Shapiro, *Perfection Salad: Women and Cooking at the Turn of the Century* (Berkeley: University of California Press, 2008).

33 Sarah Stage and Virginia B. Vincent, *Rethinking Home Economics: Women and the History of a Profession* (Ithaca, NY: Cornell University Press, 1997).

34 Mosby, *Food Will Win the War,* 34.

35 Ibid., 25.

36 Today, Pett is probably best known for the nutritional experiments he carried out at Indigenous residential schools without obtaining the consent of the children or their parents. Ian Mosby, "Administering Colonial Science: Nutrition Research and Human Biomedical Experimentation in Aboriginal Communities and Residential Schools, 1942–1952," *Histoire sociale/Social History* 46, 91 (2013): 145–72.

37 Mosby, *Food Will Win the War,* 34.

38 Ian Mosby, "Making and Breaking Canada's Food Rules: Science, the State, and the Government of Nutrition," in *Edible Histories, Cultural Politics: Towards a Canadian Food History,* ed. Franca Iacovetta, Marlene Epp, and Valerie Korinek (Toronto: University of Toronto Press, 2012), 414–15.

39 Ibid., 415.

40 Mosby, *Food Will Win the War,* 164; Harvey Levenstein, *Paradox of Plenty: A Social History of Eating in Modern America* (New York: Oxford University Press, 1993), 67; Harvey Levenstein, *Fear of Food: A History of Why We Worry about What We Eat* (Chicago: University of Chicago Press, 2012), 95–106.

41 Elizabeth Chant Robertson, "Spend Food Money Wisely to Raise Health Levels," *Health,* Spring 1939, 10. Robertson edited child health material for *Chatelaine* and worked in the Department of Pediatrics at University of Toronto. Elizabeth Chant Robertson, Medical Advisory Board 1966, March 1966, LAC, MG28, I332, vol. 106, file 2.

42 "Advanced Lectures on Nutrition," 1943, LAC, MG28, I332, vol. 125, file 4.

43 Alice MacLean, "Mr. Smith Goes to Lunch," *Health,* Winter 1941, 14.

44 *Eat Correctly for Health and Victory* (pamphlet), n.d. [c. 1941–42], LAC, MG28, I332, vol. 126, file 1.

45 *1941 Menu, Shopping List, Recipes for a Week* (pamphlet), LAC, MG28, I332, vol. 126, file 1.

46 M.R. Richardson, "Toronto Women Learn Nutrition," *Health,* Winter 1941–42, 25.

47 Health League of Canada Annual Report 1942, LAC, MG28, I332, vol. 9, file 17.

48 Minutes, National Executive Committee, 21 May 1945, LAC, MG28, I332, vol. 1, file 15.
49 Mosby, "Making and Breaking Canada's Food Rules," 409.
50 Margaret E. Smith, "High School Lunch Box," *Health,* Winter 1944, 18; Mosby, "Making and Breaking Canada's Food Rules," 417.
51 Mosby, *Food Will Win the War,* 44–45.
52 Mosby, "Making and Breaking Canada's Food Rules," 422.
53 Ibid., 418–20.
54 *1941 Menu, Shopping List, Recipes for a Week;* Franca Iacovetta, "Recipes for Democracy? Gender, Family, and Making Female Citizens in Cold War Canada," in *Rethinking Canada: The Promise of Women's History,* 4th ed., ed. Veronica Strong-Boag, Mona Gleason, and Adele Perry (New York: Oxford University Press, 2002), 306.
55 Mosby, "Making and Breaking Canada's Food Rules," 421.
56 "Doctor Gives Advice on War-Time Foods," *Toronto Telegram,* 24 January 1940.
57 *1941 Menu, Shopping List, Recipes for a Week.*
58 See, for example, E.V. McCollum and J. Ernestine Becker, *Food Nutrition and Health* (Baltimore: McCollum and Simonds, 1947); Catherine Carstairs, "'Our Sickness Record Is a National Disgrace': Adelle Davis, Nutritional Determinism and the Anxious 1970s," *Journal of the History of Medicine and Allied Sciences* 69, 3 (2012): 461–91.
59 "Cooking Vegetables for Vitamin Preservation," *Health,* Summer 1945, 26.
60 Ian Mackenzie, "Health in the Home, Health in the Nation," *Health,* Spring 1940, 7.
61 Minutes of the National Executive Committee, 23 March 1943, LAC, MG28, I332, vol. 1, file 13; *Foods for Health* and *Economical Health Menus for Every Day of the Week,* n.d. [c. 1941–42], LAC, MG28, I332, vol. 126, file 1.
62 Franca Iacovetta, *Gatekeepers: Reshaping Immigrant Lives in Cold War Canada* (Toronto: Between the Lines, 2006), 140; Mosby, *Food Will Win the War,* 190.
63 Mosby, "Making and Breaking Canada's Food Rules," 424; Mosby, *Food Will Win the War,* 187.
64 Margaret Smith, "Health Begins in the Kitchen: Is White Flour Poisonous?" *Health,* July/August 1948, 23; L.B. Pett, "Rickets: The Deformity of Ignorance," *Health,* November/December 1948, 18–19. Margaret E. Smith, "Health Begins in the Kitchen: Good Nutrition Pays, If You Can Afford It!" *Health,* January/February 1949, 25; Margaret E. Smith, "Health Begins in the Kitchen: Nutrition for the Older Citizen," *Health,* April/March 1950, 21.
65 Minutes of the National Nutrition Committee, 17 November 1952 and 4 June 1953, LAC, MG28, I332, vol. 125, file 13.
66 Margaret E. Smith, "Eat Quality – Not Quantity," *Health,* March/April 1953, 21.
67 Health League of Canada, *The Best Kind of Meals,* n.d., LAC, MG28, I332, vol. 126, file 1.
68 "Health Begins in the Kitchen: That High Cost of Living," *Health,* May/June 1948, 19; "Health Begins in the Kitchen," *Health,* March/April 1948, 25; "The High Cost of Eating," *Health,* May/June 1952, 16–17.
69 Smith, "Eat Quality – Not Quantity," 21; Margaret Smith, "Health Begins in the Kitchen: The Soil and Health," *Health,* May/June 1949, 21.

70 "Re Place Mats – 1961 National Health Week," n.d. [c. 1961], LAC, MG28, I332, vol. 121, file 5; "National Health Week 1963 Report," n.d. [c. 1961], LAC, MG28, I332, vol. 121, file 37.

71 J.E. Monagle, "Canada's Food Guide: A Route Map to Health," *Health*, October 1962, 18, 28.

72 Peter Stearns, *Fat History: Bodies and Beauty in the Modern West* (New York: New York University Press, 1997); Hillel Schwartz, *Never Satisfied: A Cultural History of Diets, Fantasies and Fat* (New York: Free Press, 1986); Helen Zoe Viet, *Modern Food, Moral Food: Self-Control, Science and the Rise of Modern American Eating in the Early Twentieth Century* (Chapel Hill: University of North Carolina Press, 2013).

73 E.W. McHenry, "Food in Canada," *Health*, January/February 1948, 15, 22.

74 Bernard Laski, "The Overnourished and the Undernourished Child," *Health*, July/August 1950, 21.

75 Margaret E. Smith, "Age Has Its Eating Problem Too," *Health*, January/February 1952, 10.

76 Harold V. Cranfield, "NO! – It May Be Fattening," *Health*, March/April 1953, 8.

77 Louis I. Dublin, "Reducing May Save Your Life," *Health*, November/December 1952, 20.

78 Corinne Trerice, "These School Lunches Give Better Health," *Health*, September/October 1957, 12; "Snacks for Santa's Helpers," *Health*, November 1958, 14–15; "Recipe for a Merry Christmas," *Health*, November 1957, 15.

79 Catharine Mahoney, "Foods for Health: Summer Salads Can Be Nutritious, Delicious," *Health*, July/August 1959, 14–15, 30–31; Catharine Hoare Mahoney, "Foods for Health: Take Time to Enjoy Christmas," *Health*, November/December 1959, 22–23, 30, 32; Catharine Hoare Mahoney, "Foods for Health: Fish Day Can Be Feast Day!" *Health*, January/February 1960, 28–30, 32, 34.

80 "Foods for Health: Basic Elements of a Nutritious Diet," *Health*, Summer 1975, 20–21.

81 Although news releases from these departments were not preserved in the league's files past 1959, those that exist included a discussion of the foodstuffs as well as recipes. Some examples are "Sandwich Time," August 1959; "Old-Fashioned Blueberry Pie Still a Favourite," August 1959; "Shoulder to Shoulder with Pork," June 1959; "The Food Basket," June 1959, all in LAC, MG28, I332, vol. 125, file 1.

82 "Foods for Health: Palatable Facts about Cheese," *Health*, December 1961, 30–31, 35; "Foods for Health: Cooking Hints on Peaches and Tomatoes," *Health*, October 1961, 22–24; "Foods for Health: Milk Can Help Your 'Prime of Life,'" *Health*, April 1962, 22, 28; "Foods for Health: Canadian Strawberries and Dairy Products," *Health*, August 1963, 20–22; "Foods for Health: Pork Can Be Tasty and Popular," *Health*, February 1964, 24–25; "Foods for Health: Cured and Smoked Pork for Springtime Meals," *Health*, April 1964, 20–21; "Foods for Health: Know Your Apples," *Health*, December 1965, 20–21.

83 "Foods for Health: Featuring Fish," *Health*, October 1962, 24, 35; "Foods for Health: Small Fry Specialty," *Health*, June 1962, 26; "Foods for Health: How to Eye and Buy Frozen Fish," *Health*, Spring 1972, 26–27.

84 "Foods for Health: Ice Cream – Nutritious and Delicious," *Health*, June 1966, 22–23.

85 "Foods for Health: Maple – Canada's Unique Sweet," *Health,* June 1967, 20–21.

86 "Food for '63," *Health,* February 1963, 20.

87 Ibid., 21–22.

88 "Foods for Health: Food Forecast/65," *Health,* February 1965, 18; "The Food Picture for 1966," *Health,* February 1966, 22.

89 John Oille, "Exercise and the Heart," *Health,* October 1933, 8. The dangers of over-exertion were emphasized until the 1960s.

90 A.S. Lambe, "'Physical Jerks' or Education," *Health,* March 1934, 19.

91 E.M. Orlick, "Mass Culture: A Russian Experiment," *Health,* September 1939, 66–67, 74; E.M. Orlick, "Czechoslovakia Is Fit," *Health,* September 1938, 65, 77–78.

92 Gordon Bates, "June Issue Is Physical Fitness," *Health,* June 1961, 6.

93 For more information, see Clarence G. Lasby, *Eisenhower's Heart Attack: How Ike Beat Heart Disease and Held on to the Presidency* (Lawrence: University Press of Kansas, 1997).

94 Paul Dudley White, "How Long Should We Live," *Health,* May/June 1962, 42.

95 Paul Dudley White, "Exercise and Aging," *Health,* May/June 1961, 16, 32.

96 Rex Wilson, "Exercise for Your Health," *Health,* Summer 1972, 10; Rex Wilson "A Doctor Looks at Health," *Health,* Winter 1973–74, 8.

97 Dorothy N.R. Jackson, "Canoeing for Health and Pleasure," *Health,* July/August 1946, 12, 26; Jerry Mathisen, "Gymnastics for Health," *Health,* December 1942, 24–25; John D. Devlin, "Learn How to Swim," *Health,* Summer 1938, 41, 55.

98 Catherine Gidney, *Tending the Student Body: Youth, Health and the Modern University* (Toronto: University of Toronto Press, 2015), 137–39.

99 Norman J. Ashton, "RX = BX: Follow This Proven Prescription for Physical Fitness," *Health,* May/June 1961, 18–20; Traute Franke-Eggeling, "Rhythmic Movement: A Way to Health," *Health,* October 1960, 21, 39.

100 Dorothy Porter, *Health Citizenship: Essays in Social Medicine and Biomedical Politics* (Berkeley: University of California Press, 2011), 67.

101 C.R. Blackstock, "To Keep Fit – Go Camping," *Health,* June 1961, 8; Ogden Hershaw, "Your Country Estate," *Health,* July/August 1948, 10, 32; D.L. MacLean, "Sanitation for the Summer Traveller," *Health,* May/June 1948, 10–11, 23; J.B. Ebbs, "Holidays for Health," *Health,* July 1941, 38; Mary L. Northway, "'If My Child Were Going to Camp ...': What Every Parent Should Know before Choosing a Camp," *Health,* Spring 1942, 16.

102 "Growing Old Successfully," *Health,* November 1955, 14–15, 31; "Successful Retirement," *Health,* November/December 1953, 17; "Your Tensions – and How to Live with Them," *Health,* October 1965, 20–21; Frank Wise, "Leisure Can Be Pleasure," *Health,* March/April 1948, 14–15, 34.

103 Karl S. Bernhardt, "Mental Health through Play," *Health,* April 1948, 13, 20.

104 "Growing Old Successfully."

105 Dr. Hartman, Dr. Irvin, and Dr. Brosin, "Industrial Health: Must Executives Suffer?" *Health,* September 1952, 27–28.

106 Harold N. Segall, "Too Many Executives Die Young," *Health,* January 1954, 9.

107 Ibid., 10; Harold N. Segall, "How to Be an Executive and Live," *Health,* January 1958, 10–11; Harold N. Segall, "Health at Work: Health of the Executive," *Health,* March 1959, 18.

108 Milton G. Townsend, "Keeping the Executive Fit," *Health*, July 1961, 18.
109 Gordon Sinclair, "Executive Health Problems," *Health*, January/February 1966, 20–21, 30–31; Segall, "Health at Work: Health of the Executive," 18.

Chapter 6: Fighting Apathy and Ignorance

1 "He Was Just Beginning to Walk," 17 October 1950, Library and Archives Canada (hereafter LAC), MG28, I332, vol. 244; also in LAC, MG28, I332, vol. 95 file 8.
2 Toxoid Week and National Immunization Week would be merged in 1953. Letter from C.C. Goldring to Dr. Gordon Bates, 15 April 1953, LAC, MG28, I332, vol. 96, file 7.
3 Jacob Heller, *The Vaccine Narrative* (Nashville, TN: Vanderbilt University Press, 2008); John Maurice, *State of the World's Vaccines and Immunization*, 3rd ed. (Geneva: World Health Organization, 2009); Jane S. Smith, *Patenting the Sun: Polio and the Salk Vaccine* (New York: William Morrow, 1990).
4 Canadian Public Health Association, "Policy Statement on Immunization," *Canadian Journal of Public Health* 56, 2 (1965): 83–87.
5 Annual Report of the Health League of Canada for the year ending 23 and 24 November 1944, LAC, MG28, I332, vol. 9, file 19.
6 "National Immunization Week," 10–16 September 1944, LAC, MG28, I332, vol. 94, file 1; G.A. McNaughton, "Here Are the Facts about Communicable Disease," News Release for Canada's Twenty-First National Immunization Week, LAC, MG28, I332, vol. 98, file 13.
7 Cynthia Comacchio, *Nations Are Built of Babies: Saving Ontario's Mothers and Children, 1900–1940* (Montreal and Kingston: McGill-Queen's University Press, 1993), 31.
8 C.A. Bourdon, "The Diphtheria Situation in Montreal and Immunization," *Canadian Journal of Public Health* 36, 8 (1945): 305–11.
9 Mona Gleason, *Small Matters: Canadian Children in Sickness and Health, 1900–1940* (Montreal and Kingston: McGill-Queen's University Press, 2013), 20, 37.
10 National Immunization Committee membership lists, LAC, MG28, I332, vol. 92, file 12.
11 "Vaccines and Immunization," Museum of Health Care at Kingston, http://www.museumofhealthcare.ca/explore/exhibits/vaccinations/profiles.html. Crawford S. Anglin, "Remembrances of an Old Infectious Disease Doctor," *Pediatrics and Child Health* 5, 3 (2000): 148–49.
12 "Report of Canada's 7th Annual Immunization Week," n.d., LAC, MG28, I332, vol. 95, file 16; "The Canadian Medical Association Endorses National Immunization Week," n.d., LAC, MG28, I332, vol. 98, file 13.
13 This practice ended in 1952. Clipping from *Toronto Telegram*, 23 September 1952, LAC, MG28, I332, vol. 96, file 1.
14 "Immunization Clip," n.d., LAC, MG28, I332, vol. 93, file 8.
15 For example, the first National Immunization Week was rescheduled due to a conflict with a Victory Loan campaign, which would have limited advertising space, and similar challenges were faced in other years. Letter from Dr. Gordon Bates to Deputy Ministers of Health, 24 July 1943, LAC, MG28, I332, vol. 93, file 4. In coming years, the timing of the week remained a challenge. Dr. Jules Gilbert of Montreal expressed

the belief that most rural Canadians immunized their children in the summer, making those months more appropriate for a campaign. Nonetheless, Bates maintained the necessity of keeping National Immunization Week in the fall in order to distance it from National Health Week in February, and thereby ensure advertiser support for both. See letter from Dr. Jules Gilbert to the Health League of Canada, 14 September 1953, LAC, MG28, I332, vol. 96, file 7. For the views of the PEI health officer, see letter from Burton Howatt to F.O. Wishart, 8 May 1957, LAC, MG28, I332, vol. 98, file 4.

16 Letter from G.F. Amyot to Gordon Bates, 27 May 1944, LAC, MG28, I332, vol. 94, file 1.

17 Various letters between Gordon Bates and ministers of health, LAC, MG28, I332, vol. 93, file 4.

18 C. Stuart Houston, *Steps on the Road to Medicare: Why Saskatchewan Led the Way* (Montreal and Kingston: McGill-Queen's University Press, 2002).

19 For example, by 1957 Christian Smith suggested that communicable disease was "under control" and that the league should instead consider promoting a dental health week. Letter from Christian Smith to Dr. Gordon Bates, 7 May 1957, LAC, MG28, I332, vol. 97, file 13.

20 Virginia Berridge and Kelly Loughlin, *Medicine, the Market and the Mass Media: Producing Health in the Twentieth Century* (New York: Routledge, 2005), 6–7; James Colgrove, *State of Immunity: The Politics of Vaccination in Twentieth-Century America* (Berkeley: University of California Press, 2006), 11.

21 National Immunization Week, 14–20 November 1943, LAC, MG28, I332, vol. 94, file 1.

22 Spot announcements suggested for use prior to and during Canada's National Immunization Week, 12–18 September 1948, LAC, MG28, I332, vol. 95, file 15.

23 This slogan was used throughout much of the league's promotional material for National Immunization Week. For example, in some years the organization arranged for it to be printed on hydro and gas bills and family allowance cheques. Letter from J. Albert Blais to Dr. Gordon Bates, 13 August 1957, LAC, MG28, I332, vol. 98, file 4.

24 Esyllt Jones, *Influenza 1918: Disease, Death and Struggle in Winnipeg* (Toronto: University of Toronto Press, 2007); Magda Fahrni and Esyllt Jones, *Epidemic Encounters: Influenza, Society, and Culture in Canada, 1918–1920* (Vancouver: UBC Press, 2012); Mark Humphries, *The Last Plague: Spanish Influenza and the Politics of Public Health in Canada* (Toronto: University of Toronto Press, 2013).

25 *War Brings Epidemics: Protect Your Child against Diphtheria, Smallpox, Whooping Cough* (pamphlet and poster), 1943, LAC, MG28, I332, vol. 93, file 5.

26 "Preventable Casualties," *Health News Service*, 20 October 1943.

27 "Safe and Snug?" (advertisement mat), n.d. [c. 1954], LAC, MG28, I332, vol. 96, file 17.

28 "Yes ... You have a very sick baby" (advertisement mat), n.d. [c. 1945], LAC, MG28, I332, vol. 94, file 9. Interestingly, this advertisement appears to have been adopted from a very similar advertisement from the pharmaceutical manufacturer Sharp and Dohme, which ran in *Hygeia* in February 1944. LAC, MG28, I332, vol. 94, file 1.

29 For discussions of vaccine development, particularly those that National Immunization Week emphasized, see Stefan Grzybowski and Edward A. Allen, "Tuberculosis: 2.

History of the Disease in Canada," *Canadian Medical Association Journal* 160, 7 (1999): 1025–28; Heller, *Vaccine Narrative;* Maurice, *State of the World's Vaccines;* Smith, *Patenting the Sun.*

30 Letter from Dr. Gordon Bates to deputy ministers of health, 19 August 1953, LAC, MG28, I332, vol. 96, file 7.

31 In 1953, the Health League endeavoured to standardize the age at which immunization was administered nationwide, collaborating with provincial ministers of health and hoping to develop a standard record form. The provinces were receptive to this, yet felt that the Health League's recommendation of immunization at six to nine months of age reflected "Toronto thinking" – most advocated for vaccination beginning at three months. The league compromised and promoted immunization at "3 to 6 months of age" within its material, but a precise consensus could not be established. See various items of correspondence between the Health League and provincial ministers and deputy ministers of health, LAC, MG28, I332, vol. 96, file 7.

32 Linda Bryder, "'We Shall Not Find Salvation in Inoculation': BCG Vaccination in Scandinavia, Britain and the USA, 1921–60," *Social Science and Medicine* 49 (1999): 1159–67.

33 Johanne Bentzen, "Memo to Mothers: The Case for BCG (Vaccination against Tuberculosis)," *Health,* March 1952, 11; Armand Frappier, "The Miracle of BCG: How BCG Vaccine Answers the Challenging Need for Protection against Tuberculosis," *Health,* March 1955, 10.

34 Summary of replies received from provinces re. BCG immunization practices, compiled by the Health League of Canada, April 1953, LAC, MG28, I332, vol. 96, file 7.

35 Letters from J.S. Robertson to Mabel Ferris, 22 December 1952, and from Mabel Ferris to Leonard Miller, 10 April 1953, LAC, MG28, I332, vol. 96, file 7.

36 In 1944, at the annual meeting, a resolution was passed instructing the Health League to discuss compulsory immunization against whooping cough and diphtheria with the provinces. The league did contact the provinces, but the consensus was that they were not in favour of compulsory immunization, and the league did not push the issue any further. See LAC, MG28, I332, vol. 93, file 1.

37 Canadian Public Health Association, "Policy Statement on Immunization as Adopted on 21 November 1964," *Canadian Journal of Public Health* 56, 2 (1965): 83–87.

38 Law Reform Commission of Saskatchewan, "Consultation Paper: Vaccination and the Law," September 2007, http://lawreformcommission.sk.ca/vaccinef.pdf.

39 Elena Connis, *Vaccine Nation: America's Changing Relationship with Immunization* (Chicago: University of Chicago Press, 2015), 101.

40 Katherine Arnup, "'Victims of Vaccination?' Opposition to Compulsory Immunization in Ontario, 1900–90," *Canadian Bulletin of Medical History* 9 (1992): 159–76; Paul Adolphus Bator, "The Health Reformers versus the Common Canadian: The Controversy over Compulsory Vaccination against Smallpox in Toronto and Ontario, 1900–1920," *Ontario History* 75, 4 (1983): 348–73.

41 Letters from Mrs. D.A. Anderson to Mr. John Fisher, 3 October 1944, LAC, MG28, I332, vol. 94, file 3; from Dr. Gordon Bates to Mr. C.R. Delafield, 7 December 1944, LAC, MG28, I332, vol. 94, file 2; and from J.J. Gamache to the Health League of Canada, 30 October 1950, LAC, MG28, I332, vol. 95, file 18.

42 Denise Baillargeon, *Babies for the Nation: The Medicalization of Motherhood in Quebec, 1910–1970*, trans. W. Donald Wilson (Waterloo, ON: Wilfrid Laurier University Press, 2009), 213–14.

43 Letter from William F. Roberts, 15 April 1921, LAC, MG28, I332, vol. 70, file 2.

44 Gordon Bates, "The Medico-Lay Affiliates of the Canadian Medical Association: 1. The Health League of Canada," *Canadian Medical Association Journal* 84, 5 (1961): 296.

45 Health League of Canada, *Report for the Year 1958*, LAC, MG28, I332, vol. 10, file 8.

46 "Canada's 11th National Health Week," n.d., LAC, MG28, I332, vol. 118, file 2; "National Health Week 1952, Sponsored Advertising Report," 1952, LAC, MG28, I332, vol. 114, file 32; "National Health Week 1959, Sponsored Advertising, 1958–1959 Report," 1959, LAC, MG28, I332, vol. 120, file 1; "National Health Week, 1961 Report," 1961, LAC, MG28, I332, vol. 121, file 8; "National Health Week, Advertising 1957," 1957, LAC, MG28, I332, vol. 118, file 10; "Ninth National Health Week," n.d., LAC, MG28, I332, vol. 10, file 4.

47 "Primitive Health Conditions Blamed on Public Ignorance," news release, 3 February 1953, LAC, MG28, I332, vol. 115, file 20.

48 "Quack Remedies Still Rob and Disappoint Canadians," news release, 3 February 1953, LAC, MG28, I332, vol. 115, file 20.

49 "National Health Week, March 12–18, 1961," 1961, LAC, MG28, I332, vol. 121, file 8.

50 "Twenty-Seventh National Health Week, 14–20 March 1971," LAC, MG28, I332, vol. 123, file 2.

51 Health Week General Report, 3–9 February 1946, LAC, MG28, I332, vol. 112, file 13.

52 Posters for sponsored advertising, n.d. [c. 1946], LAC, MG28, I332, vol. 112, file 11.

53 E.A. Hardy, *Selections from the Canadian Poets* (Toronto: Morang Educational Company, 1907). He has been written about in John A. Wiseman, "'Champion Has-Been': Edwin Austin Hardy and the Ontario Library Movement," in *Readings in Canadian Library History*, ed. Peter McNally (Ottawa: Canadian Library Association, 1986), 231–43. There are several obituaries in LAC, MG28, I332, vol. 21, file 26.

54 Letter from Gordon Bates to Dr. G.F. Amyot, 22 January 1960, LAC, MG28, I332, vol. 120, file 4.

55 "Fifth National Health Week, 1949," 1949, LAC, MG28, I332, vol. 114, file 4.

56 Letter from H.B. Wilson to T.E. Daniel, 14 April 1953, LAC, MG28, I332, vol. 116, file 8.

57 *Heroes of Health*, 1946, LAC, MG28, I332, vol. 112, file 12.

58 *More Heroes of Health*, 1946, LAC, MG28, I332, vol. 112, file 22.

59 Correspondence between educators and the Health League, 1946–47, LAC, MG28, I332, vol. 113, files 7–9.

60 Annual Report of the Health League of Canada for the year ending 20 March 1947, LAC, MG28, I332, vol. 9, file 23.

61 Report of the Thirty-Fourth Annual Meeting of the Health League of Canada, 30 November–2 December, 1953, LAC, MG28, I332, vol. 10, file 4; "Report of the Eleventh National Health Week, January 30–February 5, 1955," LAC, MG28, I332, vol. 118, file 4.

62 Council on Dental Education of the Canadian Dental Association, *Dentistry as a Professional Career* (Toronto: Canadian Dental Association, 1958).

63 Minutes of the National Health Week Committee meeting, 20 September 1949, LAC, MG28, I332, vol. 113, file 30, discuss planning for the new booklet, *Guardians of Our Health.* The booklet itself is in LAC, MG28, I332, vol. 114, file 8.

64 Letter from Gordon Bates to Mr. J.E. Atkinson, 12 February 1946, LAC, MG28, I332, vol. 112, file 10.

65 Minutes of National Heath Week Committee, 24 February 1953, LAC, MG28, I332, vol. 116, file 10.

66 Canada's Seventeenth Annual Health Week, 1961, LAC, MG28, I332, vol. 121, file 8.

67 Annual Report of the Health League of Canada for the years 1956 and 1957, LAC, MG28, I332, vol. 10 file 7.

68 "Interim Report from Public Relations Department National Health Week 1960," LAC, MG28, I332, vol. 120, file 19.

69 Minutes of the Clergy Committee meeting, 15 March 1950, LAC, MG28, I332, vol. 114, file 8; letter from Mabel Ferris to Rev. Dr. E.A. Thompson, 9 November 1953, LAC, MG28, I332, vol. 116, file 1.

70 A 1950 letter speaks explicitly of Christianity. See R.C. Chalmers and W.D. Muckle to circulate, 2 January 1950, LAC, MG28, I332, vol. 78, file 13. Bates suggests that Jewish representatives be appointed in 1950. Minutes of the Clergy Committee, 8 December 1950, LAC, MG28, I332, vol. 78, file 14. Letter from Murdoch McIver to Rabbi Dr. Stuart E. Rosenberg, 7 October 1957, LAC, MG28, I332, vol. 118, file 17.

71 Correspondence between E.A. Hardy and various denominational leaders, December 1948–January 1949, LAC, MG28, I332, vol. 113, file 26.

72 The first clergy letter was sent in 1951. Letter to the Reverend Clergy, 18 January 1951, LAC, MG28, I332, vol. 114, file 8.

73 Ibid.

74 The Health League's flies contain clergy survey responses from 1952, 1958, and 1959, LAC, MG28, I332, vol. 115, file 3; vol. 118, file 18; and vol. 119, files 17–18.

75 Reginald Bibby, *Fragmented Gods: The Poverty and Potential of Religion in Canada* (Toronto: Stoddard, 1987), 17.

76 For example, in 1951, Canada had a population of 14 million. Over 2 million Canadians identified as Anglican, over 6 million as Catholic, and almost 3 million as members of the United Church of Canada. Just over 200,000 Canadians described themselves as Jewish and fewer than 60,000 reported that they no religion. In 1961, Canada's population had increased to over 18 million. Almost 2.5 million Canadians identified themselves as Anglican, over 8 million identified as Catholic, and over 3.5 million described themselves as United Church. A quarter of a million described themselves as Jewish, and fewer than 100,000 said that they had no religion. Historical Statistics of Canada, Principal Religions Denominations of the Population, Census Dates, 1871–1971, http://www.statcan.gc.ca/access_acces/archive.action?l=eng&loc=A164_184-eng.csv.

77 Letter from Samuel Lewin to Olive Ottaway, 13 February 1964, LAC, MG28, I332, vol. 122, file 13.

78 Minutes of the Meeting of the National Clergy Committee of the National Health Week Committee, 25 September 1959, LAC, MG28, I332, vol. 120, file 4; letter from

Murdoch McIver to Montague Raisman, 6 March 1957, LAC, MG28, I332, vol. 118, file 17.

79 Letter from Murdoch McIver to Rev. J.N. Fullerton, 23 October 1959, LAC, MG28, I332, vol. 120, file 7.

80 Ian Dowbiggin, "'Keeping This Young Country Sane': C.K. Clarke, Immigration Restriction and Canadian Psychiatry, 1890–1925," *Canadian Historical Review* 76, 4 (1995): 598–627; Peter Ward, *White Canada Forever: Public Attitudes and Public Policy towards Orientals in British Columbia* (Montreal and Kingston: McGill-Queen's University Press, 1978); Mariana Valverde, *The Age of Light, Soap and Water: Moral Reform in English Canada, 1885–1925* (Toronto: University of Toronto Press, 2008); Esyllt Jones, *Influenza, 1918: Disease, Death, and Struggle in Winnipeg* (Toronto: University of Toronto Press, 2007); Isabel Wallace, "*Komagata Maru* Revisited: 'Hindus,' Hookworm and the Guise of Public Heath Protection," *BC Studies* 178 (Summer 2013): 33–50.

81 Franca Iacovetta, *Gatekeepers: Reshaping Immigrant Lives in Cold War Canada* (Toronto: Between the Lines, 2006).

82 Minutes of the National Health Week Committee, 20 October 1964, LAC, MG28, I332, vol. 122, file 4.

83 Health Week Division Report on Canada's Seventh Annual National Health Week, 4–10 February 1951, LAC, MG28, I332, vol. 114, file 22.

84 For more on the Women's Institutes, see Linda Ambrose, *For Home and Country: The Centennial History of the Women's Institutes of Ontario* (Guelph, ON: Federated Women's Institutes of Ontario, 1996).

85 Letter from E.A. Hardy to Mrs. Cameron E. Dow, 30 April 1946, LAC, MG28, I332, vol. 113, file 2.

86 Correspondence between E.A. Hardy and Miss Katharine Sheridan, January 1949, LAC, MG28, I332, vol. 113, file 16; letter from Mary Barker to Mr. Power, 28 September 1953, LAC, MG28, I332, vol. 116, file 18; and letter from Gordon Bates to Mrs. H. Petty, 23 December 1963, LAC, MG28, I332, vol. 120, file 22.

87 The Health League's letters over the years to such groups are dispersed throughout the Health League's National Health Week records, LAC, MG28, I332, vol. 113–22.

88 Letter from A. Power to Federated Women's Institutes of Canada, 23 December 1953, LAC, MG28, I332, vol. 116, file 18.

89 National Health Week 1960, Service Clubs, 1959–60, LAC, MG28, I332, vol. 120, file 21.

90 National Health Week 1958, Service Clubs, questionnaires 1958, LAC, MG28, I332, vol. 119, file 7.

91 National Health Week 1960, Service Clubs 1959–60, LAC, MG28, I332, vol. 120, file 21; National Health Week 1963, Service Clubs, LAC, MG28, I332, vol. 121, file 40.

92 A full archives of the Royal Bank monthly letters can be found on the Royal Bank webpage, http://www.rbc.com/aboutus/letter/. Letters included: "A Crusade for Health" (January 1950), http://www.rbc.com/aboutus/letter/january1950.html; "Public Health" (February 1956), http://www.rbc.com/aboutus/letter/pdf/february1956. pdf; "In Search of Physical Fitness" (January 1958), http://www.rbc.com/aboutus/

letter/january1958.html; and "In Search of Health" (February 1960), http://www.rbc. com/aboutus/letter/february1960.html. A letter from Murdoch McIver to the British American Oil Company, 25 February 1960, indicates that the bank printed 100,000 copies of the newsletter: LAC, MG28, I332, vol. 120, file 20. In 1949, the bank apparently printed 150,000 copies for the league: letter from John R. Heron to Gordon Bates, 29 December 1949, LAC, MG28, I332, vol. 164, file 15.

93 See, for example, advertisements in LAC, MG28, I332, scrapbook 236.

94 Interim Report, Canada's Sixteenth National Health Week, 31 January to 6 February 1960, LAC, MG28, I332, vol. 120, file 19.

95 National Health Week, Canadian Labour Congress, 1957–58, LAC, MG28, I332, vol. 118, file 16; National Health Week 1959, Canadian Labour Congress 1958–59, LAC, MG28, I332, vol. 119, file 11; National Health Week 1960, Canadian Labour Congress, 1959–60, LAC, MG28, I332, vol. 120, file 6; National Health Week 1963, Canadian Labour Congress, LAC, MG28, I332, vol. 121, file 23; National Health Week 1964, Canadian Labour Congress, LAC, MG28, I332, vol. 121, file 46; National Health Week 1965, Canadian Labour Congress 1964, LAC, MG28, I332, vol. 122, file 24.

96 The booklets varied slightly from year to year, but from 1948 to 1960, at least, these themes were emphasized. A selection of booklets can be found in LAC, MG28, I332, vol. 123, file 20. A *Health Facts Digest* provided an abridged version of the larger booklet.

97 "Health Week Is Shunned," *Winnipeg Free Press*, 5 January 1960.

98 Zena Cherry, "National Health Week Is On," *Globe and Mail*, 4 April 1978.

99 See "The Club," in John R. Seeley, R. Alexander Sim, and Elizabeth W. Loosley in collaboration with Norman W. Bell and D.F. Fleming, *Crestwood Heights* (Toronto: University of Toronto Press, 1956), 292–343.

100 Doug Owram, *Born at the Right Time: A History of the Baby-Boom Generation* (Toronto: University of Toronto Press, 1996); Mona Gleason, *Normalizing the Idea: Psychology, Schooling and the Family in Postwar Canada* (Toronto: University of Toronto Press, 1999).

Chapter 7: "A Malicious, Mendacious Minority"

1 "No Happy Medium in Fluoride Debate," *CBC Archives*, 7 January 1958, http://www.cbc.ca/archives/entry/no-happy-medium-in-fluoride-debate.

2 For example, see letter from Gordon Bates to the *Montreal Gazette*, 22 July 1959, Library and Archives Canada (hereafter LAC), MG28, I332, vol. 82, file 6.

3 Health League of Canada, "Financial Statement, December 31, 1963"; Health League of Canada, "Financial Statement, December 31, 1964"; Health League of Canada, "Financial Statement, December 31, 1965," LAC, MG28, I332, vol. 23 file 14.

4 H. Trendley Dean, "Endemic Fluorosis and Its Relation to Dental Caries," *Public Health Reports* 53, 33 (1938): 1443–52; Forest Ray Moulton, ed., *Dental Caries and Fluorine* (Washington, DC: American Association for the Advancement of Science, 1946); "Brantford Reports on Fluoridation," *Canadian Journal of Public Health* 47 (1956): 123.

5 Ontario, *Report of the Committee Appointed to Inquire into and Report upon the Fluoridation of Municipal Water Supplies* (Toronto: Ontario Water Resources Commission, 1962), 96–102.

6 Valeria C.C. Marinho, Julian P.T. Higgins, Stuart Logan, and Aubreay Sheiham, "Fluoride Toothpastes for Preventing Dental Caries in Children and Adolescents," *Cochrane Database of Systemic Reviews*, 20 January 2003, http://onlinelibrary.wiley.com/doi/10.1002/14651858.CD002278/full; Mark Dissendorf, "The Mystery of Declining Tooth Decay," *Nature* 322 (10 July 1986): 125–29.

7 Donald R. McNeil, *The Fight for Fluoridation* (New York: Oxford University Press, 1957), 65–84.

8 William L Hutton, Bradley W. Linscott, and Donald B. Williams, "The Brantford Fluorine Experiment: Interim Report after Five Years of Water Fluoridation," *Canadian Journal of Public Health* 42, 3 (1951): 81–87; Frank J. McClure, *Water Fluoridation: The Search and the Victory* (Bethesda, MD: US National Institute of Dental Research, 1970), 112–28.

9 "Statement of the Research Committee of the C.D.A. Regarding Fluoridation of Water Supplies," *Journal of the Canadian Dental Association* (hereafter *JCDA*) 15, 3 (1951): 165; "Supplementary Statement on Fluoridation of Water Supplies by Research Committee," *JCDA* 16, 3 (1952): 149; "Fluoridation of the Communal Water Supplies for the Partial Prevention of Tooth Decay," *Canadian Medical Association Journal* 68 (1953): 401–2; "Memorandum on Fluoridation of Communal Water Supplies for the Partial Prevention of Tooth-Decay: Avoidance of Hazards," *Canadian Medical Association Journal* 69 (1953): 214; letter from L.B. Pett to W.T.C. Berry, 18 November 1959, Pt. 2, LAC, RG29, vol. 933, file 386-4-13.

10 *Digest of Opinions on Fluoridation,* June 1954, LAC, MG28, I332, vol. 84, file 6.

11 Letter from Ewart Cather to Gordon Bates, 20 September 1954, LAC, MG28, I332, vol. 81, file 16.

12 Gordon Bates, "Health: A National and International Problem," presentation to the Annual Meeting of the Canadian Dental Association, 16 May 1955, LAC, MG28, I332, vol. 83, file 8.

13 J. Craig Baumgartner, Leif K. Bakland, and Eugene Sugita, "Microbiology of Endontics and Aspesis in Endontic Practice," *Endontics,* 5th ed. (Hamilton, ON: BC Decker, 2002), 63; Gilles Dussault and Aubrey Sheiham, "Medical Theories and Professional Development: The Theory of Focal Sepsis and Dentistry in Early Twentieth Century Britain," *Social Science Medicine* 16, 15 (1982): 1405–12.

14 Letter from Gordon Bates to Keith Box, 13 December 1960, LAC, MG28, I332, vol. 82, file 10.

15 Letter from Gordon Bates to Frederick Stare, 30 December 1974, LAC, MG28, I332, vol. 84, file 1.

16 Letter from Gordon Bates to the *Globe and Mail,* 10 March 1959, LAC, MG28, I332, vol. 82, file 9.

17 Gordon Bates, "Editorial," *Health,* June 1962.

18 John I. Ingle, "The Rebirth of Root Canal Therapy," *JCDA* 18, 10 (1955): 565–76.

19 Letter from Gordon Bates to Tom Bradley, 2 January 1975, LAC, MG28, I332, vol. 84, file 2. This was at a time when thousands of people were still dying of smallpox in

developing countries such as India. Chandrakant Lahariya, "A Brief History of Vaccines and Vaccination in India," *Indian Journal of Medical Research* 139, 4 (2014): 491–511.

20 Gordon Bates, "Fluoridation and Diet," *Health,* November/December 1958, 4.

21 Letter from E.W. McHenry to Gordon Bates, 11 December 1958, LAC, MG28, I332, vol. 82, file 9.

22 Letter from Gordon Bates to E.W. McHenry, 15 December 1958, LAC, MG28, I332, vol. 82, file 9. The idea that evidence could be provided in the form of "opinions" from practitioners reflected Bates' training in an era well before the domination of the controlled clinical trial: Harry Marks, *The Progress of Experiment: Science and Therapeutic Reform in the United States, 1900–1990* (Cambridge: Cambridge University Press, 2000).

23 Letter from Gordon Bates to Ron Haggart, 25 April 1960, LAC, MG28, I332, vol. 82, file 10.

24 Letter from Gordon Bates to K.B.C. Rowan, 8 May 1961, LAC, MG28, I332, vol. 83, file 1.

25 Letter from Gordon Bates to O.E. Laxdal, 22 October 1958, LAC, MG28, I332, vol. 82, file 5.

26 Letter from Gordon Bates to Tom Leach, 8 March 1961, LAC, MG28, I332, vol. 82, file 10.

27 Letter from Gordon Bates to Roy Farran, 15 January 1958, LAC, MG28, I332, vol. 82, file 5.

28 "Opposing Health Measures," *Health,* September/October 1956, 4.

29 The committee was briefly led by J.Z. Gillies, but Dunn appears to have taken it over by 1957. See Reports for the Years 1956 and 1957, LAC, MG28, I332, vol. 10, file 7.

30 Letter from Wesley Dunn to Gordon Bates, 9 June 1958, LAC, MG28, I332, vol. 82, file 6.

31 Minutes of a special meeting called by Gordon Bates, 4 May 1961, LAC, MG28, I332, vol. 83, file 1.

32 Re: Citizens' Committee for Fluoridation in Metro Toronto, Minutes of the Planning Committee, 10 July 1962, LAC, MG28, I332, vol. 82, file 3.

33 Letter from Gordon Bates to the editor of the *Montreal Star,* 22 January 1958, LAC, MG28, I332, vol. 82, file 6.

34 Bates, "Fluoridation and Diet," 4.

35 Mariana Valverde, *Age of Light, Soap and Water: Moral Reform in English Canada, 1885–1925* (Toronto: McClelland and Stewart, 1991).

36 Press release, 5 May 1961, LAC, MG28, I332, vol. 83, file 1.

37 Letter from Gordon Bates to Leslie M. Frost, 10 March 1961, LAC, MG28, I332, vol. 82, file 10.

38 Franca Iacovetta, *Gatekeepers: Reshaping Immigrant Lives in Cold War Canada* (Toronto: Between the Lines, 2006).

39 Letter from Gordon Bates to Leslie C. Allan, 10 November 1961, LAC, MG28, I332, vol. 83, file 2.

40 "What Is Wholesome Water," *Health,* July/August 1957, 4.

41 Catherine Carstairs and Rachel Elder, "Expertise, Health and Popular Opinion: Debating Water Fluoridation, 1945–1980," *Canadian Historical Review* 89, 3 (2008):

345–71; Gretchen Ann Reilly, "'This Poisoning of Our Drinking Water': The American Fluoridation Controversy in Historical Context, 1950–90" (PhD diss., George Washington University, 2001).

42 Comments on Fluoridation, 28 November 1962, LAC, MG28, I332, vol. 82, file 4.

43 Brief in Support of the Fluoridation of Water Supplies of Metropolitan Toronto, 4 April 1955, LAC, MG28, I332, vol. 82, file 2.

44 "Court Action Considered to Halt Area Fluoridation," *Globe and Mail*, 19 May 1955, 1; "Council in Forest Hill to Fight Fluoridation," *Globe and Mail*, 26 May 1955, 1. The concern that fluoridation might increase gum disease was particularly common in Toronto at this time, because one of the University of Toronto's leading dental researchers, Keith Box – sometimes referred to as the "father of Canadian dental research" – had expressed concern that fluoridation might harm the gums. While his views were not widely accepted in the dental community, the *Globe and Mail*, which was opposed to fluoridation, gave considerable publicity to this claim through a series of articles and a subsequent book entitled *Boon or Blunder*. See the following articles by Betty Lee in the *Globe and Mail*: "Decade of Research Needed to Decide Fluorine Benefits," 15 January 1954, 9; "Fluorine's Inroads on Teeth and Tissues," 16 January 1954, 7; "Artificial Fluoridation and Its Hazards," 18 January 1954, 6; "Long Way to Go in Fluorine Research," 19 January 1954, 6.

45 "Field of Public Health Not Council's Concern, Ruling of Chief Justice," *Globe and Mail*, 20 March 1956, 1.

46 Clark Davey, "Supreme Court Denies Metro Toronto's Right to Fluoridate Water," *Globe and Mail*, 27 June 1957, 1.

47 "Information on Fluoridation Activities," 20 March 1958, LAC, MG28, I332, vol. 82, file 2.

48 Minutes of the Fluoridation Committee, 21 April 1958, LAC, MG28, I332, vol. 82, file 2.

49 See, for example, the letter from Gordon Bates to Stuart Stanbury, 8 May 1959, LAC, MG28, I332, vol. 82, file 2.

50 "Fluoridation Literature to Home and School Associations," n.d. [c. 1958–59], LAC, MG28, I332, vol. 82, file 2.

51 Letter from Peggy Rooke to Dr. D.B. Williams, 20 March 1958, LAC, MG28, I332, vol. 82, file 1.

52 "Sample Poll Finds Water Tasters Favour Fluoridation Six to One," *Health*, May/June 1956, 26.

53 Health League of Canada Report for the Year 1959, LAC, MG28, I332, vol. 10, file 9.

54 "Anti-Fluoridationists Force Metro Plebiscite," *Toronto Daily Star*, 29 May 1961, 25; "Metro-Wide Vote on Fluoridation Predicted Late in 1962," *Globe and Mail*, 26 October 1961, 5.

55 To see Gordon Sinclair in action, see "No Happy Medium in Fluoride Debate," *CBC Archives*, 7 January 1958, http://www.cbc.ca/archives/entry/no-happy-medium-in -fluoride-debate.

56 "Freedom of Choice," *Globe and Mail*, 27 October 1961, 6.

57 See newspaper clippings in LAC, MG28, I332, vol. 85, files 1–2; also, Ron Haggart, "Fluoridation 'Poison' and How It Spreads," *Toronto Star*, 29 May 1961, 7; Ron Haggart, "Fluoridation Tragedy," *Toronto Star*, 22 November 1962, 7.

58 Minutes of the Fluoridation Committee, Health League of Canada, 21 April 1958, LAC, MG28, I332, vol. 82, file 2.

59 Letter to Dr. Alan Smith from Gordon Bates, 17 October 1962, LAC, MG28, I332, vol. 82, file 4.

60 "Metro Committee for Fluoridation: Statement of Receipts and Disbursements," LAC, MG28, I332, vol. 82, file 3.

61 The committee never paid for the newspaper advertisements, and Bates eventually paid for them with Health League funds. See correspondence with the *Toronto Telegram*, the *Globe and Mail*, and the *Toronto Star*, LAC, MG28, I332, vol. 82, file 3.

62 Re: Citizens' Committee for Fluoridation in Metro Toronto, Minutes of the Planning Committee, 26 June 1962, LAC, MG28, I332, vol. 82, file 4.

63 Report of E.T. McLaughlin, campaign coordinator, Metro Committee for Fluoridation, LAC, MG28, I332, vol. 82, file 3; cover, *Health* 30, 5 (1961).

64 Letter from Gordon Bates, 31 October 1962, LAC, MG28, I332, vol. 82, file 3.

65 Letter from E.C. Roelofson, n.d. [fall 1962], LAC, MG28, I332, vol. 82, file 3.

66 *The Fluoridation Picture*, revised, November 1961, LAC, MG28, I332, vol. 83, file 6.

67 *Fluorine: Facts and Fancies*, LAC, MG28, I332, vol. 83, file 5.

68 *Summary of Conclusions and Recommendations from the Report of the Ontario Fluoridation Investigating Committee*, n.d. [c. 1961] LAC, MG28, I332, vol. 82, file 3.

69 Literature Committee, National Fluoridation Committee Interim Report, September 1963, LAC, MG28, I332, vol. 82, file 3.

70 "Some Fluoridation Literature," May 1965, LAC, MG28, I332, vol. 84, file 13.

71 Report by B.T. McLaughlin, campaign coordinator, Metro Committee for Fluoridation, LAC, MG28, I332, vol. 82, file 3.

72 Health League of Canada Report for the Year 1962, LAC, MG28, I332, vol. 10, file 11; Health League of Canada Report for the Year 1964, LAC, MG28, I332, vol. 10, file 14.

73 Health League of Canada, Reports for the Years 1964 and 1965, LAC, MG28, I332, vol. 10, file 13.

74 Ibid.

75 J.R. Marier, Dyson Rose, and Marcel Boulet, "Accumulation of Skeletal Fluoride and Its Implications," *Archives of Environmental Health* 6 (1963): 664–71.

76 Gordon Sinclair, CFRB, 13 January 1964, LAC, MG28, I332, vol. 83, file 3.

77 Letter from Gordon Bates to Dr. Frank de N.Brent (sic), 23 January 1964, LAC, MG28, I332, vol. 83, file 3.

78 Frederick Stare, "Fluoridation and Good Nutrition," *Health*, March 1964, 32.

79 Letter from Gordon Bates to Frank de N.Brant (sic), 23 January 1964, LAC, MG28, I332, vol. 83, file 3.

80 Minutes of the National Fluoridation Committee, 24 September 1964, LAC, MG28, I332, vol. 84, file 12.

81 Letter from L.H. Bowen to Carol Buck, 23 September 1969, LAC, MG28, I332, vol. 83, file 5.

82 Letter from L.H. Bowen to P. Healy, 22 May 1975, LAC, MG28, I332, vol. 84, file 2.

83 Letter from Mabel Ferris to G.B. Armstrong, 25 March 1976, LAC, MG28, I332, vol. 84, file 2.

84 Letter from Gordon Bates to Michael Palko, 5 December 1973, LAC, MG28, I332, vol. 83, file 9.

85 See, for example, letter from Gordon Bates to Lawrence Garvie, 15 June 1973, and letter from Gordon Bates to A.T. Rowe, 15 June 1973, LAC, MG28, I332, vol. 84, file 1.
86 "A Clarion Class for Fluoridation," March 1976, LAC, MG28, I332, vol. 84, file 2.

Chapter 8: Circling the Drain

1 "Ontario TV Plans Show about Sex," *Globe and Mail,* 13 August 1975; Letter from Gordon Bates to William Davis, 15 August 1975, Library and Archives Canada (hereafter LAC), MG28, I332, vol. 80, file 24.
2 Letter from Gordon Bates to William Davis, 15 August 1975, LAC, MG28, I332, vol. 80, file 24. The letter was sent to the *Toronto Star,* the *Globe and Mail,* the Rotary Club, Toronto mayor David Crombie, the Ontario Film Censor Board, and provincial cabinet ministers and other members of provincial Parliament.
3 Bethany Philpott, "'The First Wealth Is Health': The Health League of Canada, 1935–1980" (MA thesis, University of Guelph, 2014), 3.
4 For information on tag days, see LAC, MG28, I332, vol. 25, file 14 and 15.
5 Sara Wilmshurst, "'The Dust-up Which Dr. Bates Appears Intent on Creating': Changes in the Health League of Canada's Support, Funding and Status, 1944–1975" (MA thesis: University of Guelph, 2015), 50–53.
6 Shirley Tillotson, *Contributing Citizens: Modern Charitable Fundraising and the Making of the Welfare State* (Vancouver: UBC Press, 2008), 1–3.
7 Ibid., 201.
8 Wilmshurst, "Dust-up," 52–53.
9 Tillotson, *Contributing Citizens,* 2–3; Paul G. Reinhardt, "The United Way in Perspective," *Globe and Mail,* 12 January 1974, 7, City of Toronto Archives (hereafter CTA), fonds 1040, Social Planning Council of Metropolitan Toronto Collection, box 140442, file 14; letter from Mrs. Gordon Neild to executive directors of the Financed Agencies, 29 December 1947, LAC, MG28, I332, vol. 38, file 14; letter to Herman A. Stephens from unknown writer, 11 May 1950, LAC, MG28, I332, vol. 39, file 1; letter from E.J. Spence to A.C. Ashforth, 14 December 1962, LAC, MG28, I332, vol. 41, file 6.
10 Wilmshurst, "Dust-up," 61–62.
11 Philpott, "The First Wealth Is Health," 5.
12 Eleanor Brilliant, *The United Way: Dilemmas of Organized Charity* (New York: Columbia University Press, 1990), 32.
13 Tillotson, *Contributing Citizens,* 150. Eleanor Brilliant made a similar argument in her book, *The United Way,* 32.
14 Tillotson, *Contributing Citizens,* 217.
15 Peter Desbarats, "The Great Canadian Charity Bubble: What's Really behind the Outstretched Palms and the Façade of Righteousness?" *Saturday Night,* November 1969, 40–43.
16 A submission to the Committee on Poverty of the Senate, May 1970, LAC, MG28, I332, vol. 31, file 20; Mona Purser, "Consideration for Others Key to Work of the League," *Globe and Mail,* 18 January 1948, 15.
17 Juha Mikkonen and Dennis Raphael, *Social Determinants of Health: The Canadian Facts* (Toronto: York University School of Health Policy and Management, 2010), http://www.thecanadianfacts.org/The_Canadian_Facts.pdf.

18 Unpublished article written for *Maclean's*, n.d. [c. 1962], LAC, MG28, I332, vol. 19, file 17.

19 Gordon Bates, "For the Sake of Argument," *Maclean's*, 8 August 1964.

20 Ibid.

21 Letter from Gordon Bates to R.C. Berkinshaw, 30 December 1963, LAC, MG28, I332, vol. 41, file 7.

22 Gale Wills, *A Marriage of Convenience: Business and Social Work in Toronto, 1918–1957* (Toronto: University of Toronto Press, 1995), 110.

23 Ibid., 125–26.

24 "Committee on Health League," 11 December 1952, and "Some Questions Which Need Clarification through Joint Discussion with the Health League," 26 February 1952, CTA, fonds 1040, box 146748, file 8. The Health Committee was a subcommittee within the Toronto Welfare Council that assisted with the council's planning activities, with a particular interest in health topics; "History of the Planning Committee on Health," CTA, fonds 1040, box 145642, file 2.

25 "Report of the Committee of the Health Division of the Welfare Council Concerning Matters Relating to the Health League of Canada," 14 January 1953, CTA, fonds 1040, box 146748, file 8.

26 Letter from Gordon Bates to A.D. Kelly, 11 June 1962, LAC, MG28, I332, vol. 19, file 17; letters enclosing Bates' draft article, LAC, MG28, I332, vol. 19, file 17.

27 "Guidelines for Allocation of Funds to National Organizations Affiliated with United Community Fund of Greater Toronto: Report of a Study Conducted by an Ad Hoc Committee of the Canadian Welfare Council, at the Request of the United Community Fund of Greater Toronto," July 1966, CTA, fonds 1040, box 146717, file 5.

28 Letter from John Yerger to Gordon Bates, 27 March 1962, CTA, fonds 1040, Social Planning Council of Metropolitan Toronto Collection, box 146709, file 2.

29 In a letter to Harold N. Seagall, Bates suggested that allowing the review to go forward would get the Health League "deeper" involved with the Community Chest, but this seems like a red herring. Letter from Gordon Bates to Harold N. Segall, 21 September 1961, LAC, MG28, I332, vol. 41, file 4.

30 "Draft #1: The Report of the National Agency Review Committee on the Health League of Canada," 1963–64, LAC, MG28, I332, vol. 17, file 15.

31 Tillotson, *Contributing Citizens*, 1.

32 Minutes of the Fluoridation Committee, 21 April 1958, LAC, MG28, I332, vol. 82, file 2.

33 Letter from J.H. Johnson to John Yerger, 2 October 1959, LAC, MG28, I332, vol. 40, file 15.

34 Letter from George N. Barker to J.H. Johnson, 13 October 1959, LAC, MG28, I332, vol. 40, file 15.

35 Letter from John Yerger to W.K. Long, 31 July 1961, LAC, MG28, I332, vol. 41, file 4.

36 Letter from John Yerger to Gordon Bates, 15 August 1961, CTA, fonds 1040, box 146709, file 2.

37 Health League of Canada, "Financial Statement, December 31, 1965," LAC, MG28, I332, vol. 23 file 14.

38 Elizabeth S.L. Govan, *Voluntary Health Organizations in Canada* (Ottawa: Queen's Printer, 1965), 10–12.

39 Gregory P. Marchildon, "A House Divided: Deinstitutionalization, Medicare and the Canadian Mental Health Association in Saskatchewan, 1944–1964," *Histoire sociale/ Social History* 44, 88 (2011): 309.

40 Letter from Christian Smith to Gordon Bates, 26 November 1954, LAC, MG28, I332, vol. 45, file 18.

41 Minutes of the National Executive Committee, 10 May 1951, LAC, MG28, I332, vol. 1, file 20; letter from Gordon Bates to Thora R. Mills, 31 March 1955, LAC, MG28, I332, vol. 156, file 13.

42 Thora R. Mills, "How the Health League Helped the Canadian Diabetic Association," *Heath*, Summer 1972, 28–29.

43 "We Have Moved," *Health*, Summer 1972, 23.

44 Minutes of the National Executive Meeting, 12 March 1951, LAC, MG28, I332, vol. 1, file 20.

45 Letter from Dr. J.D. Griffiths to Mary A. Clarke, 14 July 1959, LAC, MG28, I10, Canadian Council on Social Development Collection, vol. 93, file 8.

46 Minutes of the National Executive Committee meeting, 10 November 1958, LAC, MG28, I332, vol. 2, file 2.

47 Minutes of the National Executive Committee meeting, 5 January 1959, LAC, MG28, I332, vol. 2, file 4.

48 Minutes of the National Executive, Finance and Programming, 18 June 1961, LAC, MG28, I332, vol. 2, file 6.

49 Minutes of the National Executive Committee meeting, 12 December 1962, LAC, MG28, I332, vol. 2, file 8; minutes of the National Executive Committee meeting, 26 March 1963, LAC, MG28, I332, vol. 2, file 9.

50 Minutes of the National Executive Committee meeting, 4 January 1963, LAC, MG28, I332, vol. 2, file 9.

51 Gregory Marchildon, "The Three Dimensions of Universal Medicare in Canada," *Canadian Public Administration* 57, 3 (2014): 362–82. Other literature on medicare includes C. David Naylor, *Private Practice, Public Payment: Canadian Medicine and the Politics of Health Insurance, 1911–1966* (Montreal and Kingston: McGill-Queen's University Press, 1986); Malcolm Taylor, *Health Insurance and Canadian Public Policy: The Seven Decisions That Created the Canadian Health Insurance System and Their Outcomes* (Montreal and Kingston: McGill-Queen's University Press, 2009); Antonia Maioni, *Parting at the Crossroads: The Emergence of Health Insurance in the United States and Canada* (Princeton, NJ: Princeton University Press, 1998); Gregory P. Marchildon, ed., *Making Medicare: New Perspectives on the History of Medicare in Canada* (Toronto: University of Toronto Press, 2012).

52 Naylor, *Private Practice, Public Payment*, 37; Heather MacDougall, "Into Thin Air: Making National Health Policy, 1939–45," *Canadian Bulletin of Medical History* 26, 2 (2009): 283–313.

53 "History of the Health League of Canada," text of a speech delivered by Gordon Bates, 28 January 1964, LAC, MG28, I332, vol. 1, file 1; Guildford B. Reed, "Socialized Medicine in the USSR," *Health*, Summer 1936, 42; "Who Bears the Cost?" *Health*, March 1938, 16; Harris McPhedran, "The Case for State Medicine," *Health*, Spring 1934, 11. The summer issue of *Health* with the case against publicly funded health insurance is not available at the University of Toronto or Library or LAC collections of *Health*

magazine. J.A. Hannah, "Long Development Period for Health Insurance," *Health,* Winter 1939, 94, 102–3; Allon Peebles, "Health Insurance Arguments: For State Insurance," *Health,* Spring 1940, 10.

54 J.J. Heagerty, *Health Insurance: Report of the Advisory Committee on Health Insurance* (Ottawa: King's Printer, 1943), viii, xi.

55 Ibid., 3–5.

56 Heagerty wrote several articles for *Health,* one of which highlights his similarity to Bates. In a 1935 article, Heagerty argued that "no sympathy should be wasted on non-vaccinated persons who die of smallpox. The community provides vaccination without cost, and the person who does not avail himself of it is a menace to his neighbors ... The best that can be said of him is that he is a martyr to his ignorance and to anti-vaccination propaganda which is responsible for so much unnecessary suffering and unnecessary deaths." J.J. Heagerty, "Chop-Dollar," *Health,* Spring 1935, 21.

57 MacDougall, "Into Thin Air." There are examples of correspondence between Heagerty and Bates in LAC, MG28, I332, vol. 185, file 1.

58 "Report of an Interview with Dr. J.J. Heagerty, in the Department of Pensions and National Health, Ottawa, Thursday," LAC, MG28, I332, vol. 198, file 1.

59 Jacalyn Duffin, "The Guru and the Godfather: Henry Sigerist, Hugh Maclean, and the Politics of Health Care Reform in 1940s Canada," *Canadian Bulletin of Medical History* 9, 2 (1992): 194.

60 Henry Sigerist, "Health Care for All the People," *Health,* Spring 1944, 7, 23.

61 Gordon Bates, "Editorial: Health Insurance for Canada," *Health,* Winter 1943, 3.

62 "Royal Commission on Health Services, a Submission by the Health League of Canada," LAC, MG28, I332, vol. 186, file 8; W.W. Goforth, "Cost of Health and Sickness," *Health,* March/April 1956, 10–11, 15, 26–28.

63 "Thirty-Sixth Annual Meeting to Be Held March 5th, 6th, and 7th, 1956 at the Royal York Hotel – Toronto, Ontario," LAC, MG28, I332, vol. 13, file 18.

64 Gordon Bates, "Voluntary Action and Health," *Health,* March/April 1956, 4.

65 Maioni, *Parting at the Crossroads,* 123.

66 Canada, *Royal Commission on Health Services,* vol. 1 (Ottawa: Roger Duhamel, Queen's Printer, 1964), 19.

67 John E.F. Hastings, "The Report of the Royal Commission on Health Services: Implications for Public Health," *Canadian Journal of Public Health* 57, 3 (1966): 115.

68 Canada, *Royal Commission on Health Services,* vol. 2 (Ottawa: Roger Duhamel, Queen's Printer, 1965), 151–97.

69 Gordon Bates, "Editorial: Utopia Can Be Practical," *Health,* October 1964, 30.

70 Jacques Genest and John C. Beck, "Major Concern of Medical Profession in 1966," *Health,* February 1966, 24.

71 R.A. Whitman, "Give Your Doctor a Break!" *Health,* February 1968, 12.

72 Gordon Bates, "Editorial: Your Health Is Your Responsibility," *Health,* February 1968, 6; emphasis is in the original.

73 Letter from Gordon Bates to John Diefenbaker, 13 August 1970, LAC, MG28, I332, vol. 183, file 28.

74 Letter from Gordon Bates to William M. Benedickson, 19 April 1972, LAC, MG28, I332, vol. 187, file 3.

75 "The Ninety-Eighth Annual Meeting of the Canadian Medical Association," *Canadian Medical Association Journal* 93, 4 (1965): 175.

76 Robert O. Jones, "Canadian Medical Association Endorses the Health League of Canada," *Health,* December 1965, 31.

77 Gordon Bates, "The Problem of Venereal Disease," *Health,* January/February 1964, 6. For the availability of the birth control pill, see Christabelle Sethna, "The University of Toronto Health Service, Oral Contraception, and Student Demand for Birth Control, 1960–1970," *Historical Studies in Education/Revue d'histoire de l'éducation* 17, 2 (2005): 270.

78 Christopher Nowlin, *Judging Obscenity: A Critical History of Expert Evidence* (Montreal and Kingston: McGill-Queen's University Press, 2003), 88–91.

79 "Notorious and Obnoxious," *Westmount Examiner,* 2 December 1960; Gordon Bates, "The Lady Chatterley's Lover Case," *Health,* June 1960, 16, 54.

80 The *Peterborough Examiner* and *Oshawa Times* both published editorials in support of the *Kingston-Whig Standard,* which is apparently where these quotes originated. "For Investigation," *Peterborough Examiner,* 5 December 1960, and "Use of Public Funds," *Oshawa Times,* 9 December 1960.

81 "How Thomas Richard Henry Sees It," *Toronto Telegram,* 15 November 1960.

82 Jenkin Lloyd Jones, "The Decline in Morality," *Health,* December 1962, 14–16, 22–29.

83 Gordon Bates, "Magazines and Morals," *Health,* March/April 1963, 6; letter from Gordon Bates to A. Stanislav, 23 October 1923, LAC, MG28, I332, vol. 110, file 26.

84 Mary Louise Adams, "Youth, Corruptibility, and English-Canadian Postwar Campaigns against Indecency," *Journal of the History of Sexuality* 6, 1 (1995): 89–117.

85 Gordon Bates, "Science without Conscience," *Health,* August/September 1968, 6.

86 Gordon Bates, "The Venereal Disease Menace," *Health,* February 1969, 6–7.

87 R.J. Anderson, "Venereal Disease," 11 March 1971, LAC, MG28, I332, vol. 135, file 2.

88 Letter from Gordon Bates to the editor, *Toronto Telegram,* 10 May 1971, LAC, MG28, I332, vol. 20, file 11.

89 "We Need Moral Crusade, Pioneer Doctor, 85, Says," "Schools Must Teach Our Young the Perils of VD, Forum Is Told," and "Parents Advised to Tell Children all of the Facts," all *Toronto Star,* 13 October 1971, 12.

90 Gordon Bates, "Tragic Effects of VD," *Health,* Summer 1972, 6.

91 Epidemiology Division, Department of Health and Welfare, *Venereal Disease: What You Should Know* (Ottawa: Queen's Printer, 1966).

92 In 1970, there were 40 reported deaths from syphilis in Canada. In 1969, there were 41. This compares to over 900 deaths per year from syphilis in the early 1940s. In 1970, there were 15 cases of cardiovascular syphilis, 74 cases of neurosyphilis, and 51 cases of congenital syphilis. Epidemiology Division, Department of National Health and Welfare, *Venereal Disease in Canada, 1971* (Ottawa: National Health and Welfare, 1972), 5, 20.

93 Lynford L. Keyes and Henry M Parrish, "Increasing the Effectiveness of Venereal Disease Education," *Canadian Journal of Public Health* 59, 3 (1968): 119–22; Alan Meltzer, "Sexually Transmitted Diseases in Canada," *Canadian Journal of Public Health* 70, 6 (1979): 366–70.

94 Alan Petigny, *The Permissive Society* (Cambridge: Cambridge University Press, 2009).

95 David Allyn, *Make Love, Not War: The Sexual Revolution – An Unfettered History* (Boston: Little Brown, 2000); Alfred Kinsey, *Sexual Behavior in the Human Male* (Philadelphia: Saunders, 1948); Alfred Kinsey, *Sexual Behavior in the Human Female* (Philadelphia: Saunders, 1953).

96 Minutes of the Action Committee [of the Health League] meeting, 23 November 1971, LAC, MG28, I332, vol. 135, file 2.

97 "She Might Have Been Your Daughter," *Health,* Summer 1972, 6.

98 Press release, "The Venereal Diseases Require a New Campaign," 7–13 April 1974, LAC, MG28, I332, vol. 135, file 2.

99 Epidemiology Division, *Venereal Disease in Canada,* foreword, n.p.

100 The Ontario government felt that surveys would be better undertaken by the Department of Health. Letter from M.B. Dymond to Gordon Bates, 30 January 1969, LAC, MG28, I332, vol. 143, file 1. The funding was eventually obtained from Health and Welfare Canada. Social Hygiene Survey, 1974–76, LAC, MG28, I332, vol. 145, file 7.

101 C.P. Fenwick, "Venereal Disease Survey in Toronto," *Canadian Public Health Journal* 21, 3 (1930): 132–38.

102 Minutes of the VD Survey Committee, 28 January 1969, LAC, MG28, I332, vol. 132, file 11.

103 Epidemiology Division, Department of Health and Welfare, *Venereal Disease: What You Should Know* (Ottawa: Department of National Health and Welfare, 1960); Epidemiology Division, Department of Health and Welfare, *Venereal Disease: What You Should Know* (Ottawa: Queen's Printer, 1966).

104 W. Harding le Riche, *Venereal Disease: The Plain Facts* (Toronto: Photo Pix Productions, 1971).

105 *VD* (Ottawa: Health and Welfare Canada, n.d.). The pamphlet was published by the authority of John Munro, who was minister of national health and welfare from 1968 to 1972, LAC, MG28, I332, vol. 143, file 5.

106 Letters from M.B. Dymond to Gordon Bates, 30 January 1969, and from L. Norbert Theriault to Gordon Bates, 24 June 1969, LAC, MG28, I332, vol. 143, file 1.

107 See letters from J.D. Henderson to Gordon Bates, 17 July 1969, and from H.B. Colford to Gordon Bates, 18 July 1968, LAC, MG28, I332, vol. 143, file 1.

108 "Constitution and By-laws," LAC, MG28, I332, vol. 1, file 6.

109 Minutes of the CSHC Annual Meeting 1925, 11 December 1925, LAC, MG28, I332, vol. 10, file 23.

110 Letter from Gordon Bates to Lady Eaton, 15 August 1949, LAC, MG28, I332, vol. 7, file 5.

111 Letter from Gordon Bates to Burnham L. Mitchell, 10 February 1950, LAC, MG28, I332, vol. 7, file 10.

112 Peter Newman, *The Canadian Establishment,* rev. ed., vol. 1 (Toronto: Seal Books, 1979); John Porter, *The Vertical Mosaic: An Analysis of Social Class and Power in Canada* (Toronto: University of Toronto Press, 1968).

113 There were no lists available for 1927, 1931, 1932, 1951, 1953, 1970, 1971, 1980, and 1981, so when one of those years was implicated in calculating the length of

someone's membership, we erred on the side of shorter membership. For example, if someone left the board in 1970 or 1971, we have recorded their leave taking as 1970. Furthermore, for the purposes of this chapter, we focus only on Honorary Advisory Board members who resided in Canadian cities and whose city of residence appears in the sources. The board included people living in foreign countries, leaders in Canadian universities, and mayors, who were listed, respectively, by nation, under "universities," or as "mayors," but we have not included these members for several reasons. University representatives and mayors were selected as representatives of their position, not as individuals. So, while it is significant that Bates wanted municipal governments and university leaders represented on the board, the individuals representing them are less interesting for our purposes. As such, this chapter will discuss members of the Honorary Advisory Board who served in Canada and joined as individuals. These lists are undoubtedly imperfect. The Health League updated the published lists regularly, but we have not found evidence of a scheduled or particularly systematic editing process. We have obtained names from the following sources: 1929 Annual Report, CSHC Tenth Annual Report, June 1929, LAC, MG28, I332, vol. 9, file 14; minutes of the CSHC Annual Meetings for 11 December 1925, 7 May 1926, 13 June 1927, and 14 June 1928, LAC, MG28, I332, vol. 10, files 23–26; Report of the Nominating Committee, 1930, LAC, MG28, I332, vol. 10, file 31; and a list from each year of *Health* magazine (1933–81), which published the names of the Honorary Advisory Board members. These names were then compared with the following guides: Henry James Morgan, *The Canadian Men and Women of the Time: A Handbook of Canadian Biography of Living Characters*, 2nd ed. (Toronto: William Briggs, 1912); B.M. Greene, *Who's Who in Canada, Including the British Possessions of the Western Hemisphere*, 20th ed. (Toronto: International Press Limited, 1929); The Times, *The Canadian Who's Who*, vol. 1 (London: Times, 1910); Sir Charles G.D. Roberts and Arthur Leonard Tunnell, *The Canadian Who's Who*, vol. 2 (London: The Times Publishing Company of London, 1936); A.L. Tunnell, *The Canadian Who's Who*, vols. 4–10 (Toronto: Trans-Canada Press, 1948–66); A.L. Tunnell, *The Canadian Who's Who*, vols. 11–13 (Toronto: Who's Who Canadian Publications, 1969–75); Kieran Simpson, *The Canadian Who's Who*, vol. 14 (Toronto: University of Toronto Press, 1979); "Obituaries: Dr. Alfred K. Haywood," *Canadian Medical Association Journal* 67, 1 (1952): 70; "Obituaries: Dr. Harry Goudge Grant," *Canadian Medical Association Journal* 71, 1 (1954): 83; "Obituaries: Dr. Edward Salder Mills," *Canadian Medical Association Journal* 103, 2 (107): 306.

114 Newman, *The Canadian Establishment*, 438, 440.

115 The Times, *Canadian Who's Who*, vol. 1; Roberts and Tunnell, *Canadian Who's Who*, vol. 2; Tunnell, *Canadian Who's Who*, vols. 4–13; Simpson, *Canadian Who's Who*, vol. 14; Greene, *Who's Who in Canada*; Morgan, *Canadian Men and Women of the Time*; "Obituaries: Dr. Alfred K. Haywood," 70; "Obituaries: Dr. Harry Goudge Grant," 83; "Obituaries: Dr. Louis de Lotbinière Harwood," *Canadian Medical Association Journal* 31, 1 (July 1934): 106; "Obituaries: Dr. Edward Salder Mills," 306.

116 Tunnell, *The Canadian Who's Who*, 12: 33; 8: 153.

117 Ibid., 4: 261–62; 7: 46.

118 Ibid., 2: 659, 1010; 5: 783, 1068–69; 7: 89; 8: 92; and 12: 33.

119 Newman, *The Canadian Establishment*, 35.

120 "Dr. Gordon A. Bates: Founder of Health League Made Preventive Medicine His Career," *Globe and Mail*, 9 November 1971, 5.

121 Ibid.

122 "Constitution and By-Laws," LAC, MG28, I332, vol. 1, file 6.

123 Minutes of the 61st Annual General Business Meeting of the Health League of Canada, 9 March 1982, LAC, MG28, I332, vol. 6, file 17.

124 1929 CSHC Annual Report, LAC, MG28, I332, vol. 9, file 14; minutes of the CSHC Annual Meetings, 11 December 1925, 7 May 1926, 13 June 1927, and 14 June 1928, LAC, MG28, I332, vol. 10, files 23–26; "Report of the Nominating Committee," 1930, LAC, MG28, I332, vol. 10, file 31; and one list from each year of *Health* magazine.

125 The Times, *Canadian Who's Who*, vol. 1; Roberts and Tunnell, *Canadian Who's Who*, vol. 2; Tunnell, *Canadian Who's Who*, vols. 4–13; Simpson, *Canadian Who's Who*, vol. 14; and the following obituaries from the *Canadian Medical Association Journal (CMAJ)*: "Dr. Edward Bishop Alport," *CMAJ* 62, 3 (1950): 305; "Le Dr Joseph-Albert Baudouin," *CMAJ* 86, 24 (1962): 1129; "Dr. C. Noble Black," *CMAJ* 94, 5 (1966): 252; "Dr. Seraphin Boucher," *CMAJ* 55, 5 (1946): 529; "Frank De Niord Brent, M.D., M.I.H., D.P.H.," *CMAJ* 103, 2 (1970): 124; "Brown, John Reginald," *CMAJ* 117, 6 (1977): 678; "Dr. P.A. Creelman," *CMAJ* 76, 10 (1957): 904; "Dr. Douglas Verral Currey," *CMAJ* 102, 10 (1970): 1113; "Dr. Reginald Oliver Davison," *CMAJ* 100, 12 (1969): 591; "Gillies, John Zachariah," *CMAJ* 115, 11 (1976): 1173; "Dr. Frank R. Griffin," *CMAJ* 85, 8 (1961): 449; "Dr. Charles A. Harris," *CMAJ* 88, 1 (1963): 54; "Dr. Alfred K. Haywood," *CMAJ* 67, 1 (1952): 70; "Dr. John Howard Holbrook: An Appreciation," *CMAJ* 78, 9 (1958): 738; "Dr. Edward A. Keenleyside," *CMAJ* 101, 8 (1969): 114; "Dr. Albert LeSage," *CMAJ* 72, 1 (1955): 58; "Dr. Daniel. H. McCalman," *CMAJ* 38, 4 (1938): 409; "Dr. Thomas Wills Gibbs McKay," *CMAJ* 52, 2 (1945): 534; "Dr. John Harris McPhedran," *CMAJ* 89, 20 (1963): 1052; "Dr. J. Arthur Melanson," *CMAJ* 100, 11 (1969): 543; "Miller, Leonard A." *CMAJ* 126, 5 (1982): 563; "Dr. John Pettigrew Morton," *CMAJ* 76, 9 (1957): 794; "Dr. James Heurner Mullin," *CMAJ* 74, 8 (1956): 669; "Dr. Robin Pearse," *CMAJ* 76, 1 (1957): 70; "Dr. Leon A. Pequegnat," *CMAJ* 112, 12 (1975): 1434; "Dr. James Roberts," *CMAJ* 42, 5 (1940): 507–8; "Robertson, John Sinclair," *CMAJ* 133, 9 (1985): 918; "Dr. Albert J. Slack," *CMAJ* 65, 5 (1951): 499; "Dr. H.M. Speechly," *CMAJ* 64, 5 (1951): 460; "Dr. Emerson J. Trow," *CMAJ* 79, 5 (1958): 434; "Dr. Charles Vezina," *CMAJ* 72, 11 (1955): 872; "Dr. Richard G. Warminton," *CMAJ* 91, 11 (1964): 620; "Dr. William Gerald Watts," *CMAJ* 100, 9 (1969): 447; "Dr. Arthur Beaton Whytock," *CMAJ* 106, 8 (1972): 921.

126 The Times, *Canadian Who's Who*, vol. 1; Roberts and Tunnell, *Canadian Who's Who*, vol. 2; Tunnell, *Canadian Who's Who*, vols. 4–13; Simpson, *Canadian Who's Who*, vol. 14; Kieran Simpson, *Canadian Who's Who*, vol. 18 (Toronto: University of Toronto Press, 1983); Greene, *Who's Who in Canada*; Morgan, *Canadian Men and Women of the Time*; and the obituaries listed in the preceding note.

127 These files reside in LAC, MG28, I332, vol. 1, file 8, and vol. 5, file 7.

128 Ibid.

129   Tunnell, *Canadian Who's Who*, 12: 33; 7: 89; 8: 92; Obituary for "Berkinshaw, Richard Coulton," LAC, MG28, I332, vol. 6, file 10; letter from Gordon Bates to R.C. Berkinshaw, 14 February 1952, LAC, MG28, I332, vol. 6, file 6.

130   "Obituaries: Dr. John William Scott McCullough," *Canadian Medical Association Journal* 44, 2 (1941): 204; Tunnell, *Canadian Who's Who*, 12: 1193–94; "Obituaries: Brown, John Reginald," 678.

131   Tunnell and Roberts, *Canadian Who's Who*, 2: 917–918.

132   Tunnell and Roberts, *Canadian Who's Who*, 2; Tunnell, *Canadian Who's Who*, vols. 4, 5, 7, 8, 11–14; Simpson, *Canadian Who's Who*, 18: 1106–07.

133   "Majority of Canadian Women Investors are the Financial Decision-Makers in Their Households: CIBC Poll," *Globe and Mail*, 10 March 2017, https://www.theglobe andmail.com/globe-investor/news-sources/?mid=cnw.20170310.C2166.

134   "Health League of Canada Business Committee," LAC, MG28, I332, vol. 1, file 8.

135   "Mary MacNab [sic]: Fiery Unionist Was Descendent of Tory Premier," and obituary, "McNab, Mary," LAC, MG28, I332, vol. 6, file 14.

136   Minutes of the Program Division, 27 February 1961, LAC, MG28, I332, vol. 2, file 7; Minutes of the National Executive Committee, 13 May 1963, LAC, MG28, I332, vol. 2, file 9.

137   Simpson, *Canadian Who's Who*, 18: 1106–07.

138   "The Health League of Canada," *Health*, Summer 1979, 2; minutes of the 1981 Annual Meeting, LAC, MG28, I332, vol. 4, file 7.

139   Minutes of the National Executive, 10 September 1957, LAC, MG28, I332, vol. 2, file 1; minutes of the National Executive Committee, 13 May 1958 and 1 December 1958, LAC, MG28, I332, vol. 2, file 2.

140   Minutes of the National Executive Committee, 6 April 1959, LAC, MG28, I332, vol. 2, file 4; Report of Special Committee, 5 May 1959, LAC, MG28, I332, vol. 2, file 4.

141   Letter from J. Grant Glassco to J. Allan Ross, 9 August 1963, LAC, MG28, I332, vol. 2, file 9.

142   Minutes of the National Executive Committee, 11 September 1963, LAC, MG28, I332, vol. 2, file 9.

143   Income tax returns, 1956–71, LAC, MG28, I332, vol. 24, files 12–16.

144   Minutes of the National Executive Committee, 18 May 1966, LAC, MG28, I332, vol. 2, file 16; minutes of the Meeting of the Board of Directors, 20 October 1966, LAC, MG28, I332, vol. 2, file 17.

145   Minutes of the National Executive Committee, 8 June 1976, LAC, MG28, I332, vol. 2, file 14.

146   Minutes of the National Executive Committee, 12 October 1976, LAC, MG28, I332, vol. 3, file 14.

147   "Our History," *National Eating Disorder Information Centre*, www.nedic.ca/about/our-history; letter from Daniel Andreae to Jack Epp, 21 November 1985, LAC, RG29 1996–97/698, box 10, file 6751-2-7 pt. 2; Daniel Andreae, "Feature Article: The Health League Opens an Eating Disorder Information Centre," LAC, RG29 1996–97/698, Box 22, File 6751-3-7 pt. 2.

148   "Health News Digest: Special Edition," 20 August 1987, LAC, RG29 1996-97/698, box 10, file 6751-2-7 pt. 2; Sustaining Grants Program, Review Committee Meeting, 1987–88, LAC, RG29 1996-97/698, box 35, file 6751-4-6.

149 Health League of Canada, "Dr. Gordon Bates," http://www.healthleagueofcanada.
     com/founder/.
150 For example, a search of the *Globe and Mail* finds 627 mentions of the league in the
     1940s, 338 in the 1950s, 122 in the 1960s, and only 16 in the 1970s.

Index

Note: "(f)" after a page number indicates a figure; "(t)" after a page number indicates a table. CNCCVD stands for Canadian National Council for Combatting Venereal Disease; CSHC stands for Canadian Social Hygiene Council; VD stands for venereal disease.

Printed and bound in Canada by Friesens
Set in Warnock Pro and Futura by Apex CoVantage, LLC.
Copy editor: Barbara Tessman
Proofreader: Hazel Boydell
Indexer: Judy Dunlop